THE FAMILY ENCYCLOPAEDIA OF HOMEOPATHIC MEDICINE

THE
FAMILY
ENCYCLOPAEDIA
OF
HOMEOPATHIC
MEDICINE

2609 NATURAL MEDICINE REMEDIES

Compiled under the direction of Eric Meyer
Edited by J.P. LeGrand

ISBN 0-941683-25-7

Disclaimer

Education is freedom. The purpose of this book is for health education. None of the information in the book is to be used for, or interpreted as diagnosing, prescribing or treating any condition or disease. Naturally, any decision you make involving your health should be taken in consultation with your personal physician.

CONTENTS

9. ACCIDENTS, EMERGENCIES, GENERAL DISORDERS 335

APPENDIX

371

Introduction

Objectives of the Encyclopaedia

This book is intended to accompany you throughout your daily life, helping you deal with situations where your health, or the health of your loved ones, is jeopardized by disorders or disease.

Understanding Homeopathy

Whether you're already familiar with homeopathy or not, this guide will help you expand and deepen your appreciation of the alternative form of treatment called homeopathy - to use the fashionable term for a school of medicine which had already been in practice for over a century when Pasteur conducted his first successful experiments for a vaccine against rabies.

Homeopathy is undergoing a Renaissance these days. The public is turning more and more to this form of medicine, which seems ideally suited to modern needs and ways of thinking. As examples, we could mention the modest cost of homeopathic preparations, the possibilities it offers for independent action (within certain limits, of course) and the respect it holds for each individual's "personal ecology". Our troubled times have forced us to re-examine our lifestyles in the context of an environment which makes staying healthy a precarious business.

So if we want to preserve and enjoy the positive benefits our ancestors fought so hard to attain, then we must create a lifestyle for ourselves that takes our biological and ecological needs into account. This leads us to certain obvious conclusions - obvious to some, but not to all: there is still a lot of resistance out there. And we're not suggesting that we abandon the technological advances made over the last fifty or hundred years. All we're saying is that we have to be selective about our modern innovations, that we don't have to accept the bad along with the good.

The old rule of "all or nothing" - either the old or the new, the general practitioner or the specialist - does not correspond to our reality. We have the opportunity to choose what is best for us, which, in the context of this book, means recognizing the limitations of homeopathy, knowing when we can handle a situation ourselves, and when we should call in a doctor.

A Doctor's Aid

Far from being a substitute for doctors, this homeopathic guide is designed to complement conventional medicine. It will, in time, become a veritable storehouse of health information, allowing you to better understand yourself and the body you inhabit.

After all, the saying "know thyself" is not limited to your soul, but ideally includes an understanding of your physical personality and your psychological behaviour. Homeopathy teaches us, first of all, that the body and the mind are not separate, that each one of us has our own "way" of reacting to illness, according to our personality.

Develop Your Own Experience

In time, you will learn to evaluate situations, and you'll become adept at distinguishing common problems with well-known remedies from cases that can quickly become serious. So you will be able to deal efficiently with situations where a doctor is not required (to this end, the description of symptoms is always accompanied by a warning where the situation necessitates calling in a doctor). Moreover, you should ideally consult a doctor in all cases of acute symptoms.

"Doctor, it hurts..."

You will also be equipped with the tools to treat mild problems, where a doctor need not be consulted. Should you see a doctor for a persistent case of hiccups? For that black eye that won't heal, for those long-standing digestion problems? Does you doctor have the time to explain all the precautions you should take if you're diabetic, all the things you should and shouldn't eat?

If someone in your family has always been irritable and aggressive, would you dare suggest that he or she consult a doctor or a therapist (a sure way of stirring up more problems). Homeopathy will arm you against these minor problems which, although they don't merit a doctor's attention in themselves, are often precursors of more serious problems - which can make life difficult and extremely unpleasant.

Significant Advantages

Apart from the opportunity to know yourself better, to learn how to cure minor health problems and know what to do when faced with certain kinds of emergencies, you will discover that practising homeopathic medicine offers the possibility of learning all about the body and its reactions. A person who studies homeopathy in this way will learn, little by little, to evaluate symptoms, and determine the remedies that are best suited to the individual, whether it's yourself or a member of your family or circle of friends.

So, in addition to granting you a degree of autonomy, this encyclopaedia will allow you first to observe and then accurately describe your symptoms during consultation with a doctor. You will know how to distinguish between what is important and what is secondary. And if you're not already familiar with how it works, homeopathy has a few surprises in store for you!

Homeopathy

As we've already mentioned, homeopathy is not a recent discovery. Actually, the concept of homeopathy was enunciated in ancient times, three centuries before Christ. This was when Hippocrates, the father of medicine, stated that there are two ways of treating illness: using opposites and using similarities. "The remedy for most illnesses," he declared, "can be found in the series of events that caused them to appear in the first place."

Hahnemann: Founder of the Law of Similars

What Hippocrates predicted was confirmed and developed by an 18th century doctor, 2000 years later. Samuel Hahnemann became the real founder of homeopathic medicine by updating and applying the theory of "like curing like."

He was a doctor who was dissatisfied with the imprecision and inefficiencies of the medicine of his day. In 1790 - the period of his great experiments - he decided to use quinine to combat fever, after observing the effects of quinine on a healthy subject. His conclusion: "Quinine, which cures fever, actually causes fever to appear in healthy subjects."

That idea forms the basis of homeopathic medicine: the Law Of Similars. As Hahnemann said: "To cure a given disease, you must give the patient a substance which, when administered to a healthy person, would cause symptoms of that disease to appear." And he got to work, systematically documenting the effects of a large number of substances.

Infinitesimal Dilution

Hahnemann kept working on the principle of similars, expanding his research to cover infinitesimal dilution. When conducting his experiment on quinine, for obvious reasons he had used diluted doses, and quickly noticed that dilution increases the therapeutic effectiveness of the substance used (the more diluted the substance, however, the closer it must resemble the disease it is meant to cure).

Take sea salt for example, *Natrum muriaticum* (homeopathy retains the Latin names for most substances, so that they can be understood by people of any language). By taking a few grams a day, you will make yourself thirsty and increase your capacity for water retention. In infinitesimal doses, it becomes a cure for depression, melancholy, brooding. So infinitesimal dilution is the second principle of homeopathy.

A Full Life

Born in Germany in 1755, Hahnemann ended his days in France in 1843, where homeopathy had become extremely popular. He travelled throughout his lifetime, crossing Germany and Austria, always trying to build firmer foundations for the new discipline in which he had so much faith. And, despite the zealous opposition he encountered from most doctors and pharmacists of the day, he never stopped experimenting, coming up with success after success in the treatment of various diseases and spreading the doctrine of homeopathy. He wrote numerous medical textbooks, and in 1789 published one of the first treatises on body hygiene, with allusions to exercise and diet that were far ahead of their time and are only being recognized today. This shows that Hahnemann was not only interested in disease, but in the total individual and in an overall concept of health.

Courageous Research

With his disciples, Hahnemann devoted himself to unparalleled experimental work, first documenting the effects of more than 60 remedies which he tested on his own person. He took substances like *sulphur, belladonna* and *mercury* and, by applying a rigorous scientific method, uncommon for the time, observed the effects that these substances had.

In this way, Hahnemann compiled for posterity what has become the Bible of homeopathic medicine: his *Organon Of Medicine,* which expounds the fundamental doctrines of homeopathic theory. First published in Germany in 1810, the Organon has since been translated into 16 languages and reprinted in hundreds of editions. Even today it is a reliable reference text. A hundred and seventy years later, *Belladonna* still dilates the pupils and has the same effects on the body as noted by Hahnemann. That's more than can be said for conventional medicine, which seems to undergo drastic changes in approach every twenty years or so.

A Popular Success

From the 19th century on, starting with Hahnemann himself, the theories and practices of homeopathic medicine spread across Europe to Italy, Belgium, Switzerland, England, France, Germany and from there to the U.S. and Latin America. Numerous homeopathic societies were founded, and publications were distributed throughout the western world.

Hahnemann's success against diseases like typhus, which ravaged entire populations in time of war, and cholera, made him famous. Homeopathic medicine became the preferred treatment of kings, princes and a major proportion of the European upper classes, who made their way in large numbers to the little town of Coethen, Austria, for private consultations with Hahnemann who lived there for fifteen years, between 1821 and 1835.

But the progress made by homeopathic medicine was not without resistance, especially from pharmacists. They were not at all pleased by the fact that Hahnemann prepared all his remedies himself. He did this because the pharmaceutical techniques used at the time were not the most exact, to say the least. Pharmacists had the habit of occasionally modifying a prescription, or ignoring the quantities indicated. What's more, Hahnemann often gave his remedies away, instead of selling them. It wasn't until *1965* that homeopathic medicine was cited in Codex.

Homeopathy and Allopathy

Even today, medical science is still somehow resistant to Hippocrates' theory of the effectiveness of curing by similars. Actually, the medicine that is currently being practised in hospitals and clinics, and taught in medical schools, is based on the technique of treatment through opposites. Take antibiotics, for example, or sedatives, tranquillizers, laxatives or cortisone which fights inflammation. These are all substances which work against the disorder or disease.

While it might seem natural, this method is not the only way to heal, as Hippocrates stated. But we often overlook that fact and take it for granted that there is no other way. Which is why homeopaths call orthodox medicine allopathy (*allo* meaning against, and *pathos* meaning disease) as opposed to homeopathy (*homeo* meaning similar).

These two aspects of the Hippocratic theory of healing can be seen as "related enemies". Not only are they opposite in terms of theory - one proceeding on the basis of opposing substances, the other on similarities - but even to this day no common ground has been established where the two theories can co-exist and work together.

Allopathic schools of medicine have had a lot of difficulty recognizing the therapeutic validity of homeopathic medicine, and an allopathic doctor will rarely recommend that one of his patients consult a homeopathic colleague. For its part, the homeopathic school has reacted with some bitterness to this out and out rejection by the so called "official" school of medicine. Fortunately, this has not prevented it from making steady progress and from becoming more and more recognized and respected throughout the world.

Actually, the two schools both have their merits and limitations, and trying to decide once and for all which is better is not a reasonable approach and can deprive patients of a valuable therapeutic resource. On the other hand, for critical cases, for emergencies or serious problems like acute appendicitis, the effectiveness of allopathic medicine cannot be denied.

There is no homeopathic cure for acute appendicitis. So the responsibility of the homeopath would be to get the patient into the hands of an allopathic surgeon as quickly as possible. Unless he is a fanatic - which could only serve to harm his own profession - the homeopathic practitioner has no problem recognizing his own limitations, as well as the areas in which allopathic techniques are superior.

On the other hand, homeopathic medicine specializes in treating health problems before they reach a critical stage where recourse to the scalpel is the only way out.

Popular Recognition

To a large extent, the public is responsible for the important role homeopathic medicine plays today. It's the public who has appreciated its merits and most directly benefits from its discoveries. And it's the public who will continue to support it, for the sake of its own well-being.

Allopathy

One could then ask why official (orthodox) medicine has so much trouble recognizing the effectiveness of so-called "alternative medicine" in general, including disciplines like acupuncture, osteopathy, reflexology, yoga and other holistic approaches to health. Since the self-proclaimed mission of orthodox medicine is ostensibly to experiment and discover (new treatments and cures), why then is it left up to the public to bear the cost of such experimentation? How can we avoid concluding that this outright rejection of all new forms of therapy is motivated by fear, on the part of allopathic medical associations, of seeing the validity of their own basic principles questioned?

What are the basic principles of today's orthodox medicine? Without getting into a serious criticism of allopathic medicine as a whole, we can observe the way it functions, if only in a general way.

Omnipresent Technology

Technology plays a role in almost every area of human endeavour, and medicine is no exception. Technology can be compared to the Sirens of antiquity - mythical beings who exerted an irresistible attraction for anyone who encountered them. This fascination with technology can easily lead us to forget that what we're really interested in is the health of the patient, and not the patient's disease or the methods used to conquer it. We literally expect miracles from technology, forgetting that the real protagonist in the drama of illness is the sick person.

If you observe the great majority of modern medical discoveries, you will see just how central a role technology plays. X-rays, lasers, chemotherapy, surgical interventions - in short, all kinds of medical equipment (and techniques) - are becoming ever more complex, sophisticated and costly.

Each new technological discovery - whether it's a miracle drug or a machine - is proclaimed with a great fanfare of publicity. A few spectacular cures tend to monopolize our attention and make us forget that these are most often exceptions and that a host of more ordinary illnesses remain untreatable. This is not to say that real progress has not - and cannot - be made by following this route, but is it the only route open to us?

Every year, pharmaceutical companies put new products on the market. They stay in fashion a while (usually four or five years) until some unknown side-effects begin to appear, at which point the product is quietly withdrawn, with no hue and cry about its defects.

Sometimes, the side-effects have to be treated as if they were a new form of disease. This has happened often enough to warrant the creation of a new order of diseases - called iatrogenic diseases (from the Greek *iatros* for medicine) - i.e. illnesses which are the result of actual treatments. At the present time, about 10% of all hospital patients are suffering from these types of complications.

We should also mention the increased trend towards specialization in allopathic medicine, which divides treatment of the human body into separate and unrelated disciplines, often with little or no communication between them. Such fragmentation, as well as the way in which larger hospitals are organized, leaves little room for compassion, patience and tender loving care, which is so essential to the effective treatment of disease.

Patients are shuttled between filling in forms, undergoing various procedures and tests and being examined by different specialists, and do not always have the feeling that they're really being taken care of. Instead, it's the disease, and the disease alone, that seems to interest everyone around them. Yet it has been proved beyond a shadow of a doubt that the confidence patients feel is an essential factor in their recovery.

This leads us to another unfortunate characteristic of allopathic medicine: the atmosphere in which consultations and treatments take place - clinical, impersonal, unfriendly - so that most often the only thing patients can do is be patient, usually without knowing what they're really suffering from, nor what the cause is. Of course, not all doctors work this way. Some take the time (and trouble) to treat patients like people rather than objects - simple carriers of a given disease - and to explain the origins of the illness and the treatment he or she considers necessary. But the diagnostic procedure usually has more to do with finding the characteristic signs of the disease than with the patient as an individual.

We must also mention that allopathic medicine systematically uses surgery as the only way to cure a problem. This is because success, for traditional practitioners, is based on the concept of making the symptoms disappear by fighting the disease directly.

Once more we wish to state that it is not in any way our intention to refute the undeniable advances made in the field of allopathic medicine. But we do feel that it is better to understand where the traditional approach may have gone wrong, that it is far from being perfect and that there are other approaches which can also make valuable contributions to the progress of humanity as a whole.

The Homeopathic Method

Homeopathy is a discipline whose basis is essentially experimental. This means that, although we may develop all kinds of theories and explanations, it is still difficult to determine exactly how homeopathic remedies work. Rest assured, however, that all the remedies used in this encyclopaedia have been thoroughly tested on human subjects (administered orally) and not on laboratory animals. It's very difficult to ask a rat if it feels dizzy, if it has a headache, if it slept well, etc. In addition, results of experiments carried out on animals do not necessarily apply to humans.

Similitude

Each substance tested produced a collection of clinical signs, which resulted in a symptoms picture (or pathogenesis - a complete repertory of sensations and physical and mental problems). Every specific substance mentioned in this book has its own drug or remedy picture. When you or I get sick, we present a symptoms picture - i.e. a collection of signs and symptoms. Homeopathy will then prescribe the remedy with the drug picture that most closely corresponds to that symptoms picture. In other words, it prescribes a remedy which, in a healthy person, would produce the same reactions as those detected in the symptoms.

The experiments on which the body of homeopathic knowledge has been built were carried out on people of both sexes, of all ages, coming from different backgrounds, and under highly controlled conditions. Research subjects did not know what substances they were being given, or even if the substances were active or not. This was done to control and maintain the accuracy of the experimental findings.

The result of this is that during a consultation, a homeopathic therapist can often determine the personality of the treatment by examining the symptoms, because the drug picture for each of these remedies takes the complete personality of the patient into account, rather than just the illness.

Let's look at an example to illustrate this theory and learn more about the characteristics of one such personality, associated with an important homeopathic remedy - *Nux vomica*.

> ### NUX VOMICA
> - Individuals who are hyperactive, short-tempered and easily upset, who get angry about little things and exasperated at the slightest provocation.
> - People who are meticulous, authoritarian, jealous and impatient.
> - People who have trouble dealing with any kind of pain, who are extremely intolerant of exterior disturbances (like noise). They are also very susceptible to cold and draughts.
> - From a physical point of view, their greatest weakness is their digestive system. They often have trouble digesting their food, they are constipated and frequently suffer from hernias and/or haemorrhoids. They also tend to overeat, and abuse substances like alcohol, tobacco and other stimulants. They feel nauseous after eating and usually need to rest and loosen their clothing. The back half of their tongue is often coated.
> - Waking up is difficult for people with a *Nux vomica* personality. They are often stiff, in a bad mood and nauseous just after waking.

Nux vomica is, therefore, well suited to the times in which we live. It has even been called an antidote for the "the restlessness of modern times." Whether it's a question of appetite, sexual habits, sleeping habits, or the way people instinctively react to certain situations, the symptoms can be related to certain traits and/or idiosyncrasies which serve to make up a personality, in the same way as an author creates a character in a book by describing his or her characteristics.

Another Concept of the Sick Person

This is how we look at the personality of a remedy, at least for a certain time, taking the characteristics of a Mr. or Mrs. Sulphur, Arnica, Lachesis, etc. into account. In this way, homeopathic therapists learn to distinguish the characteristics of various medications, and will talk about a case that is "very Ignatia" or a "Phosphorus personality."

Of course, human beings present a much more diverse spectrum of personality traits than the two thousand medications included in the homeopathic repertory. Each person is a blend, a multi-faceted synthesis of characteristics, some of which become more dominant at various times during the progression of an illness. It's up to the homeopathic doctor to determine which remedy is appropriate at any given time - a task which can sometimes be very arduous, especially when treating chronic illnesses. Therefore, a number of different illnesses may be treated with the same remedy, in so far as that remedy provokes a reaction in patients which is similar to the symptoms of the disease.

Thus, the homeopathic method involves seeking harmony between a sick person and his/her remedy. When one of our organs malfunctions - the stomach or liver for example - it isn't just that organ which is affected, but our whole being, including our personality. That's why we say, "I am sick."

In addition, every person reacts differently to an illness, depending on their personality. So while allopathic medicine looks for a few symptoms which are common to all people (say in a case of gastro-enteritis), homeopathy is more concerned with individual signs.

Beyond diagnosing illnesses, homeopathic therapists also have to find remedies, and will therefore look for the sign, or group of signs, that are likely to put them on the right track. That is why you won't find a group of remedies which correspond to each illness in this guide, but rather a series of remedies, accompanied by descriptions designed to help you choose the one that best corresponds to the person you wish to treat.

Simillimum

When the symptoms which we describe are the same as or correspond to a given remedy on the following levels:
- The affected organ (same kinds of pain, for example)
- Symptoms
- Personality

...then we can rely on that single remedy. In homeopathic terms, this is called a *simillimum*. A *simillimum* is, therefore, the remedy with which a patient has the largest number of affinities, at a given time. In fact, it is rare for people to exhibit all the symptoms or all the characteristics associated with one remedy. This is because there is also a hierarchy of symptoms that must be taken into consideration. And this is what has led to an understanding of an essential aspect of all homeopathic treatment - the importance of a patient's individuality.

To summarize what we've said up to this point: each remedy corresponds to a collection of symptoms, and the homeopathic method is based on the principle of establishing a correspondence between the state of the sick person and one or a number of remedies. It must be stressed that we are more interested in the sick person than in the sickness itself. This may be disconcerting at first, especially if we are used to the orthodox, allopathic approach where doctors first make their diagnoses, and then, once the illness is determined, write out prescriptions for ready-made medications which are the same for all cases.

Stimulating the Body's Defences

This is the basic difference (and the major bone of contention) between the "allo" and "homeo" -pathic approaches. The reason allopathic doctors prescribe antibiotics in cases of infection is that they count on the medication to combat the disease. And of course this seems to be perfectly normal. What else can be done, you may ask, since the body, in its weakened condition, has allowed the infection to become established?

This just goes to show how far we allow ourselves to be lulled into false beliefs through force of habit, thinking that there is only one possible approach. However, there is another approach, which involves stimulating the body's natural defences. And that is exactly what the infinitesimal dosages prescribed in homeopathic medicine try to do.

Infinitesimal Dosage

The Discovery of a Continent

As we saw earlier, during the initial experiments carried out on his own person with products like quinine, Hahnemann used very small dosages to avoid poisoning or intoxicating himself. Realizing that the substances he used remained active, he discovered the process of dilution, called Hahnemannian Dilution, which led to the technique of preparing the substances used in homeopathic medicine. This is based on the fact that the same substances have diametrically opposite effects, depending on whether they are ingested in small or large dosages. So while coffee is a stimulant which often prevents people from sleeping, Coffea is a homeopathic remedy for insomnia. Opium, which is a well-known soporific, becomes a homeopathic preparation (Opium) used to treat cerebral and sensory torpor. Digitalis, which in large doses slows down the heartbeat, is used as a homeopathic remedy (Digitalis) to speed up cardiac rhythm.

The Process of Hahnemannian Dilution

In the past, homeopaths prepared their remedies themselves. Today, specialized laboratories usually do it for us.

Starting with a given substance (say a plant like belladonna, for example) an initial extract is prepared, called a Mother Tincture (T.M. or Ø). One part of the mother tincture is then mixed with 99 parts of a solvent (distilled water or 70° alcohol) in an absolutely sterile container. This solution is agitated in a process called "succussion" - which is essential if the preparation is to remain active. This produces the first centesimal dilution, also called the first Hahnemannian Centesimal (represented by the abbreviation 1 C).

One part of this solution is then used to make a second dilution by following the same procedure: one part is again mixed with 99 parts solvent, then agitated (succussed), producing the second dilution (2 C). The process is repeated in exactly the same way a number of times, resulting in various concentrations of the same substance, up to 30 times (30 C) which is the maximum level of dilution authorized in most countries.

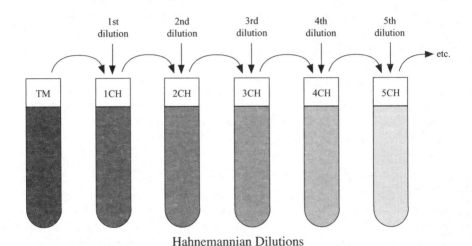

Hahnemannian Dilutions

An Unknown Factor

One criticism often aimed at homeopathic medicine by its allopathic counterpart is the fact that we are still only able to speculate as to why the process works.

However, as the saying goes, the proof is in the pudding, a pragmatic outlook to say the least. Just because science does not completely understand how things function at the molecular level (which is no doubt the level at which homeopathic remedies take effect) does not mean that we cannot use those remedies (and we should add that a good pudding is worth more than a bad recipe).

In Hahnemann's time, the concept of infinitesimal dilution caused a great stir. Today, accustomed as we are to very small numbers and to the fact that there are invisible forces all around us (atoms, X-rays, bacteria etc.), we don't find the concept unusual at all.

There is still, however, a factor which baffles so-called observational scientists: somewhere between the seventh and ninth dilution (7 C to 9 C) all traces of the original homeopathic substance disappear, even under scrutiny by the most sophisticated scientific instruments. It seems not to be present at all, and yet we know it is, since it is precisely at these higher levels of dilution that the substance most strongly affects the mind.

Hypothesis: The Infinitesimal Effect

One of the principles that governs organisms is that all foreign substances (except food, which is transformed by the body) are rejected and eliminated. This is what happens in organ transplants, for example, where the main problem is getting the host body to accept the foreign organ. This law, which in a sense maintains the integrity of our inner boundaries, is active no matter what substance is introduced, whether beneficial or harmful.

That is why patients must absorb huge quantities of an allopathic medication, flooding the body with millions of molecules so that the drug can overcome the body's natural tendency to reject it. But such massive intervention also produces side-effects - the body is forced to modify its equilibrium in order to adjust to the new substance, and this is precisely what causes problems.

This method of treatment, the allopathic approach, therefore consists of compensating for the body's deficiencies. As such, patients do not really regain their health, since they remain vulnerable to further attacks of the same type. At best, the germ or virus is destroyed or its reproduction is halted, allowing patients to build up their strength after the aggression is over. However, a germ or virus can also take refuge in some part of the body to avoid being destroyed by the antibiotic and then re-emerge in force to launch another attack. In other words, the battle-field (the body, with its weaknesses and strengths) has not been changed. The aim of homeopathy, on the other hand, is to restore the body to a true state of equilibrium.

Small Cause, Large Effect

Since the internal workings of this enormous factory of chemical products we call the body take place at a molecular level, i.e. through the transfer of electrons, the introduction of an infinitesimal quantity of a substance does not result in a similar kind of rejection. Homeopathic remedies act more like regulators. Their effects are gentle, working from within to stimulate the body to build up its own defences. In French, homeopathy forms part of what is called "médecine douce" which literally translated means "gentle medicine." And in this sense, it corresponds perfectly to Hahnemann's objective, which was to eliminate the toxic effects of medication.

A Military Analogy

Suppose a small country is invaded by an enemy. A third power, desiring to help, has two choices. It can intervene directly, for example, by bombarding the invading army. However, by so doing, it will also inevitably destroy a part of the country that was invaded in the first place. This may even lead to the smaller country resenting its benefactor because of the destruction and disorder it has produced.

However, there is an alternative. The country wishing to help can send an emissary who offers help in reorganizing and building up the smaller country's own defences. Little by little, with the help of its ally, the smaller country increases its resistance until it is able to defeat the invading army and reassert sovereignty over its own territory. And if the aggressor tries to attack again, the smaller country will already have the necessary forces to resist, this time without having to depend on its ally for help.

The second scenario is a good illustration of the way homeopathy functions, both in its infinitesimal intervention (sending a single emissary) and in its strategy (reinforcing the country's own defences). However, it must always be remembered that emissaries have to be acceptable to the country they are visiting: they must, so to speak, talk the same language as the people they are hoping to help. In homeopathy, this would correspond to the concept of *similitude*.

Note that, strictly speaking, it is not the homeopathic remedy itself that cures the patient. Rather a cure is achieved by mobilizing the patient's own resources, which are then able to react and fight the invader. In other words, homeopathic remedies help patients cure themselves. As the saying goes, "it's better to show a man how to fish than to give him a fish to eat every day."

So the homeopathic remedy works on the internal environment, i.e. the host body which is being attacked by disease, and tries to cure it first by eliminating the toxins which are weakening its defences and then by reinforcing those defences and making it less receptive to disease. In this sense, an illness can be seen as a negative event which leads to a positive result - a step towards attaining a higher level of evolution.

Limits of Homeopathy

Homeopathy can do nothing to cure severe lesions, except perhaps ease the pain. If a person has an accident, *Arnica* can be prescribed for this purpose. If an operation is absolutely necessary, the only thing homeopathy can do is ease the patient's fears, or help speed up the recovery process.

Use common sense when consulting this guide, and always be aware of your own limitations. If you feel you're out of your depth, then by all means obtain professional help.

Substances Used in Homeopathy

At present, homeopathy makes use of about two thousand possible remedies. You may wonder where all these medications come from. We can say, without risk of exaggerating, that they are taken from more or less all types of material - animal, vegetable and mineral. In fact, any substance has the potential to become a homeopathic remedy. All you have to do is transform it according to the homeopathic rules.

When substances are not soluble, they are ground into fine powders (trituration) before being diluted and agitated (succussion), in the same way as soluble substances are handled.

A majority of substances are plant extracts, whose diversity and unexpected properties say a lot about the powers of homeopathic dilution and agitation explained earlier. For example, take *Aconite* which becomes *Aconitum napellus*. When administered in large dosages (in its TM or mother tincture form), it is certain to cause paralysis of the heart, followed by death. But in its homeopathic form, *Aconite* is a remedy either against hot flushes, or against haemorrhage and anxiety, depending on its dilution.

> ### *A Mythical Plant: Belladonna (Deadly Nightshade)*
> As an illustration of how homeopathy borrows from nature, we should mention the use of *Atropa belladonna* (literal translation: beautiful woman, perhaps because of its cosmetic effect on the pupils of the eyes, which it causes to dilate), originally dreaded because of its toxic properties, but which amply demonstrates just how diverse and multi-faceted nature can be. In infinitesimal dosages, *belladonna* is very effective in fighting cases of infectious disease, such as measles and scarlet fever, whooping cough and conjunctivitis (on condition, of course, that the symptoms manifested by the patient correspond to those which an infinitesimal dosage of *belladonna* would provoke in a person in good health - i.e. according to homeopathic law).

Homeopathy looks to the plant kingdom for a host of other active substances, such as digitalis, opium, drosera and aconite. It also makes use of substances like camomile, black radish, sarsparilla, peony, etc.

There's no lack of diversity in the mineral kingdom either. Carbonate of soda, carbonate of magnesium, sea salt, iron, lead, silica, silver, copper, mercury, gold, graphite - all these substances, and more, are used to make powerful homeopathic remedies.

The animal kingdom plays its part as well. Snake venom (cobra, rattlesnake, etc.) is a well-known cure, as well as serum drawn from eels, powders made from cuttlefish, red ants and crayfish. Organ extracts (from thyroid glands and ovaries, for example) are also common, although these properly belong to a discipline called opotherapy instead of homeopathy.

Various organic substances are also exploited, some of which may seem a little scary, for example *Tuberculinum* which is prepared from an extract of the tuberculosis bacteria culture. But it should be remembered that homeopathic medication is never toxic.

Forms of Homeopathic Remedies

Homeopathic remedies appear in different forms, which are prescribed depending on the situation and the patient's needs.

- Tablets or pills: these are the most popular and widely used form - small tablets impregnated with the correct amount of the remedy, in its appropriate dilution. They are usually placed on the tongue and allowed to dissolve.

- Granules: small grains the size of a pinhead, which homeopaths usually prescribe in "doses" - about half a dozen granules per dose.
- Powders: these can be placed straight onto the tongue, like pills, or taken with water.
- Mother Tincture (TM): a liquid mixture of equal parts of fresh plant juice and alcohol, diluted to its appropriate degree and taken in the form of drops.
- Ointments, salves, creams, etc. are designed for external use, especially in treating wounds and skin disorders.

Consultation

The homeopathic consultation deserves special attention. It does not coincide with our usual understanding of what a consultation is, since it is not looking for the same kinds of symptoms.

The objective of homeopathy - what the homeopath is looking for - is not so much the character of the illness as that of the patient. As we have seen earlier, people react differently to the same disease and to the same remedies. An effective remedy for headaches for one person may be no more useful than a cube of sugar to someone else.

Homeopathic consultation assumes that every person must be the object of an individual investigation. In this age of ever increasing standardization, where everyone seems to be in a hurry to jump to conclusions, the least that can be said is that the homeopathic approach is unusual. The consultation, the nature of the observations and the questions asked may seem disconcerting to those of us who are not familiar with homeopathy.

For homeopathic therapists, illnesses do not arise because of chance or bad luck - they observe people's attitudes as well as their behaviour to find clues about each person's individual personality and reaction patterns, in order to put them on the road to recovery. Each person forms a totality whose parts are all interrelated. Our mind and our emotions act on our physical body, and vice versa - there is no separation between these levels. One informs us about the other, and all of them inform the homeopath.

Types of Constitutions

The importance accorded to mental signs does not mean that the body is ignored. Over time, homeopaths have identified a number of different physical types which exhibit certain constant features: different constitutions are more susceptible to different illnesses, and react differently to those illnesses. In relation to *Calcarea,* for example:

Carbonic type

People who are well-built, big-boned, stiff-jointed. Teeth are square and white, with few cavities. They have short fingers and broad hands. They are orderly, patient, methodical, opinionated, reasonable and respectful of conventions. Sociable and good-natured, they tend not to take care of their health because they are so robust. Because of this, they usually develop health problems at an older age - problems with digestion or with increased stiffening of the joints.

Phosphoric type

Of a frail appearance, tall, supple and slender, these people usually have yellowed teeth, rectangular in shape, often with many cavities. Sensitive and nervous, they are also very imaginative and tire easily. They have trouble staying in confined spaces. They are vulnerable to cardiac disease and disorders of the nervous system. They also often suffer from calcium deficiency.

Flouric type

These people have an asymmetrical constitution: ligaments which are too supple, and lax joints which often result in sprains. Teeth are crowded together, and they often have to wear orthopaedic devices. They have long fingers and thin hands. They are intuitive and their character is often unstable, disordered and feverish.

These brief descriptions are meant primarily to illustrate the relationship which exists between our physical type, our attitudes and the kinds of diseases we are susceptible to. Like all attempts at classification, they refer to "ideal" types, which do not necessarily correspond exactly to the individuals we all are. But for homeopathic doctors, this kind of classification can be used as a supplementary source of information.

This doesn't mean that homeopaths do not attempt to diagnose the illness, or that they don't use any other means of investigation, like laboratory tests, X-rays, etc. On the contrary, by combining all these techniques, they are able to come up with a much more accurate diagnosis. They then rely on their knowledge of homeopathy to choose an appropriate remedy.

What Is Health?

As we have seen, different medical approaches are not necessarily based on the same notion of what health is. Therefore, it may be of benefit to our readers if we try and explain what we mean by health and specify what the various schools of medicine understand the word to mean.

St. Augustine presented no less than two hundred and eighty-nine opinions about the meaning of the word happiness. In other words, everyone has his or her own definition. It's much the same for health. For some people, good health means being able to work hard all day long, while for others it means getting through a winter without catching cold, even if they find themselves out of breath after climbing a flight of stairs.

Staying Healthy for the Rest of Your Life?

If we had to give a quick answer, we would say that health is simply the absence if illness. But this apparently simple proposition leads to conclusions which are difficult to accept. Because if you carry this vision of health to its extreme, you will see that it is an impossible and unattainable ideal, and that it is, in fact, harmful to even want to attain it! In fact, until humanity regains its place in paradise, life is hardly conceivable without disease.

This is why a view of health which excludes disease, which tries to ignore the natural order of things, is nothing more than an illusion.

Allopathy tends to define health in functional terms - in appearance, everything seems to be going well. It's a little like a shoe salesman saying, "These shoes suit you very well, the proof being that you're walking in them!" In other words, this medical approach will evaluate people's health in terms of their ability to go to work, to carry out their daily occupations without too much difficulty and/or suffering.

This doesn't mean that allopathic doctors don't care about the people they treat. It just means that they are often not prepared because of the way they have been trained. If they can't see a clearly defined illness, with obvious symptoms, calling for some drug or operation, then their training leaves them perplexed and their remedies are useless as long as the problem remains vague - i.e. until it has reached a stage of crisis.

We can easily see that the two approaches (homeopathic and allopathic) are far from being incompatible. Together, they could form a global medical approach, because despite all the prevention and preparation offered by homeopathy, accidents still happen and defects in nature still occur. And it is in those kinds of situations that allopathic techniques play an important role. The obstacle to co-operation perhaps lies in an unwillingness, on the part of the allopathic establishment, to share its power, and this obstacle can only be overcome by public pressure.

The Body Has Its Reasons

This failure on the part of allopathy explains, in part, its frequent recourse to sedatives (drugs which soothe physical pain and dull the mind, alleviating anxiety) as soon as a patient complains of pain or a problem that does not seem to be related to a specific illness. Sedatives can ease the symptoms, but they do nothing to eliminate the cause. And the abuse of tranquillizers and other sedatives ignores the fact that pain, like fever, is a signal that is being sent to us by our body.

Why not try to understand these signals as a language through which the body expresses itself, telling us about some harmful condition or habit, about some past or imminent event, or even about our personality?

In addition, tranquillizers usually have harmful side-effects. People who depend on them to get through the day or night are generally very far from meeting our third requirement for health.

Being Healthy Means Sometimes Getting Sick

Advocates of this third definition can be seen as more realistic and at the same time more demanding than others. What they are saying, in fact, is that health is something completely different from a simple absence of disease. It is the presence of something much more than that. What is that something? Well, fortunately it isn't anything extraordinary, but simply a desire to accept life as it is - with humour, spirit, drive, energy and joy - in other words a simple love of life.

This doesn't mean that illness has no place. It is part of life, just like death, and even in the happiest of lives, difficult moments must be faced and overcome. Illness is one of those difficulties, but it can also be useful. Firstly, it makes us aware of just how important and pleasurable being healthy is. Secondly, it tests our ability to adapt, to modify our behaviour and adjust to our situation. When not caused by an external agent like a virus, illness in many cases is due to an adjustment of the body to some new, and often difficult, situation.

It may be a question of having to change diet, or adapting to difficult weather conditions, which happens every winter. Sometimes it means getting used to a new environment, where the body goes through a transition phase - a period of temporary disorder. Although such periods may be difficult, they are nevertheless essential to the process of adaptation.

New Habitat, New Habits

In terms of environment, consider the city, for example. In its history, which stretches back over three million years, the human race has rarely had to adapt as rapidly, and to such radically new conditions, as to those presented by modern cities. Because if you compare human existence to a 24-hour day, the appearance of cities as we know them would occupy only the last two minutes! Two minutes of radically different conditions and circumstances, with no precedents upon which to base our reactions. So it is no wonder that we often look back with nostalgia at the good old days, when we lived close to nature, when the air was clean and the water was pure.

In other words, human bodies must adapt to new sets of conditions. Let's enumerate just a few:

1. The disappearance of nature, and its replacement by a world of concrete, designed to be functional, and nothing more.
2. Daily cycles extended by the introduction of artificial light.
3. More and more sedentary and intellectual work (with rapid growth of the service sector, which is fast becoming the principal source of employment).
4. A radical change in the relationship between the individual and the community - which has become more a collection of individuals than a real community per se - so that even the family, which represents the last bastion of emotional exchange, is disappearing.
5. Changes in the food we eat, most of which now contains chemical additives.
6. New sources of stress: less space, constantly growing populations (especially in urban centres), more cars, etc. Dangers to health are no longer obvious and direct, but abstract and intangible. Money, for example, is a great cause of stress, depending on rates of interest and inflation, taxes, etc.
7. Add to this the instability of today's marriages, frequent relocation due to availability of jobs, loss of belief systems (religion) so that our values may undergo a number of changes in one lifetime - all these result in a

certain sense of worry and insecurity, which is perhaps reflected in our obsession with acquiring material instead of spiritual wealth.

That, in a few words, is the kind of world we have to deal with. Will we have the courage, will we find the power to adjust this new environment and to make it more... human? (Homeopathy can help us do just that - we'll be talking more about this later on.) Only time will tell.

Of course, it isn't fair to say that stress started with the creation of cities. New sources of stress (much less physical now than in the past) appear all the time, and are more and more the result of human endeavours, over which we should have some control, which we should be able to direct according to our needs.

So while we have conquered a host of diseases that plagued our ancestors, our modern lifestyle has created a whole new category of diseases - diseases of modern civilization - such as arteriosclerosis, cancer, mental disorders, etc. to name just a few. We are not saying that homeopathy can cure all these problems. It's simply that homeopaths are trained to observe and understand the language of the body as it reacts to these diseases. And they know that the answer does not always lie in new forms of medication, new surgical interventions or technological devices. We also have to make "choices about civilization."

What To Do

In the meantime we are all, as individuals, faced with a life choice which will have an impact on our health. We can opt for the third definition, which supposes that life is an inspiring force that we should accept with energy and enthusiasm, or we can resign ourselves to suffering and disease.

In terms of choosing the way we live, there are three areas that come immediately to mind, over which we have obvious and direct control: the food we eat, the level of physical activity we engage in and the quality of our relationships with our fellow human beings.

This means that health is not just a question of illness and medication, but rather the way a person behaves in all aspects of his or her life. It means seeing the person as a whole entity, where activities (work and play), environment (city, home, workplace), situations (stress, emotions), habits (exercise, diet) and background (physical, mental and emotional) are as important in understanding and combating disease as identifying a virus or a malfunction.

To Fight - Or Not To Fight Disease?

It is one of these aspects of our lives which opened the door to disease in the first place. But as we've seen, homeopathy doesn't fight the disease directly - it tries to stimulate the body, to make it capable of defending itself. That's why it has so much to do with diet, with breathing clean air, with exercising - in short with anything that serves to help people regain their health.

However, not everyone agrees with the definition of health as a state of well-being. But what would happen if, instead of earning a living because of people's illnesses, doctors and health care professionals in general (maybe we should call them disease professionals) had their income regulated according to their patients' state of health? They'd probably do all they could to prevent us from getting sick in the first place. This brings us back to our first definition of health - the absence of disease - with one subtle condition: a complete absence of disease is an impossibility, and we cannot hold the medical profession responsible for all our health problems.

Why Health?

Being actively occupied with our own health (not preoccupied, which makes you sick!) is not some kind of moral obligation, which is precisely what people who regard health as a question of "good or bad" think it is: it's bad to eat harmful foods, it's good to eat foods that are beneficial for our health (even if such foods sometimes taste very bad).

If we take no pleasure in doing healthy things (whether taking exercise, feeling good after a well-balanced meal, realizing the harm of some foods and automatically avoiding them), then how can we expect to attain the inner strength and discipline needed to separate us from those who just follow the pack?

Harvest the Benefits Each Day

The immediate reward - the instantaneous result of our effort to improve our lifestyle and pursue our efforts at improving health, is simply that we feel better. We feel more comfortable in our own bodies, we get sick less often, we're less tired and in better overall shape. We have more vitality when we're in good health. And all this places us in a much better position to enjoy life, or to face difficulties (which we can be sure will arise in any case). But the problems we face will not be the same.

And little by little, as we begin taking care of our bodies, we become more sensitive, and learn naturally to avoid foods (as well as situations and behaviour patterns) which may cause us harm. The idea is not necessarily to live to a ripe old age. What would be the good of that, if we're unhappy? No, the idea is to live better. And in most cases, living better means living longer.

Instant Healing in the Age of Speed

When stricken with an illness, we're not always ready to let our body take the time it needs to cure the problem on its own. We may have to get back to work, or take care of some important business. So we look for an instant cure. Even machines break down from time to time, and if we fight against our own biological rhythm, we run the risk of having to keep on fighting our own bodies for the rest of our lives.

This doesn't mean that relying on homeopathy necessarily requires a long waiting period. *Aconite* can soothe an earache in a few minutes, and remedies which include *Sulphur* can do a lot to speed up convalescence. But certain chronic illnesses which are "cured" very rapidly can result in more problems the next time around. Because it's one thing to get rid of the symptoms and quite another to urge the body to reorganize itself and regain its strength so that it can resist a new attack.

With this in mind, we must learn to respect the ecology of our own person. Homeopathy works to reorganize the body. The small dosages act as a signal and set off a series of subtle reactions. Its effect is not limited to a single organ or part of the body, even if the prescription corresponds strictly to a single problem experienced by one individual. On the other hand, we obviously have to take our day-to-day routines into account. There are some things we have to do that just can't wait, in which case we are forced to resort to quicker methods.

How To Observe Yourself

This manual does not pretend to be complete. However, it should be very useful in many cases, by helping you to become familiar with the homeopathic approach and its remedies.

To start with, you should treat problems that are not serious, where you run no risk of causing harm to yourself or someone else. Don't forget that it takes time to develop your faculties of observation, your understanding of homeopathic remedies and the way they work.

Recognizing Symptoms

Making an accurate observation of symptoms is essential, since it is on that observation that you base your choice of a remedy.

How to recognize a symptom? Well, symptoms are, in fact, anything new - any changes in the body - that occur from the outset of a disorder: unusual (even strange) reactions; the circumstances under which the disorder appeared; personality changes; physical sensations like thirst, the craving for - or aversion to - certain foods; the appearance of the skin; pains. In short, you must make a list of all unusual signs, even those that do not seem to be directly related to the disorder.

- A symptom should be clear and precise.
- It should be constant.
- The absence of a usual condition is also a symptom.

The way you feel, your impressions about what is happening to your body and any behavioural anomalies you notice are also signs which can point to the right treatment. To illustrate what we mean, here are three groups of possible symptoms:

- *Arsenicum album* (arsenious acid) would be administered to people who have a phobia about death, tunnels, coffins, etc. and who are afraid of being alone. They suffer from acute burning diarrhoea, which usually has a very bad odour and which is soothed by hot drinks. Their symptoms are usually aggravated between one and three o'clock in the morning.
- *Aconite* (monkshood) would be given to people who are agitated, who suffer from breathing pains, and who are unstable, fluctuating rapidly from states of calm to extreme anxiety. They are also afraid of dying, even when the disorder they have is not serious. Their symptoms seem to

be at their worst around midnight.

- *Ambra grisea* - for people who are easily upset by the slightest thing, who are extremely timid, who lose their train of thought easily, who are indifferent and seem to experience no joy in life. Music seems to aggravate their symptoms, as does everything else that bothers them.

Keep in mind that symptoms are not the only things to be considered. However, it is possible to classify symptoms into a kind of hierarchy of important signs.

Major Signs

These concern changes of personality, behaviour, sleep patterns, rhythms, preferences and aversions to various foods, general reactions, sensitivity to heat or cold and the times of day when symptoms are worst.

Mental symptoms set the tone (intentions, desires, passions, etc.). Then come attitudes (worry, anger) and symptoms related to intelligence (imagination, phobias, comprehension), behavioural clues (sleep patterns, dreams, sexuality), and finally more general signs (sensitivity to heat or cold, craving for or aversion to foods, etc.).

One must not underestimate the importance of psychological changes which take place during the course of an illness. For example, *Pulsatilla* (wind flower) signifies uncontrolled crying, *Sepia* (cuttlefish ink) signifies sadness, *Kali phosphoricum* (potassium phosphate) signifies hypersensitivity where the symptoms are alleviated by eating.

Identifying the Right Remedy by Referring to This Encyclopaedia

In this guide, each disorder is accompanied by a collection of possible remedies, and each remedy corresponds to a collection of symptoms. When you suspect a particular disorder, check the symptoms, then read the indications for all the possible remedies. In this way, you will be able to determine which remedy is best suited to a given case.

Note that the same disorder at different stages of development often requires different remedies.

Many remedies are accompanied by a qualification such as "Aggravated" or "Soothed" as in "aggravated by heat. . ." or "soothed by cold. . ." Such remarks are not meant to be therapeutic instructions, but rather an aid to observing symptoms more accurately.

It is not essential for all symptoms described to be present in each case. The important thing is to determine the most significant symptoms, in order to find the appropriate remedy.

Simillimun

In certain cases, a symptom is so obvious that its presence alone indicates which remedy to use, even if all the other signs do not necessarily correspond to it. As we have explained earlier, when the concordance between a remedy and the symptoms it is meant to cure is very high, we are dealing with the *simillimum* ("the most similar").

For example, in a case of infant diarrhoea, a child who is constantly seeking sugar would lead us to the remedy *Argentum nitricum*.

To make identifying the remedy which best corresponds to a given set of symptoms easier, each medication is accompanied by a description which is as complete as possible. If you've never consulted a homeopathic doctor, you may find the precision of certain details troubling at first. How can a remedy differentiate between a right and left ovary? What is the good of knowing whether a person is agitated or calm?

In fact, this is where the strength of homeopathy lies: in the precision of its effects, through which we can act on a specific part of the body, or on one symptom in particular, without disturbing the body as a whole.

For this reason, homeopathic doctors are interested in details which may seem innocuous to the untrained observer, but which may provide them with important indications as to which remedy is best suited to a particular case. Remember that homeopaths treat the person and not the disease - what they're interested in is the way a patient reacts to the disorder, rather than the symptoms the disorder produces.

Read the Entire Section

This is why, after identifying a disorder from its general description, you should read the entire section devoted to that disorder, in order to clearly identify the group of symptoms which correspond to that particular case. If there is some overlap between the symptoms related to various remedies, you can combine remedies. If you are unable to find certain symptoms - which is possible since the cases described are inevitably limited by space - and if you're dealing with an acute disorder, then do not hesitate to ask for outside help. However, in some cases, you'll find a seemingly insignificant detail that will put you on the right track.

Unresponsive Cases

In some cases of recurring disorders, you may find that a remedy which worked the first time becomes less and less effective the more it is used. This means that a basic remedy is required - something that modifies the entire body. A homeopath is in a better position to prescribe such a radical remedy than you are. The same goes for cases where an obvious symptom cannot be found in the descriptions. This may happen, since it isn't possible to cover all remedies for all symptoms within the confines of this book.

A Word of Advice

When dealing with an acute disorder which progresses rapidly, or when the remedies you choose do not produce positive results, do not hesitate to consult a doctor. The same goes for chronic illnesses and/or difficult or delicate cases.

Homeopaths base their evaluations on a collection of symptoms. Their observations are in no way mechanical. They feel out their patients and use their years of experience to come up with treatments that often border on the "inspired."

Homeopaths: Looking for the Link

In addition to his or her experience and knowledge, a homeopath is completely separate from your life, and therefore has a much greater chance of being objective, of seeing something in your character which corresponds to such and such a remedy, or to a specific disorder. Because as we've already stated, the homeopathic viewpoint is based on the assumption that a very strong link exists between our disorders, the remedies which are best for us, and ourselves.

In fact, these are the three basic links in the homeopathic chain. For a homeopathic practitioner, the illness is a language, and its symptoms are his allies.

For that reason, this manual is limited. It cannot replace the practitioner, nor does it try to. In acute, complex or chronic cases with long histories and recurring symptoms, you'd be better off consulting a doctor straight away, instead of wasting your time experimenting with procedures that you're not sure will work. Even if homeopathic remedies do not harm you, and only take effect when they are appropriate to the patient and the illness, absorbing a number of remedies, especially at high levels of dilution can, in the long run, reduce your body's ability to react positively and make it insensitive to future treatment.

Practical Guide

Choice of Dilution

In this manual, dosages are almost always indicated, and hardly vary from one person to another, whatever their age. For very young children and infants, you would use a different method of administering the medication (see Directions for Use - Infants).

As for the indicated dosages, they can be considered as reference points, which are subject to modification. If you think a remedy is appropriate, for example, but you haven't got the exact dilution required, you can still use it without worrying, because a homeopathic remedy is only effective if it is indicated for the condition and the person being treated. And it is the choice of remedy which is important, more than the choice of dilution.

The directions for use are generally indicated, as follows:

- *Weak dilutions* (4 C or 5 C) are generally used for acute disorders or very localized pains.
- *Medium dilutions* (7 C) are aimed mainly at functional disorders.
- *High dilutions* (9 C to 30 C) are designed for psychological problems or for treating chronic disorders.

How Often Should the Medication be Taken?

You are in the best position to judge how frequently a homeopathic medication should be taken. You just have to follow a few simple directions:

- *The principle of applying a homeopathic remedy* is as follows: as symptoms improve, you gradually increase the time between administering medication, until you can stop altogether. This is why increasing the interval when an improvement in the condition is observed is usually recommended.
- *For stable states,* administer the medication more frequently, the more pronounced or acute the symptoms. This can be as frequently as every five minutes, for extremely acute cases.

You can also rely on an average interval:

- *For low dilutions* (4 C or 5 C) take two or three granules or pills, two or three times per day.
- *For medium dilutions* (7 C) take two or three granules or pills once a day, or once every two days.

   –   *For high dilutions* (8 C and up) take five to ten granules or pills at a time, once a week or once every two weeks.

When Should You Take the Medication?

Medication should be taken at mealtimes, and as regularly as possible.

What To Avoid When Taking Medication

There are no substances which are dangerous to take with homeopathic medication. However, there are some which may hinder the effects of the remedy. For this reason, you are usually advised not to use camphor in any form (drops, creams, vapour etc.) when undergoing treatment. Also, avoid storing homeopathic medicines in places where camphor is kept.

Toothpaste containing mint and/or fluoride should also be avoided during periods of homeopathic treatment (in order to avoid saturating thyroid activity, which is responsible for changes in metabolism).

How To Handle the Medication

Avoid touching pills or granules directly with your hands as much as possible. Simply pour them into the cap of the bottle or tube, and then drop them onto your tongue where you let them melt. It's a little hard to prevent children from chewing the medication. However, this does no harm because the remedy will enter the system through the digestive tract.

Which Homeopathic Remedies Should You Keep at Home?

There's a list of about thirty remedies which should be kept in the home at all times, since they are the ones most often prescribed.

You'll find them in the section on Emergencies. Of course you can add to this list, depending on your particular needs, or those of your family. The contents of an Emergency Kit are only a general indication of remedies most frequently used, and may not correspond to the needs of every individual.

Also, as time goes on, you will develop your homeopathic skills and along with it the elements you need to complete your personal medicine chest.

Remarks About This Guide

You will encounter the following qualification: "Most general remedy." This is the remedy which corresponds to the general description of symptoms in the first paragraph of the section.

Each section generally contains a brief description of symptoms, and a list of possible remedies. It sometimes includes practical advice which, although not necessarily part of homeopathic theory, may be useful in soothing or curing a disorder.

List of abbreviations:

C	centesimal dilution
X	decimal dilution
g	grams
gr	granules
h	hour

Chapter 1

General Disorders

Allergies
(See Also Asthma, Eczema, Rashes)

For some people, it may be flower pollen, for others strawberries. For others it may be seafood, or wheat or white flour, or certain beauty products. Some people are even allergic to trees! The range of allergies is almost infinite.

An allergy is a state of hypersensitivity, where people react as they would to a poison: they may develop gastric problems, or skin disorders (breaking out in a rash, for example).

Allergy-causing Environments

In some cases, allergies are developed by children living in flats or houses where the heating dries out the air and a lot of dust accumulates. The resulting night-time coughing is taken for nasopharyngitis and the child is given antibiotics, cough syrup or drops - none of which work. Some doctors will go as far as removing the child's tonsils, which doesn't help either.

If you are suffering from an allergic reaction, the first thing to do is try to identify the food or substance that triggers it off.

Obviously, you'd then try to avoid that substance. For example, you may find that you cannot live with a pet, not because you don't like animals, but because their fur causes an allergic reaction (which may sometimes last for months, even after the animal is gone). This is often caused by protein left on the fur when the animal licks itself.

Vaccinations

Vaccinations are costly, and not always effective, although they can ease the problem in certain acute cases. Homeopathy bases its approach on *isotherapy (iso - the same)*. The method works as follows: first the guilty substance is identified; this substance is then treated like any other used to make homeopathic remedies - i.e. it is extracted in a laboratory, and then ground up, diluted and agitated (see the section on Vaccinations).

The advantage of this method as opposed to allopathic injections, is that it takes effect in just a few months, and is ingested orally instead of by injection. Homeopathic isotherapy also makes use of substances which come from the patients themselves - blood, urine, faeces, etc.

- *Antimonium crudum 4 C.* 2 granules four times per day. For gastrointestinal allergies triggered by drinks, foods or medication, which cause mouth ulcers, swelling of the stomach, digestive problems, intestinal cramps.

- *Isotherapy 9 C.* 3 gr. To be taken at the moment of contact.

Allergies: Eyes and Nose

Choose from the following remedies to deal with crises whose cause is already known, while waiting for a specific isotherapeutic treatment (for example, reactions caused by spring pollen, animal fur, etc.) These treatments are more effective if taken as a preventive measure.

3 granules once a day:

- *Allium cepa 5 C.* The tip of the nose burns and there is abundant nasal drip.
- *Euphrasia 5 C.* Here the eyes, rather than the nose, run profusely; eyelids are red.
- *Kali iodatum 7 C.* Extremely runny nose.
- *Rhus tox 5 C.* Intense inflammation, eyes are painful.
- *Sabadilla 9 C.* Sneezing, runny nose and watery eyes.

Other Allergies

- *Apis mellifica 7 C.* Runny nose, itching pains accompanied by swelling (oedema) and reddening of the skin.
- *Cantharis 9 C.* Skin rash forming blisters.
- *Ipecac. 5 C.* The allergic reaction takes the form of coughing fits and asthma.
- *Nux vomica 7 C.* For those suffering from coughing fits, especially in the morning.
- *Rhus toxicodendron 7 C.* Red marks around tiny blisters which form on the skin (vesicles) causing itching which can be soothed by hot compresses.

Antibiotics (Reaction to)

Antibiotics are a powerful weapon in the fight against disease, and homeopathy has no objection to their existence as such. But they do sometimes have harmful effects, because they attack useful, as well as useless bacteria, and the body needs its flora of bacteria to survive. Antibiotics can cause digestive problems, vitamin deficiencies, allergies, blood disorders, and skin disorders (dermatosis, Quincke's oedema). However, their effectiveness is undeniable, and the good they do often compensates for the inconvenience of any harmful side-effects. But over the last few years, they seem to have been prescribed with a little less discernment. One risk is that they will become less and less effective over time; another risk is the fact that patients become dependent on them - their body relies on antibiotics like a kind of therapeutic crutch. Antibiotics combat infections directly, whereas homeopathy tries to stimulate the body's natural defences.

If a major problem arises, it's best to interrupt the antibiotic treatment and consult a doctor as quickly as possible.

While waiting to see a doctor, we recommend taking 1 to 4 capsules of *Ultra-Levure* (Saccharomyces boulardii) every 24 hours, before meals. To compensate for vitamin deficiencies caused by antibiotics: a multivitamin preparation in syrup form for children and tablets for adults.

- *Penicillum 9 C.* 5 granules. Taken once, or the same dosage of a homeopathic medication extracted from the antibiotic (isotherapy).

Appetite
(See Also Anorexia)

Homeopathic remedies can be used to treat various disorders related to appetite. Of course, resolving the problem "naturally" is always the best method - nothing can replace fresh air and exercise to stimulate the appetite.

A brisk, so-called "active" walk, is a simple and effective way to stay in shape and regulate your appetite at the same time: you'll be less hungry than if you don't do any physical exercise, and if you lack appetite, regular walks will stimulate it.

In addition, your stomach is constantly being affected by your emotions; getting angry can have a strong negative effect on digestion. That's why your state of mind plays an important role in regulating your appetite. A relaxed atmosphere, good friends, and an attractive table laid out with nutritious food goes a long way towards stimulating appetite and aiding digestion.

- *Cina 9 C.* 3 granules, once a week. For cases where anorexia alternates with excessive appetite. Also for people who are still hungry after eating, or who get up to eat during the night.
- *Lycopodium 7 C.* 5 granules every ten days. For lack of appetite. Not advisable for people suffering from otitis (ear infection).

- *Natrum carbonicum 7 C.* 2 granules, once a day. For people who are frequently ravenously hungry.
- *Sulphur iodatum 9 C.* 3 granules per week. For people who feel full as soon as they start eating.

Arthritis

Although heredity plays an important role in this disorder, arthritis has often been called a disease of modern civilization, encouraged as it is by our sedentary lifestyle and the food we eat, which is processed and refined to excess.

This is why the real "remedy" for arthritis is essentially preventive. It consists of doing everything you can to avoid the disorder, which can be so destructive to older people and which sometimes even cuts short a working life.

Prevention, once again, is based on developing healthy habits: leading a healthy life, breathing lots of fresh air (which means getting out into the country as often as possible if you are a town dweller), eating a little less food and avoiding toxic chemical additives - all these combine to combat the development of arthritic symptoms.

Diet

A healthy diet forms the basis for treating arthritis. Don't use refined products (sugar, flour, tinned foods, etc.). Replace them with potatoes, rice, cereals, fresh fruit and vegetables.

The Secret of Potatoes

Drink a glass of fresh potato juice each morning (grated or squeezed). Before eating lunch, slowly chew on two or three juniper berries, and after the meal swallow two or three mustard seeds. Use the water you cook your potatoes in to quench your thirst throughout the day. Cabbage and carrot juice are also highly recommended.

What To Avoid

Reduce the amount of sodium salts (like ordinary kitchen salt) that you use. By retaining water in the system, they prevent adequate elimination of uric acid.

Drink infusions of *Solidago, green aniseed* or *dandelion*. Finally, researchers have established a correlation between arthritis and eating foods which are rich in saturated fats, found in animal fats and in hydrogenated oil. So try to avoid hydrogenated oils, replacing them with natural, non-hydrogenated fats and oil - fortunately these are getting easier and easier to find - and especially cold-pressed sesame oil.

Local Treatment

Apply compresses made of cabbage leaves or clay every day, alternating between them. You can also make a poultice with boiled maize and millet (cook without seasoning and apply while warm).

- *Urtica urens mother tincture,* 10 drops diluted in a glass of water - drink a mouthful from time to time throughout the course of the day. At the same time, take *Solidago 5 C.* 2 granules, twice a day, to stimulate kidney function. This is a general remedy.

The following remedies do not cover all cases of arthritis, and it's up to an experienced physician to prescribe the most appropriate one (or combination) for more complex cases, which are not mentioned here.

- *Ammonium muriaticum 7 C. 3* granules, twice a day. For those who are rather overweight, who have flabby skin and are subject to fits of mental depression and irritability. Their problems seem to worsen in cold weather.
- *Causticum 7 C. 5* granules every ten days. For cases where pains are aggravated by cold, dry weather.
- *Ledum palustre 7 C.* 3 granules, twice a day. Pains are aggravated by heat and movement, and seem to get worse at night.
- *Pulsatilla 7 C.* 3 granules, twice a day. For cases where aches and pains move from one part of the body to another.

Brain

Since the brain regulates all internal and unconscious physical activity, it deserves some passing mention. If we had to carry out consciously all the functions that the brain does in a single second -controlling respiration, digestion, cellular exchanges, combating harmful bacteria, etc. - we'd need months of calculating, by which time we'd be long dead.

Blood nourishes the brain, which is why a healthy balanced diet and fresh air are so important for regulating brain functions. Another factor is also very important - sleep - a source of renewed energy, during which the brain goes through a decompression stage, so to speak, and is thus able to carry on regulating our various states of activity, all of which are essential to our equilibrium.

Cancer
(See Also Longevity)

This dramatic illness, which costs so many lives every year, could well be included in the chapter on psychological disorders, so important is the role of attitude in the process of combating it. Being constantly worried, fearful, tormented, etc. can only make you more susceptible and vulnerable to certain types of cancer, just like smoking makes people more susceptible to throat or lung cancer.

This doesn't mean that you'll never get cancer if you're always happy and in a good mood, or that you'll be overcome by the disease if you're melancholy and unhappy. But the fact is that, if you live in a constant state of nervous tension, where you get upset about the least little thing - if you're always nervous, uptight, tense etc. - you make your body more vulnerable: your body becomes a much more favourable breeding ground for the development of those anarchic, destructive cells that we call cancer.

American researchers have demonstrated the effectiveness of garlic in preventing the formation of cancerous tumours. On the other hand, refined salt is being closely monitored as a possible cancer-causing agent. Also it is in the USA, the country where the highest levels of animal fat are consumed, that the highest incidence of cancer is found (as well as other diseases like arthritis, diabetes and heart disease). Finally, some people believe that large doses of vitamin C do a lot to slow down the development of cancer.

Although cancer is still a mystery, there are certain clues which can help us, if not to cure the disease completely, then at least to create conditions which are unfavourable for its appearance. It's rare for only one factor to be the cause of cancer. Usually a collection of factors work together, such as bad nutrition, lack of physical activity and/or clean air, general mental condition, and in some cases heredity.

Diet must certainly be taken into account when looking for the cause of many types of cancer. Vitamin deficiencies, problems caused by regular intake of processed foods that contain chemical additives and/or colouring, diets which are loaded with animal fat, chronic constipation are all factors that, over time, contribute to the formation of various types of cancer.

Other substances are also at fault: cooking fat that smokes on the fire becomes carcinogenic; insecticides used to protect plants against parasites; certain medications used in chemotherapy (like tar derivatives); some fertilizers which disturb the biological balance of plants; radioactive emissions, gas emissions. . . the list goes on and on.

The Curse of Modern Civilization

Faced with such an avalanche of information on products suspected of being carcinogens, many people fall prey to a sort of defeatist attitude, or even become completely negative and pessimistic. "What the hell - everything causes cancer these days!" says the pessimist, taking another puff of a cigarette. And to some extent, it's true. Every year, two and a half million people around the world die from inhaling other people's smoke. We are still ignorant and insensitive about matters concerning the environment, indifferent to the long-term consequences of our inventions, fascinated as we are with their novelty and practicality. Just look at food preservatives. These days, a loaf of bread lasts six weeks!

Health for Health's Sake?

But being actively occupied with the state of your health (instead of preoccupied, to the point where you get sick worrying about getting sick!) does not provide any kind of moral comfort - and this is what pessimistic people don't understand: taking care of your health produces an immediate or at least very rapid effect - you simply feel better! You're more in tune with your body, you stop getting ill so often, you're less tired, in a much better position to enjoy life, and leave it serenely, whatever the cause.

A Natural Process

Little by little, as we learn to take better care of our body, we become more sensitive, and learn spontaneously to avoid foods (as well as situations and behaviour patterns) which are harmful to health. Learning to relax, for example, as a way of dealing with cramps and other forms of tension (which slow down all functions in the body and thus make it more susceptible to the appearance of cancer) constitutes an excellent preventive measure. And at the same time, learning to relax makes us feel better.

The idea of living a healthy life does not necessarily mean living longer. What would be the point of that, if we are unhappy? The real aim is to live better.

And if illness prevails, despite all our precautions, we must not give in to despair. It would be more useful to take certain measures. And don't forget it has been shown conclusively that the attitude of people suffering from a disease is often a decisive factor in remission of the illness - even prayer (if it is heartfelt) can become a remedy and a powerful healing agent. It will be a long time before researchers, working in their laboratories, are able to find this psychic medication!

Anti-Cancer Foods

Certain foods are reputed to have anti-carcinogenic properties. Prominent among them are garlic (mentioned above), beetroot, raw grated carrots, raw chopped spinach, tarragon, fresh fruits, parsley. Other recommended substances include brewer's yeast and wheat germ, not to mention all other foods which are grown as naturally as possible, without chemical additives or artificial colouring. As for cooking oil, opt for cold-pressed corn or sunflower oil.

Foods To Avoid

All foods rich in cholesterol should be avoided. Here are some examples, to mention just a few: offal, game, sausage, brains, sweetbread, smoked meats (which contain carcinogenic tar), meat from immature animals, egg yolks, seafood, sardines, anchovies, eels, lard, butter, fresh cream, cheese, mushrooms, chocolate - as well as any foods which contain colourants and chemical additives which are likely to be carcinogenic agents.

Petasite - A Cancer Deterrent

Although not a remedy that cures cancer per se, *Petasite officinalis* is reputed to be an anti-cancer and antispasmodic agent that eliminates cramps and eases pain. You can consume massive doses of this completely non-toxic plant. Also *mistletoe* is said to have a positive influence on all levels of metabolism; *Celandine* is effective in healing the liver; and *Echinacea* helps soothe inflammation. Larkspur (*Delphinium consolida*) is said to have a beneficial effect on stomach and bowel cancers.

Here are some guidelines concerning homeopathic remedies which help people fight various forms of cancer, even though homeopathy - like allopathy - does not have any miracle cures or short-term solutions to the problem.

3 granules, once a day:
- *Arsenicum album* 5 C. Patients exhibit anxiety and are extremely agitated; rapid weight loss; pale face, swollen eyelids; bedridden; various pains, burning sensations, aggravated at night; for patients who think

they are incurable.

- *Calcarea flourica 5C*. For very hard, persistent tumours.
- *Carbo animalis 5 C*. When tumours develop in people with bluish skin, lined with little varicose veins, or in cases of cervical cancer. Patients are very susceptible to cold.
- *Condurango 5 C*. This remedy is reputed to have cured inoperable stomach cancers, marked by constant burning gastric pain and vomiting. Fissures appear around the corners of the mouth.
- *Conium 5 C*. For cancer of the testicles or uterus. Also for tumours which are the result of some kind of trauma. A characteristic sign is the yellowing of palms and fingernails.

Cataracts

- *Arnica 7 C*. 3 granules, three times per day. For cataracts resulting from a blow or injury.
- *Causticum 5 C*. 2 granules, once a day. For older people who are nervous, choleric, paralytic.
- *Magnesia 5 C*. 2 granules, once a day. For women with gynaecological disorders.
- *Phosphorus triiodatus 5 C*. 2 granules every three days. For people who bleed easily, and who are susceptible to haemorrhoids.
- *Silicea 5 C*. 2 granules, once a day. For older people, or people who read a lot and strain their eyes.

Cellulite

We don't have to give a detailed description of this well-known condition which affects women's hips and thighs, giving their skin that "orange peel" look. It seems that women suffering from asthma, urticaria (hives, rashes), gout and liver troubles are more likely to develop cellulite.

Lifestyle is also an influencing factor: lack of fresh air, rich food, late nights, and jobs that force women to remain standing for long periods of time. In addition, birth control pills can also cause cellulite.

Foods To Avoid
Processed meats, bread and pastries, biscuits, margarine, fried foods, alcohol,

sugar and very sweet fruits, salt.

Fruits That Fight Cellulite

Pineapples and strawberries, peaches, melons, grapefruit.

Drink a lot of demineralized water, especially between meals. Drink infusions of *Palthe, Santane O1 or Obeflorine Lehning*. Also take seaweed baths (*Thalgo, Sargasso*) and aromatic baths (*Lehning A or Seaweed Essence*). Complete the treatment with regular massages. Keep active!

- *Rhus tox 9 C and Arnica 8 C*. 2 granules when you awaken in the morning, on alternate days.
- *Badiaga 6 C* and *Pulsatilla 7 C*. 2 granules when you wake up, on alternate days. For skin that has hardened, and legs that have taken on a bluish red tint.

Cold (Sensitivity to)

Being sensitive to cold is often one of a group of symptoms which can be treated effectively by homeopathy.

3 granules, once a week:

- *Asarum Europum 7 C*. These people are sensitive to cold, and also can't stand noise, even slight noise. Nervous and emotional, they are so sensitive even their clothes bother them. They cough a lot - a kind of nervous coughing. Women have their periods early. Sunny dry weather, as well as pregnancy, aggravates the symptoms.
- *Calcarea silicata 7 C*. These people are pale and weak, and lack moral strength. They are irritable, hypersensitive, and want to be alone; they have equal difficulty dealing with hot or cold weather; they retain their appetite, but symptoms are aggravated by extreme heat or cold.
- *Petroleum 7 C*. For people who are sensitive to cold, usually thin, with dry, dull skin that cracks easily. They usually don't eliminate waste products regularly - perspiration is particularly insufficient. At times, such people can be irritable and depressed.

Conjunctivitis

The mucous membrane of the eyes turns red, and the tiny blood vessels in the whites of the eyes dilate. Consult a doctor. While waiting to see a doctor:

External Treatment

Bathe the eyes and eyelids with sterilized cotton-wool pads, dipped in *Camomile solution* (3 heads of camomile infused in a cup of boiling water).

- *Aconite 5 C.* 2 granules, four times a day. When conjunctivitis re*sults from exposure to dry cold*.
- *Allium cepa 7 C.* 3 granules, three times per day. For cases where conjunctivitis is accompanied by non-irritating dripping.
- *Apis mellifica 4 C.* 2 granules, four times per day. Eyelids are swollen and red, people are very sensitive to light.
- *Euphrasia 5 C* and *Belladonna 5 C.* 2 granules every hour, alternating. This is the most general remedy.
- *Mercurius corrosivus 9 C.* 3 granules, three times per day. Cases where irritating pus forms.
- *Pulsatilla 9 C.* 3 granules, three times per day. Cases where non-irritating pus is present.
- *Thuja 9 C.* 3 granules, three times per day. For conjunctivitis that recurs, or persists for a long period of time. Often the eyes are encrusted with dried mucus when the person wakes up.

Convalescence

Convalescence is an in-between state - the illness has regressed, but you aren't healthy yet. Your body is working to rebuild its strength, so this is not the time to treat it roughly, especially if the illness was serious.

Don't force people who are convalescing to eat - instead you should offer a varied diet. Foods like cabbage, apples, raw spinach and juices stimulate the appetite at the beginning of a meal. Serve fruits and nuts like apricots, almonds, dates, strawberries, hazelnuts, apples, prunes and grapes. Add green vegetables, green salads, eggs, lean red meat, offal, cereals and honey.

- *Wheat 1 C. Barley 1 C* and *Oats 1 C.* 10 drops in a little water, before meals.
- *Alfalfa 1 X* (one decimal). 20 drops in a little water before meals. For convalescing patients who are slow in recovering - they feel tired, discouraged, and think they'll never regain their health.
- *Calcarea phosphorica 5 C.* 3 granules, three times per day. For convalescents who have lost their appetite.
- *China 5 C.* 3 granules, three times per day. For persistent sweating.

- *Gelsemium 5 C.* 3 granules, three times per day. For cases where the lower limbs have lost all their strength.
- *Zincum 5 C.* 3 granules, three times per day. For convalescents suffering from insomnia; they have cramps in their lower limbs, sometimes accompanied by trembling.

To Get Back Into Top Shape

- *Arnica 9 C* and *Kali phosphoricum 9 C.* 3 granules of each, once a day. The combination of these two remedies helps regain the strength needed to carry out daily activities. They are also helpful in restoring memory.

Cysts

There is an alternative to surgery for getting rid of cysts, which are either hard or filled with liquid, and which usually appear around joints.

Cysts can have numerous causes: a sprain, bruise, rheumatism (consult the section on rheumatism). Wrap the affected joint in warm clothing, which you only remove to wash.

- *Benzoicum acidum 5 C.* 3 granules, three times per day. Especially for synovial cysts, in those suffering from rheumatism or uricaemia, and who are sensitive to cold air.
- *Kali iodatum 5 C.* 3 granules, three times per day, for people who are more sensitive to humid cold.
- *Sticta pulmonaria 4 C.* 3 granules three times per day, in cases of cysts accompanied by synovitis.

Decalcification

If your nails break easily and have little white spots on them, or if your teeth hurt when you're eating, and the tooth enamel starts breaking off, then it's high time you added some calcium to your system.

To prevent decalcification, you can use *Calcium flouratum,* a biochemical remedy used to fight tooth decay. Get out in the fresh air, take some sun, add foods to your diet that are rich in calcium (powdered milk, cheese, dried almonds, watercress, egg yolk, semolina, cabbage, endive, spinach, wheat germ, lentils, leeks, sole and yoghurt, for example).

- *Natrum muriaticum 9 C.* 5 granules, once a month; *Silicea 7 C* and

Baryta carbonica 7 C. 2 granules when you wake up, on alternate days. Also *Calcarea carbonica 7 C* and *Symphytum 7 C.* 2 granules around noon, on alternate days.

Dental Cavities
(See Also Teeth)

We all know that sugar is bad for young teeth. But we should specify that this refers to refined sugar and not to honey, dried fruits, figs, dates etc. - all of which are sweet but do not produce cavities. (Research has also shown that the sugar contained in sweets and soft drinks makes people more aggressive).

- *Belladonna 7 C.* Gums are red, inflamed and very sensitive to the touch. Abscess is possible.
- *Bryonia 7 C.* Any movement of the jaws aggravates the pain.
- *Chamomilla 7 C.* For cases where heat aggravates the pain.
- *Coffea 7 C.* For people who are over-excited and nervous.
- *Kreosotum 9 C.* 3 granules, three times per day, when the decayed tooth has become black.
- *Mercurius solubilis 9 C.* 3 granules, three times per day - if the decayed teeth are grey.

Diet
(See Also Cancer, Longevity)

Breathing air and eating food are the two fundamental and constant exchange processes that take place between ourselves and our environment. For the most part, we have inherited eating habits which have not been tailored to the sedentary lifestyle most people lead in these modern times (see Introduction).

The food we absorb is transformed into fuel for our bodies through a series of chemical reactions which occur during digestion. And that's why the combinations of foods we ingest are so important, whether we are aware of it or not.

One Heavy Afternoon

A delicious lunch in the best tradition - meat and potatoes washed down with a couple of beers or a glass of wine, and mop up the gravy with bread and butter. . . top it all off with a piece of sugary sweet dessert and a good strong cup of coffee.

And there you are, ready to face the rest of the day. . . except that you suddenly feel so tired. Not even the stimulation of a good strong cup of coffee is enough to overcome this combination of starch and sugar which is so heavy to digest, not to mention the red meat. We'd be much better off with a salad instead of potatoes, and we should forget about dessert altogether.

That would be a good first step, and the difference would be enormous. Take *Nux vomica 5 C* (3 granules) to help deal with any over-eating, until you can modify your eating habits to include lighter meals.

Change Is in the Air
We absolutely must learn to explore new types of food, put together new combinations and stop being afraid of change. We have to develop our curiosity and depend more on our instinctive desire to seek out foods that agree with us, instead of relying on outdated formulas. And we must pass these new habits on to our children. After all, who's to say that in the twenty-first century, our diet may not be based on seaweed? The best way to proceed is to gradually explore and integrate new foods and eating habits, without relying on our old prejudices.

Find the Right Rhythm
We sometimes underestimate the power of tradition and acquired habits. It's better to make a gradual change than suddenly attempt a complete transformation, where you run the risk of falling back into your old habits once the novelty wears off, or you have some unpleasant experience.

However, we now know that some diseases, like cancer, are not simply hereditary but are caused, at least to some extent, by the food we eat, the emotions we feel and the kind of lifestyle we lead. This is not the place to try and develop an "ideal diet" - the study of diet merits a book in itself. But to put it simply, if you succeed in gradually modifying your eating habits to include lighter, high-energy foods and reduce the number of foods you eat which contain chemical additives (for example, replacing tinned vegetables with fresh ones whenever possible) then you'll go a long way towards increasing your store of "vital energy."

Losing Weight
So many people dream of finding a miracle pill that would allow them to indulge in all kinds of culinary excesses without endangering their health, or their waistline! Obviously, anyone who could develop such a drug would become a

millionaire overnight.

But in the meantime - and if we look at the problem with a little perspicacity we'd realize that this kind of miracle product would do us more harm than good, since we'd lose touch with an essential aspect of reality - we have to learn to control our desire to overeat, or continue to pay the price.

Controlling your appetite is fine, but there's one important condition: never endanger your health. So avoid slimming pills which are synthesized from chemicals or from iodine (although iodine is an essential substance for our body, it becomes a poison if taken in large quantities).

A Natural Diet

Choose a diet that is low in protein, and reduce your intake of carbohydrates (potatoes, pasta, noodles, bread, rice). Avoid sugar-based products and refined flour (e.g. pastries). Green vegetables, salads, yoghurt, lean meat and fruit are the best foods to keep your waistline trim, provided you keep the amounts down to a reasonable level, of course. Doing a carrot juice cure from time to time is also excellent. Another method is to replace rich foods with raw vegetables, juices and salads. Avoid all animal fat, and reduce the amount of butter you use. Spices like horseradish and curry, and brewer's yeast are also excellent for stimulating the glands. Kelp, a form of seaweed, helps you lose weight gradually, and stimulates the glands at the same time - it also makes you feel better overall.

However, your appearance isn't all that counts. You have to know if you are really overweight, or if you are making a vain attempt to conform to certain fashionable and purely aesthetic standards - to fashion, which values the body more than the person inhabiting it.

Finally, we should remind you that exercise regulates the appetite and does not stimulate it is the popular belief. So, taking a brisk walk before eating will actually diminish your appetite, whereas being a "couch potato" will make you want to eat more.

- *Antimonium crudum 9 C.* 3 granules, 10 minutes before meals, it curbs appetite.

Abnormal Weight Loss

This can happen during the course of an illness - a patient loses so much weight that she/he becomes too weak to recover, or simply causes undue worry to the people caring for him or her.

3 granules, one dosage (repeated if necessary):

- *Abrotanum 4 C*. For infants who lose weight, especially in the lower limbs. They have trouble standing up, their face is wrinkled, their eyes are dull and have dark rings around them. Continue the treatment with *Natrum muriaticum 5 C*. If the condition persists, see a doctor.
- *Natrum muriaticum 7 C*. One dosage, repeated 15 days later if necessary. Combine it with another medication. For cases where a child is sick, and continues losing weight even though she/he eats well. She/he is also depressed, always moody; any physical or mental effort is almost impossible; she/he is intensely thirsty.
- *Arsenicum album 5 C*. Sometimes excited, sometimes depressed, these patients exhibit signs of anxiety; they are afraid of dying; the condition worsens during the night. They experience itching sensations, which are aggravated by heat.
- *Calcarea phosphorica 5 C*. Children who grow very quickly often get headaches, especially when they have to make a mental effort; they show signs of sexual arousal; their appetite is good, but they usually eat a lot between meals; sleep is agitated.
- *Iodum 5 C*. Patients who may eat a lot but are never satisfied, and continue losing weight; constantly agitated, they seem to be exhausting themselves.
- *Silicea 5 C*. Patients are so thin they cannot stay warm; they catch colds and develop bronchitis, as well as other respiratory problems; in children, development is below normal; in adults, there is a pronounced lack of energy.

Ears
(See Also Hypersensitivity)

These remedies concern disorders of the auditory canal and the outer ear, and pains which are specific to the ear (otalgia). Except for otitis, such pains are often caused either by a boil, by eczema in the auditory canal, or by the presence of a foreign body (insect, dust, etc.)

- *Belladonna 5 C*. 2 granules every hour. Patients feel exhausted, and the pains are very intense.
- *Calcarea picrata 5 C*. 3 granules every three hours. For boils in the inner auditory canal.
- *Capsicum 5 C*. 3 granules once every hour. A burning sensation spreads

from the throat to the ears, which are swollen and sensitive to the touch.

- *Chamomilla 4 C.* 2 granules every hour. For violent, intolerable pain which affects the ears in cases of sore throat or infections of the nose and/or throat. You can also administer a few drops of *Plantago tincture* directly into the ear.
- *Oscillococcinum 200* - a single dose (a tube of the remedy in powdered form) dissolved in a small glass of water. For ear-ache with or without fever, even for cases of otitis.
- *Petroleum 5 C.* 3 granules three times a day. For chapping caused by exposure to dry cold.
- *Picricum acidum 7 C.* 3 granules every three hours. For boils of the exterior auditory canal.
- *Malandrinum 5 C.* 3 granules three times a day. For chapping caused by exposure to humid cold.
- *Nitricum acidum 5 C.* 3 granules, three times a day. For clean, bleeding fissures. Use *Sepia* if the edge of the fissure is not clean.

Fever

Fever in itself is not an illness, but a defensive reaction of the body against some form of aggression. That is why you are actually hindering your own immune system when you take an aspirin or some other medication at the first sign of fever.

This is obviously also true for antibiotics which, although they don't act on the fever itself, attack the bacteria which cause it. By so doing, they usurp the role of the body's immune system, which should be able to defend itself. And it is precisely that capacity which homeopathy stimulates and encourages, while antibiotics make the body dependent on external protection, which reduces its own ability to detect problems and react accordingly.

Of course, the fact that fever is a desirable reaction of a body against aggression does not mean to say that very high fever cannot be dangerous. Remember that the body's average normal temperature is 98.6° Fahrenheit (37° Celsius).

Different Degrees Of Fever
Up to 100.4°F (38°C) - very slight fever
From 100.4° to 101.5°F (38 - 38.5°C) - slight fever

From 101.5° to l02.2°F (38.5 - 39°C) - moderate fever

From 102.2° to 104°F (39 - 40°C) - high fever

Above 104°F (40°C) - very high fever

Ideally you should take a person's temperature while they are lying down, using a rectal thermometer (if you prefer to use an oral thermometer, add about one degree to the reading), in the morning when the person wakes up, and in the evening around six o'clock. Make a note of the reading each time; this can be very useful information if a doctor is called in.

A fever that subsides naturally does so at a very slow pace, burning the substances in the body that it is supposed to get rid of. But once it starts going down, it will hardly ever start rising again. This is a sign that the toxins have been eliminated. In fact, for fever to do its job properly, the three main elimination routes - intestines, kidneys and skin - must be functioning smoothly and play their part.

To be assured of proper elimination, administer natural laxatives (use anal suppositories if they have no effect orally) and intestinal stimulants as soon as the fever appears. Diuretics, especially *Solidago or Golden rod,* stimulate the kidneys. Infusions of parsley, onion and juniper also have a diuretic effect.

Note that animals, when they fall sick, stop eating altogether. You should not try to ease your conscience by force-feeding someone who is ill. If the patient isn't hungry, don't insist, at least for a few days. Offer fruit juices, or infusions with a little honey. These are a kind of cure in themselves, and can only speed up recovery.

And if the patient wants to eat, serve light foods that are easy to digest.

In cases of high fever, you can administer lukewarm baths, cooling the water down little by little; or wrap patients in damp, cool sheets or towels; or wash them with cool or cold water. Make sure patients change position in bed at least once every four to six hours.

Administer 2 granules of one of the following remedies, every two hours (note that quinine, in homeopathic remedies, is a veritable antidote):

- *Aconitum 5 C.* After catching a cold, fever mounts rapidly. Patients are agitated, nervous; their skin is dry and burning, the pulse is strong and occasionally irregular.
- *Belladonna 5 C.* Patients feel exhausted, and are sensitive to light. Their faces are flushed, their skin is clammy and they perspire from all parts of

the body which remain covered.

- *Bryonia 5 C*. For fever which rises after a sudden change in temperature. Accompanied by chest pains (and especially between the ribs) or in one or a number of joints. Patients prefer to remain immobile.
- *Eupatorium perfoliatum 5 C*. Thirst is an important characteristic in these cases. Patients ache all over, and suffer from violent shivering and nausea, which gets worse when they drink. They often develop headaches, especially around the eyes.
- *China 5 C*. Intermittent fever, which appears only during the day. However, the night before the fever appears, patients' sleep is agitated. They shiver, are not thirsty unless they sweat a lot during the night. The upper right side of the abdomen is especially painful.
- *Chininum sulphuricum 5 C*. Intermittent fever, especially mid-morning and afternoon. Violent shivering and pain in the middle part of the spine. Intense thirst, flushed face.
- *Ferrum phosphoricum 5 C*. For moderate fevers.
- *Gelsemium 5 C*. Patients feel as if their head is being squeezed in a vice. Congestion and hot flushes to the head, eyelids are heavy and almost closed, abundant sweating and shivering. Pulse is slow. Absence of thirst is a characteristic sign.
- *Ipecac. 5 C*. Intermittent fever, especially early morning (between 9 and 11 a.m.) or late in the afternoon. *Ipecac*. produces abundant sweat, which is cold and viscous, as well as nausea and digestive problems. Often one cheek is red while the other is pale. Patients are very sensitive to heat.
- *Rhus tox 5 C*. For people who get caught in the rain, for example. After an initial sensation of cold (more marked on the right side of the body) they start shivering and coughing. Patients cannot stay in the same place for long periods. In addition to excessive perspiration, they develop herpes sores around the mouth area, and a red triangle on the tip of the tongue.
- *Sulphur 4 C*. This is a convalescent remedy. *Sulphur* is an excellent preventive measure, in cases of impending relapse. Patients feel very weak - they absolutely must eat around eleven in the morning, in order not to become too weak. Hot flushes, feelings of oppression, burning sensations in the palms and feet; temperature between 99.5°F (37.5°C) and 100°F (37.8°C) completes the *Sulphur* picture.

Fortifiers

(See Also Convalescence, Aches and Mental Fatigue)

Strictly speaking, there are no fortifiers in homeopathic medicine, but certain remedies can sometimes act as temporary stimulants.

Take three granules, three times a day, of one of the following medications:

- *Arnica 9 C.* For cases of fatigue after excessive physical exertion, or some kind of trauma.
- *Calcarea phosphorica 9 C.* For children going through a period of rapid growth.
- *Calendula 7 C.* For wounds - this remedy stimulates healing.
- *China officinalis 9 C.* Cases where people have lost a lot of liquid (because of diarrhoea, profuse sweating, excessive menstruation or vomiting).
- *Cocculus Indicus 9 C.* When sleepless nights and prolonged insomnia undermine strength.
- *Gelsemium 9 C.* Bad news can sometimes sap our energy.
- *Iodum 9 C.* Patients are tired and lose weight even if they eat well.
- *Kali phosphoricum 9 C.* When fatigue becomes a permanent state of lassitude, and develops into a psychological disorder.
- *Rhus tox 9 C.* For getting rid of aches and pains caused by over-activity or sports.

Gingivitis

(Inflammation of the Gums)

Patients are pale, weak and lack appetite. But the principal symptom is that their gums are inflamed, sometimes to the point where they can no longer close their mouth or chew their food. So because of their swollen, sensitive gums, they are forced to fast, and grow weak.

There are numerous possible causes of gingivitis: it can, for example, result from teething, tooth decay, the growth of a wisdom tooth, a lack of vitamins, smoking or an infection of the kidneys, liver or intestines.

After each meal, patients should brush their teeth with toothpaste containing 30% hydroxydase. They should rinse their mouths with *Calendula mother tincture* (10 drops in a glass of water which has been boiled and then cooled) and with lemon juice a few times a day. They should avoid eating nuts and abstain almost completely from meat. For infant cases, make sure not to overfeed, and sterilize all teats and bottles.

2 granules of the appropriate medication, every two hours:

- *Agave 5 C.* Patients are anaemic and have dark blue pustules on the legs.
- *Ammonium carbonicum 5 C.* Patients are even weaker than for Agave treatment; they tend to haemorrhage easily and suffer from pains in their joints.
- *Arsenicum album 5 C.* Gums bleed and this form of gingivitis occurs during a serious illness, where patients become anxious and exhausted.
- *Kali phosphoricum 5 C.* Patients are depressed; their tongues have a brownish coating, their mouth is dry and a red line can be observed around the edge of the gums.
- *Kreosotum 5 C.* For bleeding gingivitis; in addition to being inflamed, gums are dark bluish red and very painful (burning pain); they bleed easily; patients' breath is putrid, and teeth may show dark splotches and break easily.
- *Mercurius 5 C.* The tongue is moist and flabby, and retains marks made by the teeth; bad smelling breath and occasionally ulcers around the mouth; gums are more painful at night or when drinking hot or cold liquids.

Halitosis
(Bad Breath)

Bad breath is an embarrassing condition, both in social and personal life, and has resisted treatment by so-called modern scientific methods.

- *Antimonium crudum 4 C.* 3 granules, every three hours. When people belch and taste the food they have recently eaten; this condition is often caused by badly digested food, which has been eaten too quickly.
- *Chelidonium 4 C and Taraxacum 4 C.* 3 granules, every three hours. Both remedies help alleviate symptoms due to a poorly functioning liver. Typically, these people are obsessed by their bad breath, which they find tastes like faeces.
- *Graphites 5 C.* 3 granules, every four hours. Bad breath is accompanied by constipation. People have trouble digesting; flatulence and belching smell like rotten eggs; symptoms are aggravated during menstruation, sometimes producing mouth ulcers or skin rashes.

- *Nux vomica 4 C*. 3 granules, every three hours. When overeating leaves a bad taste in the mouth, and people are in a very bad mood when they wake up the next day.
- *Pulsatilla 5 C*. 3 granules, every four hours. Fights bad breath in those with weak stomachs, who have trouble digesting fatty foods and pastries; they also feel the need to rinse their mouth very frequently.

Hernia

This term describes a condition where part of the bowel falls into the scrotum (in men) or into the outer vaginal lips (in women). Hernias may be congenital, or they may result from occasional but violent exertion or a particular physical activity. Repeated physical exertion can also produce a hernia.

A strangulated hernia, which is very painful and impossible to push back up into the abdomen, is a real problem. The hard, painful ball formed by the hernia, usually situated at the base of the anus, is easy to locate.

For some strange reason, people at both ends of the age spectrum are most often affected - i.e. infants and old people. Intense local pain is accompanied by colic, nausea and vomiting; small amounts of blood may flow from the anus - in such cases, consult a specialist as quickly as possible.

While waiting to see a doctor:

- *Belladonna 4 C*. 2 granules every 20 minutes, if the region is extremely sensitive and pains are acute (cutting, searing pain).
- *Opium 5 C*. 2 granules every 20 minutes, when the stomach is swollen and hard.

Hiatus Hernia

After some traumatic event (a fall or an accident) or sometimes in cases of obesity or pregnancy, a part of the stomach penetrates the chest cavity. After meals, people experience pains and nausea and become short of breath very easily.

Precautions

Physical activity is all right, but in moderation. Avoid tight-fitting, restrictive clothes and do not lie down after meals - stay sitting, or get up and walk around. Make sure the food you eat is easy to digest. Avoid sauces, coffee and acidic fruit juices.

- *Argentum nitricum 5 C.* 3 granules, three times per day. For cases where the hernia is accompanied by burning sensations in the stomach and aggravated by sweets.
- *Kali carbonicum 5 C.* 3 granules, three times per day. Burning sensations in the stomach are accompanied by nausea and acidic belching; patients feel as if their stomach is full of water.

Hunger
(Also See Appetite)

Sick people often find that their appetite is disturbed in one way or another; the form of this disturbance may be a clue in choosing the appropriate remedy.

Choose the remedy which most closely corresponds to the patient's condition (Dilution: 5 C) and administer 3 granules, twice a day.

- *Abrotanum, Iodum* and *Natrum muriaticum.* Although the patient eats well, she/he continues losing weight.
- *Anacardium.* For patients whose appetite is good and whose symptoms are eased by eating.
- *Cina* and *Lycopodium.* For those who are still hungry after eating.
- *Colchicum, Sepia* and *Stannum.* For those people who lose their appetite as soon as they see or smell food.
- *Ignatia* and *Sulphur.* People who are hungry towards the end of the morning, and experience feelings of inadequacy.
- *Natrum carbonicum.* For those who are excessively hungry during the day, between 5 in the morning and 11 o'clock at night.
- *Psorinum, Lycopodium* and *Petroleum.* For people who suffer from excessive hunger at night.

Hypoglycaemia

This disorder is due to an insufficiency of sugar (glucose) in the blood, which results in various kinds of problems: weakness, dizzy spells, sweating, muscular spasms, etc. Below a certain threshold, people may become depressed and even suffer blackouts, accompanied by visual problems and mental confusion.

People who suffer from hypoglycaemia (e.g. diabetics) often carry some form of sugar around in their pocket at all times, which they take at the least sign of a crisis. However, it seems that this method produces only very temporary benefits.

Strangely enough, the most effective and natural way to combat hypoglycaemia is to stop eating sugar altogether, especially refined sugar, and to rely on the glucose contained in fruits.

An episode of hypoglycaemia can also result from some excessive physical exertion or from fasting.

- *Insulinum 5 C.* 2 granules per day, with *Nux vomica 5 C* and *Cocculus Indicus 5 C,* 2 granules of each, once a day.

Incontinence (Urinary)

Opotherapy can be very helpful for people who have reached old age, and who find that their reflexes have lost some of their acuteness, and that they have trouble controlling their sphincter and bladder. Opotherapy is a medical process which consists of taking tissue from healthy organs, then diluting and dynamizing it to form a homeopathic remedy.

- *Sphincter, Neck of the bladder, Ligaments, 4 C* trituration. Take a pinch of powder twice a day.

Kuhne Baths

Kuhne baths are a useful treatment for a large number of disorders, such as headaches, cerebral congestion, anorexia, frigidity, hypersexuality, and many more (depression can also be soothed sometimes with regular application of Kuhne baths).

Place a board across a tub of cold water, sit on it and wrap yourself in hot sheets or towels, leaving your abdomen exposed.

Rub your skin around the genital area with a sponge or bath brush, which you dip into the tub from time to time. The idea is to change the temperature of one single part of the body. Continue the procedure for about an hour, making sure to keep the rest of your body warm, wrapped in hot towels.

Longevity

"The best way to prolong your life is not to do anything to shorten it," said Herbert Spencer. That's all very well, but how are we supposed to know what is harmful and what isn't?

Observations of populations who are remarkable for their longevity have determined three factors which always seem to be present in cultures where people reach very advanced ages while remaining in excellent health (and after all, what would be the use of spending your last ten years of life confined to a hospital bed, being fed via an intravenous tube?).

The Three Secrets of Longevity

1. People who reach very old age remain physically active all their lives, and in a natural way. For such people, exercise is not an end in itself - an effort they have to make to stay in shape. Instead, it becomes part of their lives, as they engage in activities like gardening, working in the fields, walking in the mountains, etc.

2. Have you ever seen an obese centenarian? As a general rule, these people eat little - they maintain a frugal diet (the famous Bulgarian Hundred-Year-Old diet is cited as an example later on).

3. Finally, these people remain integrated into the communities in which they live, right up to a very old age. They continue to play an active role in community affairs - to assert their place, so to speak. They have a very developed sense of belonging, and feel useful (at least symbolically).

We need not emphasize the fact that these customs are precisely those which are lacking in modern western societies. They only exist in small villages, or in isolated rural or mountain communities in Bulgaria or in the Himalayas. Another factor is certainly the purity of the air these people breathe, and of the food they eat, which is not contaminated with pollutants or transformed and processed in factories.

Even if we cannot clean up the air we breathe overnight (see the section on Pollution) or modify the social habits of the community in which we live, having access to a certain amount of information is nevertheless essential if we want to live longer. Most important is information concerning what we eat.

Longevity Diet

- Grains, nuts and cereals are excellent for a highly nutritious diet. Rice and millet, sesame and sunflower seeds and soya beans contain complete protein nutrients with very high nutritional value.
- Sprouting increases the nutritive value of grains and cereals: wheat germ, mung beans, alfalfa and soya seeds make excellent sprouts. Millet, rice and oats are delicious and nourishing cereals.
- Vegetables are an excellent source of protein, enzymes and minerals.

Most vegetables can be eaten raw. Garlic, onions, condiments and natural spices should also be a regular part of your diet.

• Fruits, like vegetables, are an excellent source of vitamins, enzymes and minerals, and also play a role in cleaning out the body. Eat fresh fruit as often as possible.

How To Eat Half as Much

Ideally, three quarters of your food should be eaten raw. It has been proved that it is possible to reduce your intake of food by half if you eat raw foods. This is because their nutritive value is so superior to foods that are cooked. Also drink lots of vegetable juice (one vegetable at a time, not mixed with fruit). A good juicer is far from being a luxury - it is a necessity if you want to maintain a healthy diet.

Make sure you buy natural or organic products which are not processed or refined and are grown without chemical fertilizers, as far as possible.

Dairy Products

Milk constitutes a complete nutrient, especially in its more acidic forms, like kefir, yoghurt, buttermilk etc. All these products help maintain your gut flora - bacteria which are essential for proper digestion - and this has the effect of preventing constipation. Goat's milk is superior to cow's milk. Use honey as a sweetener as much as possible.

Oils: Cold-Pressed

Use only cold-pressed vegetable oils - unrefined and non-hydrogenated. Choose oil made from sesame seeds or sunflower seeds. Since consumers are demanding these products more and more, they should be readily available.

Meat: Moderation Is the Key

Avoid eating too much protein, especially from animal sources. You can eat eggs, fish and meat, but none of these are absolute necessities. A diet that contains a lot of animal-based protein is harmful to your health and can cause - or at least predispose you to - various disorders like arthritis, heart disease, cancer, schizophrenia and kidney problems. Eating a lot of meat also causes premature ageing, and shortens life expectancy in general.

In addition, older people who are less active, and whose organic functions have slowed down, should consume even less protein.

Water: Lots of It!

Drink pure, non-contaminated water, either spring water or well water. Studies have shown that people who regularly drink water which contains minerals suffer less from heart disease, have fewer cavities and are less susceptible to diabetes and arteriosclerosis. (Also avoid drinking too much distilled water.)

And From Time to Time - Nothing at All!

You should fast periodically, in order to give your system a rest and a chance to clean itself out. Fasting allows you to eliminate accumulated toxins and to re-establish your vital functions. We recommend fasting at least once a year, for seven to ten days, preferably in spring. During your fast, drink liquids like vegetable broth (unsalted), mineral water and fruit juice.

You can eat a piece of fruit from time to time, if the idea of not eating at all worries you. Another suggestion: fast for three days a week (Wednesday, Friday and Saturday) after each full moon.

Juice Cures

Juice cures are more effective than traditional water cures. They strengthen the body's organs of elimination (lungs, liver, kidneys, intestines and even the skin - a very important eliminatory organ). You'll feel the beneficial effects throughout your body, and on all levels - physical, mental and sexual.

Five Pointers for Better Health

1. Eat slowly, in a relaxed atmosphere, and chew your food well.
2. It's better to eat a number of light meals throughout the day, rather than one or two heavy meals.
3. Don't mix raw vegetables and raw fruits in the same meal.
4. When you eat foods that are rich in protein, start the meal with those foods.
5. Eat only when you're really hungry, and stop before you're completely full. The less you eat, the less hungry you'll be.

What To Avoid

You probably already know the list of harmful substances, but they're worth repeating:

Coffee, tea, chocolate, fizzy drinks and excessive amounts of salt; tobacco; alcohol in excess; white sugar, white flour, and any foods that contain them;

refined, processed, or prepared foods or food that is cooked in a factory; any rancid or rotten food.

Remember that many foods may contain hidden amounts of sugar. These include sausages, powdered milk, tinned vegetables, white bread, savoury biscuits, etc.

Daily Physical Activity

Feeding your body isn't enough - you also have to make it move. The best exercise, which is absolutely risk-free, is simply to walk for at least an hour each day.

The Bulgarian Hundred-Year-Old Diet

The diet in question is largely lacto-vegetarian (based on dairy products and vegetables). It includes many cereals grown in the region and freshly ground (barley especially), fruits and vegetables often grown in local gardens by the people who eat them, many of whom have aged way beyond conventional retirement.

These centenarians also eat a lot of honey. Fermented foods, like pickled cabbage, are often included in a meal (sauerkraut is rich in vitamin C and lactic acid, which is why it is reputed to be an excellent anti-cancer agent). In addition, sunflower seeds are usually part of their daily diet.

Lumbago

It's a very familiar problem: you make one of those awkward movements, and there you are, twisted in pain afflicted with lumbago. Both the cervical region and the spine at the level of the kidneys, are often placed under a lot of strain when you make some heavy physical effort.

It isn't the effort itself that's dangerous, but the sudden movement or misplaced burden that causes this kind of painful muscular contraction. As with torticollis (stiff neck) the condition often persists, preventing us from carrying out even the simplest daily activities. Depending on the case, the problem may be of recent origin, or chronic, resulting in a prolonged involuntary contraction of the muscles either side of the spine.

Lumbago can also result from a simple cold, a fall or accident, or rheumatism. If the pain is related to some specific muscular effort, consult an osteopath. But whatever the cause, it's better to heal yourself and not allow the problem to become permanent.

Relaxing Your Muscles

Practising one of the various forms of relaxation (yoga, autogenic training, isolation tanks, etc.) can help loosen up "twisted" muscles. Also, use a soothing balm to rub your muscles (as you would do for a stiff neck).

Take 2 granules, twice a day, of one of the following medications:

- *Cimicifuga racemosa 5 C*. Cramps or back pains are seemingly caused by a uterine disorder; they are aggravated by cold and/or humidity, and eased by movement, fresh air and heat.
- *Arnica 5 C*. For cases of injury: sudden shocks, false moves, intense or repeated exertion (at work, for example); people feel that their bed is hard, and their whole body seems to ache along with the localized back pain; they are irritable; the pain is aggravated by touching and by movement.
- *Dulcamara 5 C*. After exposure to cold, humid air, especially in summer and autumn; pain is soothed by exposure to heat.
- *Calcarea flourica 5 C*. For chronic lumbago caused by rheumatism; reappears after physical exertion, but diminishes when the exertion is continued for some time; veins are dilated, and varicose veins appear on the chest.
- *Calcarea phosphorica 5 C*. Pains in the joints accompany the lumbago; psychological symptoms include feelings of anxiety and some mental confusion.
- *Kali carbonicum 5 C*. A basic remedy for chronic lumbago; people often experience acute pains at night; they are weak and have cold sweats; this type of lumbago can occur after sexual relations, or when you catch a cold, even a mild one.
- *Nux vomica 5 C*. Resulting from excessive exertion, this type of lumbago is marked by (involuntary) contraction of the affected muscles; patients have to sit up in bed in order to turn around; they are often irritable, anxious and find the pain intolerable; pains seem to increase when patients have to remain still, and are alleviated by moving around.
- *Rhus tox 5 C*. A basic treatment for all cases of lumbago, which worsens especially after exposure to humidity and cold; characterized by stiff muscles and pains; accompanied by rheumatic ankylosis (numbness, stiffening), and general aches, especially in the morning and when

patients have to move; they are hypersensitive, both physically and mentally; they despair of ever recovering; gentle movement and rest ease the pain.

- *Ruta graveolens 5 C*. For cases of lumbago caused by lifting heavy objects with the arms; characterized by a sensation of something having broken; when asleep, patients are agitated; weakness and pain is felt in the lower limbs, as well as pressure in the bladder; patients are at their worst before getting up, and the symptoms are eased if they remain lying on their back.
- *Natrum muriaticum 5 C*. People awaken each morning with pains caused by their lumbago. Here the cause is organic; it often appears in people who tend to develop eczema, and are inclined to be depressed.

Meningitis

The symptoms of meningitis are relatively easy to identify. Firstly, there are violent and incessant headaches; then pains in the nape of the neck, which becomes stiff, as if it were made out of a block of wood; fever rises to between 102°F (39°C) and 104°F (40°C) and is accompanied by intense shivering; there may be herpes sores around the mouth, the skin develops blue blotches; vomiting completes the picture.

In its tuberculous form, this illness remains very serious, despite the advances made by orthodox medicine in treating it, which have reduced the number of deaths attributed to the illness by a third and in some areas by one half. In any case, if you see these symptoms developing when fever occurs, consult a doctor as soon as possible. In addition, this is a notifiable disease by law, since it can be very contagious - patients usually have to remain in isolation for a period of 20 days after recovering.

While waiting to see a doctor:

- *Aconitum napellus 5 C*. 2 granules every two hours. Symptoms have just begun to appear, and the patient is very agitated.
- *Apis mellifica 5 C*. 2 granules every two hours. This is an initial remedy. The patient is in a state of stupor, the face is bloated, she/he is agitated, and may even go into convulsions, accompanied by piercing shrieks; she/he cannot drink or urinate. Symptoms are aggravated by heat.
- *Belladonna 5 C*. 3 granules every three hours. An initial remedy, when the fever is very high. Patients are delirious and may start writhing and

throwing their head back against the pillow; they can't stand noise, light or any kind of movement; the face is red and hot. Stop administering this medication at the first sign of effusion.

- *Cicuta virosa 4 C.* 2 granules every three hours, in cases of cerebrospinal meningitis. Headaches are accompanied by what is called Kernig's sign: patients cannot extend their legs, which flex automatically when they are seated on the edge of the bed, or when you try to get them to stand up.
- *Crotalus horridus 4 C.* 2 granules every hour. Alternate with Cicuta virosa, if purple blotches appear in addition to the symptoms described for that remedy.
- *Helleborus 5 C.* 3 granules, three times per day. Patients stare into space, pupils are dilated, they are in a state of complete torpor. They do not react to any stimulation, their jaw hangs loose, and they move their head in a mechanical way.
- *Veratrum viride 4 C.* 3 granules every three hours. Fever rises and falls, the head is congested, pulse is weak and intermittent, the patient is agitated and goes into convulsions.

Mental Retardation

- *Aethusa cynapium 7 C.* 2 granules upon waking up, alternated with *Bufo 7 C.* 2 granules.
- *Agaricus muscarius 9 C.* 5 granules each week. For children who are mentally weak or slow, usually at its worst in the morning. They have trouble with comprehension, their memory is weak, and they are moody.
- *Baryta carb 9 C.* 5 granules once every ten days. For people who are slow, timid and susceptible to cold.
- *Rana bufo 9 C.* 3 granules once a week. These cases don't seem able to control their thoughts or reactions; they appear dazed and apathetic; they often lack control over their sexual impulses and exhibit a very weak memory.

Migraine

Migraines are distinguished from ordinary headaches by their intensity, which is sometimes intolerable. They occur in the form of attacks and are accompanied by a general feeling of unease, as well as nausea and vomiting.

We could easily write a whole chapter - indeed a whole book - on the subject of migraine. However, space limits us to citing only a few sample remedies.

Avoid Migraines

Eat light foods and chew well. Abstain from chocolate, cooked fat and fried foods, alcohol, processed meats, wild game, marinated fish, blue cheese, white wine. Drink spring water or water that has a low mineral content.

- *Belladonna 5 C*. 3 granules every two hours. For cases where the face is flushed and hot, pupils are dilated; pain is intensified by noise, light, any jolting movements or when the head is tilted forward.
- *Bryonia 5 C*. 3 granules every two hours. The migraine gets worse as night approaches, and the slightest movement - even moving the eyes - aggravates the pain. Patients are very thirsty, their tongue is coated white, they feel dizzy if they try to get up.
- *Cyclamen 7 C*. 3 granules every three hours. Pain is concentrated in the forehead, with a sensation of heaviness above the eyes, which affects vision. When vision improves, the pain increases. Menstruation also intensifies the pain.
- *Gelsemium 5 C*. 3 granules every two hours. As well as being preceded by problems with vision, this type of migraine is accompanied by trembling and depression. The face is red and congested, people feel exhausted, their pulse is slow. Although they are not thirsty, passing a lot of urine usually signals the end of the attack. *Gelsemium* is also recommended for migraines which are accompanied by eye problems that are brought on by some kind of bad news.
- *Iris versicolor 5 C*. 3 granules every two hours. Vision problems, in particular sensitivity to bright lights, marks the beginning of each attack. Localized in the forehead, this type of migraine is accompanied by acidic vomiting, or a burning sensation in the stomach, which can rise up into the throat and mouth, where it is felt on the tongue. If it occurs on a regular weekly basis, notably at weekends, administer *Iris versicolor 15 C* and *Lac defloratum 9 C*, 3 granules of each, once a week, to complete the treatment.
- *Melilotus 5 C*. 3 granules every three hours. The face is red and congested. A characteristic of this type of migraine is the fact that bleeding (menstrual or a nosebleed) seems to alleviate the pain.
- *Natrum muriaticum 7 C*. 2 granules, three times per day. Preceded by

vision problems, this migraine is accompanied by intense thirst and weeping. Herpes sores often form around the mouth. *Natrum muriaticum* is also effective in treating migraines made worse by intense mental effort, when you feel like there's a grain of sand lodged under your eyelids, you're extremely thirsty and you feel depressed, especially in the morning.

- *Nux vomica 7 C.* 3 granules, three times per day. This migraine follows a bout of overeating, which produces digestive problems. The back of the tongue is coated with a yellowish-white substance, cheeks are red; these people are irritable and often short-tempered, cannot stand bright lights or noise and are frequently constipated.
- *Sanguinaria 5 C.* 2 granules every three hours. For recurring migraines, which strike about every two weeks. The face is red, people suffer from hot flushes, and the pain radiates out from the nape of the neck to above the right eye. Although hungry, these people feel an aversion to food.
- *Silicea 5 C.* 2 granules every two hours. People are more sensitive to cold than usual and feel pain in the nape of the neck, starting in the early morning. Keeping the head warm by wrapping it in a hot towel seems to ease the pain. Those who suffer from this type of migraine usually lack energy and self-confidence.
- *Sepia 5 C.* 2 granules every two hours. Concentrated under the left eye, pain seems to ease off in the dark; eyelids are heavy, the complexion is muddy and patients seem to have no energy at all.

Neuralgia
(See Also Pain)

Neuralgia is distinguished from ordinary pain by the fact that it is felt in areas where nerves are concentrated. Only a specialist can ascertain the cause of the disorder, and prescribe an appropriate remedy. However, for temporary relief, when a doctor is not available, you can choose from among the following list of remedies:

- *Aconitum 4 C.* 2 granules every half an hour. Radiating, tingling pain appears in those who are anxious, after being exposed to dry cold.
- *Arsenicum album 4 C.* 2 granules every 8 hours (maximum). Burning prickly pains, worse at night. People are agitated and can't sit still.
- *Belladonna 5 C.* 2 granules every half an hour. Cutting, throbbing pains,

stronger in the middle of the night, or if there's any noise, draughts or movement; also for pains centred around the eyes.

- *Chamomilla 4 C.* 2 granules per hour. The face is red, people are very thirsty, and unsociable. Pains, which are intense, seem to worsen at night, and are accompanied by a numbing sensation.
- *Cedron 7 C.* 2 granules twice a day. Pains are peculiar in that they occur periodically, always at the same time of day.
- *Gratiola 7 C.* 2 granules three times per day. When pains are caused or aggravated by coffee.
- *Mezereum 4 C.* 2 granules every hour. Pains are aggravated by heat and get worse in the middle of the night; accompanied by shivering.
- *Paris quadrifolia 7 C.* 2 granules three times per day. Only one side of the body is affected at a time; acute pains, accompanied by sensations of heat and numbness around the nape of the neck; aggravated by light physical contact, but alleviated by firm pressure, these shooting pains usually strike the left side of the body.
- *Platina 5 C.* 2 granules every two hours. For those who are nervous, or even hysterical; numbness, accompanied by pain as if being squeezed in a vice; pain is localized in the back, the waist area or the teeth (aggravated if teeth are touched by the tongue).
- *Ranunculus 7 C. 3* granules twice a day, for cases of intercostal pain, after exposure to cold, or remaining seated for long periods; people feel pinching and shooting pains; pains are frequently intensified by cold and humidity or when the person changes position.
- *Spigelia 9 C.* 2 granules once a day. For neuralgia of the eyes (aggravated by the slightest movement), the teeth (soothed by lying down and eating), the base of the nape (radiating out to the left eye) and the chest (feeling of heaviness, lack of breath, worse when lying on the left side with the head down).

Facial Neuralgia

- *Aconitum 5 C.* For pains that occur after exposure to dry cold; itching and tingling beneath the skin.
- *Actaea racemosa 9 C.* 2 granules, twice a day, in cases of cardiac neuralgia (pinching pains around the heart spread to the left arm, as if it were numb or paralysed); ocular neuralgia (aggravated by jolts, walking and light); pains in the chest wall (spasms of the left pectoral muscles).

Patients experience a sensation of having a cloud around their heads, and spasms are intense.

- *Arsenicum album 5 C.* 2 granules three times per day. Pain is burning, but soothed by heat; patients fluctuate between periods of irritability and prostration.
- *Belladonna 5 C.* Facial muscles twitch spasmodically, especially on the right side, and pupils are dilated.
- *Bryonia 5 C.* 2 granules twice a day. Movement aggravates the pain, while firm pressure (massage), rest and heat applications soothe it.
- *Coffea 5 C.* 2 granules twice a day. Pain, which is soothed by cold applications, is localized around the ears and forehead.
- *Iris versicolor 5 C.* 2 granules twice a day. Pain is centred above the eye sockets, on both sides.
- *Kalmia 5 C.* 2 granules twice a day. Pains are piercing, resembling electric shocks, spreading to the tongue and teeth, usually on the right side.
- *Magnesium carbonicum 7 C.* 2 granules twice a day. The neuralgia gets worse at night, or when the affected area is touched.
- *Paris quadrifolia 7 C.* 2 granules three times a day. Only one side of the face is affected at a time; pains are acute, accompanied by sensations of heat and numbness; they are aggravated by light contact, but soothed by firm pressure; pains are generally on the left side.
- *Rhus tox 5 C.* 2 granules twice a day. After exposure to humid cold, pains and cracking develop in the jaws.
- *Spigelia 7 C.* 3 granules three times per day. For cases of pain in the trigeminal nerve, usually on the left side, aggravated by coffee, movement or physical contact.

Nose

Homeopathy can be used to treat certain isolated parts of the body directly.
- *Antimonium crudum 7 C.* 3 granules once a day. For those who are constantly picking their nose.
- *Arnica 5 C.* 3 granules, three times a day. The tip of the nose is cold, while the skin on the rest of the face is warm.
- *Borax 5 C.* 3 granules three times per day. The nose is red and shiny.
- *Causticum 5 C.* 2 granules, three times per day. For cases of small,

painful tumours. Can also be taken with *Psorinum 5 C* and *Sepia 5 C,* for dry wrinkled skin.

- *Cina 5 C.* 3 granules, three times a day. For those (and especially children) who rub their noses raw (because of itching due to worm infestation).
- *Petroleum 5 C.* 3 granules, three times a day. For fissures and cracking caused by exposure to dry cold.
- *Malandrinum 5 C.* 3 granules three times a day. For fissures and cracking caused by exposure to humid cold.
- *Nitricum acidum 5 C.* 3 granules, three times a day. For cases of clean, bleeding fissures. Use *Sepia* if the edge of the fissure is not clean.

Obesity

(See Also Diet, Losing Weight and Appetite)

Carrying around two pounds of excess weight shortens life expectancy by two months. Various glands play an important role in obesity, as they do in cases where people lose too much weight. We have already mentioned the thyroid gland, the ovaries, testicles and the pituitary - when they become sluggish and function at lower than normal rates, obesity results.

To this can be added a number of psychological factors like emotional trauma, as well as various neuroses which generally require the help of a specialist (psychiatrist, psychotherapist or psychologist), before patients can hope to achieve a lasting cure. One thing is certain: so-called miracle diets, even though they may produce spectacular results in the short term, do nothing to solve the real problem and will only have a very temporary effect.

And, in fact, it is useless and even harmful to lose a lot of weight one week, only to put it back on again the next week. This kind of behaviour produces a series of shocks to the system which can be detrimental in the long run. A lasting change can only be achieved through regular and persistent work, since it takes a considerable effort to change old habits, which is the only way to gain lasting results. Don't fool yourself - there's nothing easy about losing weight.

There's No Hurry

Your lifestyle is the issue here, and you will obtain reliable results only when you transform your basic day-to-day habits. This is why gradual change is the surest way to make progress. Another essential factor is motivation - you really have to want to change - without which even the best methods will only prove to be temporary, becoming an eventual source of disappointment. Be especially wary of iodine-based slimming pills (see Losing Weight).

All or Nothing

American studies have shown that the best way to lose weight consists of combining the following techniques: putting yourself on a strict diet; following some kind of exercise programme and consulting a professional psychotherapist. And there are other methods, which perhaps haven't been as fully explored.

Hot mineral baths (sitz baths) are external applications which help take off extra pounds. Also vitamin C (as in wheat germ) fights obesity by stimulating ovarian activity. Oil made from cereal germ also helps people lose weight. Reinforce the oil's effect with something like *Kelpasan* - a product made from seaweed.

Eight Things You Should Know

1. Don't drink when you eat; start meals with a food that doesn't contain a lot of calories - green salad, cucumber, grapefruit, etc.
2. Try to avoid going shopping when you're hungry.
3. Opt for a diet that is mainly vegetarian.
4. Reduce your salt intake (you can replace salt with aromatic herbs).
5. Abstain from creamy salad dressings.
6. Replace alcohol with mineral water.
7. Forget about chocolate and pastries altogether.
8. Eat four meals instead of three and don't make lunch the big meal of the day.

Obviously you have to control how much you eat; cut down on pasta and bread, but remember that, like rice, pasta and potatoes, bread is okay as long as it's not fried, or dunked in a creamy sauce, or smothered with butter.

Finally, recent studies have shown that, contrary to popular belief, physical activity reduces appetite to some extent. Taking brisk walks is an excellent way to exercise and to reduce appetite.

- *Ammonium carbonicum 7 C.* 2 granules twice a day, for overweight people who show a general lack of energy.
- *Aurum 30 C.* 5 granules, once a week. For people who are congested, very tense and disgusted with life in general.
- *Capsicum annum 7 C.* 2 granules, twice a day. These people are sensitive

to cold, flabby and indolent, both physically and mentally; they're often irritable; their face is red and cold to the touch.

- *Calcarea carbonica 5 C*. 3 granules, three times a day. These people are flabby and indolent, and are particularly sensitive to damp cold.
- *Graphites 7 C*. 2 granules, twice a day. For cases where glands (especially the thyroid) function badly. These people are sensitive to cold. Women are often frigid, they menstruate late and are often constipated.

Odour

Our sense of smell can sometimes be disrupted, giving us unpleasant impressions.

- *Chelidonium 15 C*. 3 granules, once a week. A person detects an odour which is really present, and then becomes obsessed with it, believing she/he can smell it all the time.
- *Paris quadrifolia 7 C*. 2 granules, three times per day. For those who smell unpleasant odours which aren't really there; they are often over-excited and very talkative.
- *Paris quadrifolia 5 C*. 2 granules, every two hours. The symptoms are the same as for the higher dilution of *Paris,* but the olfactory problem is caused by a head cold.

Pollution

Unfortunately, we have no cure for people who prefer to take advantage of a temporary benefit and pay for it by sacrificing the future of their children and of the species as a whole - not to mention themselves.

However, even where pollution is concerned, homeopathy may have a role to play. In fact, infinitesimal dosages help build up a degree of immunity to the effects of pollution.

- *Plumbum tetraethyl 15 C* and *Petroleum 15 C*. 5 granules, once every fortnight. These remedies restore organs affected by exposure to lead and oil respectively.
- *X-ray 15 C*. 5 granules every fortnight. To ease the effects of X-ray therapy.

Premature Ageing
(See Also Longevity)

- *Lycopodium 7 C.* 2 granules, three times a day.

Respiration (Breathing)

Respiration is life. There's nothing simpler and more natural than breathing. Yet very often, people breathe only superficially, without realizing that they are missing something.

For example, in certain cases of emotional trauma, some people develop the habit of using only a fraction of their lung capacity. It's as if they want to inhale only the amount of air which is absolutely necessary for survival, because they are afraid of asserting their right to exist.

An American, Leonard Orr, has developed a technique designed to liberate our respiration, along with our emotions - the two usually go hand in hand - called the "Rebirth" method.

Doing a few minutes of breathing exercises each day is helpful in relieving constipation and alleviating symptoms of angina pectoris. It can even help you get rid of that spare tyre or pot belly. The exercises are also useful during pregnancy and childbirth, since they force you to strengthen your abdominal muscles. Start with five minutes a day, increasing the time gradually until you reach fifteen minutes a day. Concentrate on your breathing, contracting your stomach as you exhale, and releasing it as you inhale.

Rheumatism

Rheumatism is comprised of a number of important disorders, which are still not well understood and which affect the joints.

Fighting Rheumatism

One way to fight rheumatism is to drink half a glass of fresh *potato juice,* mixed with hot water, every day. You can also chew on two or three *juniper berries* half an hour before your mid-day meal (they are especially helpful in eliminating uric salt). Also, swallowing a few *mustard seeds* after meals is excellent.

For local relief, apply various compresses: one day use *cabbage leaves,* the next day use clay, and the day after prepare a poultice using *quark* (i.e. curd cheese). Take *seaweed baths,* and rub your body with a stiff brush.

As for your diet, try to stick to natural foods as much as possible, such as those suggested in the diet for Longevity, for example.

Make sure you eat celery regularly, and also porridge made from corn and millet, which are reputed to have a very beneficial effect both in cases of rheumatism and arthritis. You can also prepare hot cereal poultices (with no seasoning added) - these will stimulate the flow of blood. To quench your thirst, drink only the water you use to cook potatoes in.

A Sample Menu

For lunch, you'd have some kind of vegetable soup to which you can add raw cabbage juice (after cooking); then some brown rice accompanied by salad (use lemon juice instead of vinegar). Drink raw potato juice at both lunch and dinner, and include some whole rye or oat bread. Also, drink fresh fruit juice.

Exercise regularly, and get out in the fresh air as much as your workplace and/or home allow. Avoid humid places as much as possible, and be careful of sudden changes in temperature.

- *Caulophyllum 5 C.* 2 granules, every two hours. Pains tend to move around from one part of the body to another. The smaller joints are the ones most often affected (fingers, wrists, toes, ankles, vertebrae). Pains are intermittent, with occasional crises which are more intense. The condition is aggravated by cold, and soothed by heat and during menstruation.
- *Dulcamara 9 C.* 2 granules, once a day. Pains are caused or aggravated by humid cold, which mostly affects the muscles and joints. Affected areas are cold, and the person feels the need to move them frequently. Pains are dull, and in cases of muscular rheumatism, affected limbs are weak and heavy.
- *Formica rufa 5 C.* 3 granules, once a day. A remedy for problems with smaller joints - fingers and feet.
- *Ledum 7 C.* 2 granules every two hours. Rheumatic pains are aggravated by bed heat, and soothed by the cold and by cold compresses. Also prescribed when urine shows traces of red sediment. The skin around the affected area is often swollen, purplish and marbled in appearance. Rheumatic pains start in the feet, and work up towards the top of the body; they are prickling and tearing pains, which mostly affect smaller joints.

- *Kali iodatum 7 C.* 2 granules every three hours. Pains are aggravated by warm, damp wind, especially at night, and eased by continual movement.
- *Kali sulphuricum 7 C.* 2 granules every three hours. For chronic rheumatic pain, aggravated by staying indoors, and soothed by fresh air. Unlike *Ledum,* cold applications do not ease the pain.
- *Natrum sulphuricum 7 C.* 2 granules every three hours. Pains are chronic, intensified by changes in temperature and humidity in all its forms. People experience more pain when they change position, and usually become irritable.
- *Kalmia 9 C.* 2 granules every three days. Shooting pains which affect all joints, but which do not remain fixed in one area.
- *Rhus tox 9 C.* 3 granules every two hours. Chronic pain of the tendons and joints. Particularly painful after getting up in the morning. People feel a constant need to change position. Pains are more intense after midnight, and in dull, cloudy weather and are soothed by massages.

Acute Articular Rheumatism

- *Abrotanum 7 C.* 2 granules every three hours. These people are weak and extremely thin; affected joints are stiff and swollen; symptoms are more frequent in cold humid weather and especially during periods of fog.
- *Bryonia 4 C.* Affected joints are inflamed (generally pale and shiny); pains are aggravated by the least movement, by heat and by touch; sweating and a cool room temperature seem to alleviate the symptoms somewhat. Patients have fever and sweat profusely.
- *Causticum 9 C.* 2 granules, once a day. Affected joints are stiff, deformed and weak, and tend to become slightly paralysed. Symptoms are aggravated in cold weather. In many cases, the muscles are also stiff.
- *Colchicum 7 C.* 3 granules every three hours. Joints are inflamed, and very sensitive to the touch; any movement causes patients to suffer; pains are soothed by hot compresses, and by heat in general; patients are often prostrate, with aches all over their body.
- *Ginseng 7 C.* 2 granules twice a day. Patients are weak, stiff, and their joints are constantly contracted.
- *Lithium carbonicum 7 C.* 2 granules, once a day. Chronic articular pains are often accompanied by a state of depression, abundant urination, sometimes problematical. In some cases the skin is dry and rough. Smaller joints in particular may be deformed. The tip of the nose is often

red and inflamed.

Rheumatism may be accompanied by various other problems: cardiac disorders (aggravated when a person leans forward and while urinating); urinary problems (frequent need to urinate during the night, with reddish brown sediment in the urine itself); headaches (worse in the morning after waking up); ocular troubles (dry eyes); gastric and intestinal problems.

- *Magnolia 9 C.* 2 granules, once a day. When rheumatism is accompanied by cardiac problems. Pains, which are acute, move around; affected joints are stiff, especially in the morning and in humid weather. Constant movement seems to ease the pain. When cardiac problems arise, the pain spreads to the back and the left shoulder; sufferers are often short of breath, or cannot breathe properly, their pulse is weak and rapid. Palpitations often occur after meals.

Crippling Rheumatism

- *Actaea spicata 7 C.* 3 granules, twice a day. The rheumatism attacks small joints, especially fingers, wrists and the top of the feet; these become deformed and inflamed (more so if the person is even slightly tired).
- *Guaiacum 7 C.* 3 granules, three times per day. Affected joints are stiff, contracted and deformed; symptoms are aggravated by heat; these people are often sad or even depressive, and suffer from headaches. Urine, which is abundant, has a very strong odour. Pains are also aggravated by touch.

Ringing in the Ears (Tinnitus)

For chronic cases, you'd be wasting your time if you did not treat the cause, which only a specialist can determine. It could be the result of arterial hypertension, arteriosclerosis, or some other benign problem with the inner ear.

Turning a Deaf Ear

To some extent, ringing in the ears is a psychological phenomenon. It's not that the cause is in any way imaginary. It's simply that you're better off not getting too concerned about it - you don't want to sit there waiting and listening for the ringing to start.

Try to forget it as much as possible, until you are able to consult a specialist.

Tinnitus is a sign, a warning which you should not neglect. While waiting for a consultation, one of the following remedies may help soothe the condition.

- *Chininum sulphuricum 9 C.* 3 granules three times per day. For buzzing, throbbing, whistling, ringing in the ears.
- *Glonoinum 9 C.* 3 granules, three times per day. Ringing is preceded by acute cerebral congestion which is heavy. Ringing in the ears may occasionally be caused by arterial pressure or sunstroke. Also for tinnitus that sometimes accompanies the menopause.
- *Natrum salicylicum 9 C.* 3 granules, three times per day. Use with *Chininum sulphuricum* or *Glonoinum,* depending on the case.

Sciatica

This rheumatic pain spreads from the kidney area down to the feet, passing through the back of the thighs or sides of the legs. It starts with a numb sensation in the lower limbs, and then the pain starts. It can be caused by a herniated disc, tuberculosis, diabetes or blennorrhagia (copious mucous discharge, gonorrhoea).

- *Ammonium muriaticum 9 C.* 3 granules every three hours. Leg muscles are permanently contracted, right down to the feet; pain is localized on the left side and worsens when seated or lying down, especially at night, as well as in a cold, damp room.
- *Arnica 5 C.* 3 granules every three hours. When a blow or fall causes sciatica; the condition is accompanied by a general aching sensation; patients cannot sleep, even though they feel very tired.
- *Bryonia 9 C.* 3 granules, three times a day. For cases of acute sciatica, when a person is immobilized, often lying on the painful side of the body.
- *Magnesia phosphorica 9 C.* 3 granules, three times a day. People pace the room to try and ease their pain, which becomes less intense with movement.
- *Mandragora 9 C.* 3 granules, three times a day. An afflicted person needs to move around; pains are worse in the morning and when they are resting, standing or sitting down. Walking and heat ease the pain.
- *Valeriana 9 C.* 3 granules, three times a day. Person is nervous, extremely sensitive, and pains get worse when he/she remains immobile, whereas movement and changing positions eases the pain.

Scurvy

People with scurvy are pale and anaemic; they lack appetite and their gums are inflamed and often bleed. Tumours and ulcers develop in the mouth, and teeth are loose. In addition you may observe dark bluish pustules, especially on the legs.

Preventing Scurvy

The best diet to prevent scurvy is one which is rich in vitamin C; orange juice, lemons, almonds, seaweed, wheat, apricots, garlic, carrots, cabbage and cheese are just a few examples of foods which contain high levels of vitamin C. Two or three teaspoons of orange or grape juice will help young children, especially those who have been fed with artificial formula.

- *Ammonium carbonicum 5 C.* 3 granules, three times a day. Patients are weak, their joints are painful, and they tend to haemorrhage easily.
- *Agave (American aloe) 5 C.* 2 granules three times a day. The most general remedy for scurvy.
- *Citric acid 4 C.* 2 granules every two hours. Symptoms are intensified by bleeding gingivitis, pains in the joints, and marked weight loss.
- *Kreosotum 5 C.* 3 granules, three times a day. Gums are painful and bluish in colour, breath smells bad. Patients sometimes also suffer from diarrhoea.
- *Mercurius 4 C.* 2 granules, three times a day. The tongue is flabby and moist, and retains marks made by the teeth. Ulcers appear on the gums; patients are parched with thirst.

Sense of Smell - see Odour

Sleep
(See Also Insomnia)

Sleep has a curative and therapeutic value, just like forgetting; it is certain that each day we must wipe clean our minds, cluttered as they are with millions of details and impressions gathered during the course of each day. The next day, our minds will fill up again with details just as important as the day's before.

Sleep accomplishes this task of cleaning out the mind marvellously well.

If you have trouble sleeping, learn to control it; camomile tea, for example, is an excellent soporific. Also avoid thinking about disturbing events or problems, or getting into heated discussions, before going to sleep. You should know that five hours of sleep induced by sleeping pills is worth less than two hours of naturally induced sleep.

The Best Sleep

Biologically speaking, our habits run counter to our interests. We usually eat the heaviest meal of the day in the evening, shortly before going to sleep, and we often go to bed late (after midnight). Our stomach is digesting while we sleep, which diminishes the restorative quality of our hours of rest. Ideally, you should have supper around 6 o'clock, and get to bed before midnight - the hours of sleep before midnight count for double.

Sleep with the window open as often as possible - you'll soon notice how much more rested you feel when you wake up. Avoid taking sleeping pills altogether, unless absolutely necessary.

- *Apis 9 C*. 3 granules, three times per day. For people who are agitated and cry out in their sleep.
- *Belladonna 9 C*. 3 granules, three times per day. For people who grind their teeth or talk a lot when sleeping.
- *Chamomilla 9 C*. 3 granules, three times per day. For people who perspire or weep when sleeping.
- *Cocculus 9 C*. 3 granules before going to bed. For people who have not had enough sleep for some days.

Teeth
(See Also Dental Cavities)

Taking good care of your teeth will pay off your whole life long, while neglecting them results in untold torment and suffering (not to mention expense!). So there is every reason to adopt good dental hygiene habits starting from a very early age.

You must be firm and help children avoid all those tempting displays of sweets and chocolate bars found in so many shops - above all, don't buy your children's co-operation with little treats. If you help them to avoid developing a taste for sugar (making it the exception rather than the rule), then you're doing them a great service. As you will come to realize, a child's need for sugar is artificially created and by no means inevitable.

Good Habits Starting at an Early Age

Children get used to chewing their food at a very early age (around nine months old) as they are weaned off so-called baby food, which informed parents can now avoid altogether thanks to the invention of blenders. In this way, children learn to share their parents' food and receive all the nutrients they need.

Refined white bread, like white sugar, contains nothing that nourishes the teeth. As for soft white bread, it doesn't have the crunch that teeth need to build resistance. Whole wheat bread, cornbread and chewing firm foods - especially raw vegetables like carrots and celery - strengthen the teeth.

Meat

This is the problem with diets that are centred around meat: very often, the meat is the only thing that has to be chewed - vegetables are overcooked and need hardly any chewing at all. So it's always a good idea to accompany a meal with some raw vegetables. Apart from containing all their nutrients - many of which are lost in cooking - they're crunchy and good for the teeth.

If we get used to brushing our teeth regularly at an early age (ideally after each meal), it quickly becomes a habit which we hardly think about at all. Brushing even becomes a pleasure - it's great to feel your teeth all clean and shiny. It's hard to understand people whose teeth are yellow and full of cavities, who still don't think they need to practise better dental hygiene.

You can also chew gum (containing no sugar, of course) to clean your teeth after eating.

Problems With Teeth

Three granules when there is pain. Repeat once every hour, spacing out the dosages as the pain diminishes.

- *Chamomilla 5 C.* 3 granules. When a toothache is accompanied by green diarrhoea.
- *Cheiranthus 5 C.* 3 granules. For pain caused by wisdom teeth.
- *Magnesia carbonicum 5 C.* 3 granules. When a toothache is accompanied by acute diarrhoea.

In Cases of Surgical Intervention

- *Arnica 5 C.* 3 granules immediately after surgery, in case of bleeding gums.
- *Gelsemium 9 C.* 3 granules, the night before surgery, or even shortly

before (up to fifteen minutes). This remedy helps soothe apprehension.

Rinse the mouth with solutions using 20 drops of *Plantago* tincture, *Calendula tincture* and *Phytolacca tincture*. These act as a sedative and help speed up healing.

Thirst

Exaggerated thirst - or its opposite, lack of thirst - can sometimes be cured by homeopathic means. Check if a person's incessant desire for water is not simply caused by an excessive intake of salt (contained in some processed meats, crisps, salted peanuts, etc.). Fever or diabetes can also cause intense thirst.

- *Apis mellifica 4 C.* 2 granules every two hours. For absence of thirst.
- *Arsenicum album 5 C.* 2 granules every two hours. For intense thirst (sometimes followed by vomiting).
- *Arsenicum album 5 C.* 3 granules every two hours. People feel a frequent need to drink small quantities of cold water.
- *Capsicum 4 C.* 3 granules every two hours. For cases of intense thirst which, once satisfied, is followed by shivering.
- *Natrum muriaticum 4 C.* 3 granules every four hours. For people who feel the need to drink large quantities of cold water, but at longer intervals.

Tobacco

There are enough victims of smoking for most of us to know its harmful effects. Yet smoking continues to play an important role in many people's lives. A report has shown that no less than two and a half million people around the world die from passive smoking each year.

What smokers don't seem to realize is just how much they suffer from day to day. You only have to stop for a day to feel the difference. Food tastes better, you can breathe more deeply, your head is clearer and you generally feel a lot better. Experiencing these things can help people who lack the motivation to stop smoking. Because first and foremost, you have to want to get rid of this ridiculous form of slavery.

A number of different methods are available to help people stop smoking. Tablets or chewing gum, for example, which make cigarettes taste bad; nicotine supplements which let you rid your body of toxins gradually; acupuncture, which can serve as a powerful aid.

Each cigarette destroys 2 milligrams of vitamin C in your body; if you smoke one pack of twenty cigarettes a day, you should take a vitamin C capsule every night before going to bed. You should also not smoke in the morning before eating, and preferably smoke filter-tip cigarettes.

- *Caladium 5 C.* 3 granules every two hours. For cases of tobacco intoxication; those suffering from it avoid moving as much as possible, preferring to remain lying down; they suffer from memory loss, and their minds do not function clearly. *Caladium* is also useful for people who want to stop smoking completely.
- *Ignatia 5 C.* 3 granules, three times a day. For tobacco abuse; also for people who have stopped smoking, and can't stand other people's smoke, or who become hypersensitive and nervous.
- *Nux vomica 7 C.* 2 granules, twice a day. Very useful when stopping smoking; people are irritable, can't stand noise or bright lights, and are often short-tempered.
- *Spigelia 5 C.* 3 granules every three hours. Palpitations are strong enough to prevent people from sleeping; in addition, they frequently experience bouts of nausea.

Also consult the section on Cancer.

Torticollis (Stiff Neck)

Rheumatism, some sudden movement, exposure to cold - there are numerous possible causes for this highly unpleasant condition.

Osteopathic techniques can be used to relieve a stiff neck, especially when caused by a fall or an injury. Keep the neck warm, wrapping it in a woollen scarf, for example. You can also rub the affected areas with a suitable liniment.

- *Lachnanthes 4 C.* 3 granules every three hours. This remedy is indicated for all cases, especially when the head is tilted to one side.
- *Aconite 5 C* is recommended for people who develop torticollis after exposure to cold, dry wind. In such cases, the pain appears suddenly, and gets worse at night; sometimes accompanied by headaches in the morning.
- *Actaea racemosa 5 C.* 3 granules every three hours, for women whose torticollis gets worse during menstruation.
- *Agaricus 4 C.* 3 granules every three hours. People are susceptible to

arthritis; they suffer from headaches in the morning and feel as if the base of their neck is ice cold.

- *Arnica 15 C.* 3 granules every three hours. For torticollis due to some kind of shock or jolt.
- *Bryonia 5 C.* 2 granules every three hours. Pain and stiffness is alleviated when the person stays as still as possible.
- *Cimicifuga 5 C.* 3 granules every three hours. For pain caused by muscular contractions, resembling cramps; people are highly agitated.
- *Dulcamara 5 C.* 3 granules every three hours. For cases of rheumatoid torticollis, caused by exposure to humid cold, and soothed by heat.
- *Lachnanthes 4 C.* 3 granules every two hours. Muscles are permanently contracted, and the head is inclined to one side.
- *Rhus tox 5 C.* 3 granules every three hours. For cases of torticollis caused by arthritis, and triggered by exposure to humidity and cold.

Underweight

(See Also Diet, Abnormal Weight Loss, Appetite)

For people who are underweight (as in cases of obesity), the amount and kind of food you eat, as well as the amount of exercise you do, are not the only factors you have to be concerned with. The secretions of certain glands, notably the thyroid, pituitary, testicles and ovaries, have an important effect on our weight.

Hyperactivity of these glands causes people to be thin. On the other hand, if the function of these glands is sluggish (or at least below average), then people generally become overweight.

In certain cases, homeopathy can have an effect on excessive thinness. People who are suffering because their weight is too low can improve their condition by regularly incorporating wheat germ oil into their diet.

- *Abrotanum 7 C.* 3 granules, twice a day. People are too thin, especially in the lower limbs, despite a voracious appetite; their skin is flaccid, and seems to be ageing prematurely; they feel sad and lethargic; a bloated stomach, and an extreme sensitivity to cold completes the picture of this type.
- *Iodum 7 C.* 3 granules, twice a day. People have a hearty appetite, but are thin, nervous and agitated; they have trouble digesting milk and fats, and suffer from pale diarrhoea.
- *Natrum muriaticum 7 C.* 3 granules three times per day. For cases of

weight loss due to dehydration, despite a normal, hearty appetite; people are often thirsty; they lack strength, get tired easily, but seem to need to move around all the time; the face is pale, they are sensitive to cold, and oversensitive to noise.

Chapter 2

Childhood

Childhood

You'll find this chapter very useful for dealing with the first signs of normal illnesses in children, so that you can successfully check the development of illnesses as quickly as possible. However you should acquire some experience in prescribing homeopathic remedies before attempting to treat children - never use them as guinea-pigs!

When treating children, keep the following recommendations in mind.

Recommendations

1. It's best to prescribe only one medication at a time, in order to observe its effects better.
2. For the same reason, avoid mixing homeopathic and allopathic medication as much as possible, although doing so is not dangerous.
3. A homeopathic remedy should produce rapid results. If there is no improvement in 24 hours, try another medication in mild cases, or consult a doctor if the case is serious. If the child's condition worsens, consult a doctor as soon as possible.
4. As for the dosage and directions for use, follow the instructions in the section on Directions for Children and Infants.

Draw On Your Own Experience

When in doubt, do not hesitate to consult a doctor. However, don't forget that, in time, your ability to recognize conditions that present no danger will improve - in other words, as your experience grows, you'll be able to distinguish symptoms easily and you'll become more and more familiar with a wide range of homeopathic remedies.

For more information on children, you can also consult the sections on Pregnancy and Breast-feeding.

Behaviour Problems

You can turn to homeopathy to help overcome many psychological problems associated with childhood. As with all homeopathic treatments, choosing the right remedy requires careful observation of the child's reactions and behaviour.

These observations are also essential for understanding what other measures you can take, on a more general and human level, to help your children. In fact, children's behaviour, like that of adults, is inherently linked to the environment in which they live. Excessive reactions are usually triggered by some disturbing event: our own impatience, anger, indifference, overprotection, anxieties - even our absence may be the cause of certain problems.

However, we should not over-simplify matters and systematically blame parents or teachers. The real causes are sometimes very difficult to identify, even with the help of a professional (psychologist or psychiatrist). Yet we can sometimes solve a problem, even though we only have an intuitive understanding of the cause.

Remember that life is a complex collection of simple things. But one truth is certain - we all need the attention and affection of others. And this is even more true for children.

Our Friends the Plants

To help children who have trouble sleeping, or whose sleep is agitated, you can use three sedative plants which induce sleep: lime blossom, passion-flower and orange blossom. Valerian is also effective for such cases.

Choice of Dilution

Administer these remedies in 9 C dilutions, 5 granules once a week. As usual, stop the treatment as soon as you notice an improvement in the symptoms.

Agitated Children

- *Agaricus*. Children can't stop touching things, are unstable and weak. Symptoms are worse at school but are alleviated after a good night's sleep.
- *Anatherum*. When a child plays the fool, she/he is really trying to attract attention. Such children need more affection.
- *Kali bromatum*. Children are always restless - they can't stop moving (especially their hands) yet they are slow. They get mixed up easily and

don't seem able to finish what they start.

- *Luesinum*. Children sleep badly and seem to have memory lapses; they're afraid of the dark. They have trouble with mathematics; symptoms seem to ease off during visits to the seaside.
- *Medorrhinum*. Although bright, these children have trouble concentrating; they are undisciplined and their minds are foggy.
- *Zincum*. Their feet shift constantly, as if they had a life of their own. The children are slow to adapt and have trouble dealing with authority at school.

Anxious Children

- *Borax*. In households where everyone else seems to be happy, these children are afraid. And in general, their fear prevents them from doing things.
- *Causticum*. Children who are always wary of others, fearful and have trouble sleeping in the dark.
- *Gelsemium*. For children who are inhibited and have trouble concentrating.
- *Kali carbonicum*. For children who suffer from general anxiety.
- *Stramonium*. These children cannot sleep without a light on (they suffer from night terrors). During the day they are generally fearful, but easily get excited to the point of becoming violent.
- *Phosphorus*. Children can't sleep without a light; they are subject to abstract anxieties beyond their age group.
- *Pulsatilla*. For children who cannot sleep in the dark.

Aggressive Children

- *Hepar sulph*. These children have no qualms about biting in a fight; they are the type who take pleasure in tearing off insects' wings, tormenting kittens, etc.
- *Nux vomica*. These children do their best to be coarse and disgusting; they enjoy quarrelling - everything seems to upset them and they "fly off the handle" at the slightest provocation.
- *Tarentula*. For children who can't stand being touched - you have to find other ways to show them that you care for them and love them. When angry, they hit out and scratch, and will destroy anything they can.

Talkative Children

- *Actaea racemosa.* For children who can't stop talking; they jump from one topic to another, without really understanding what they're saying.
- *Hyoscyamus.* For children who are always distorting the truth to suit themselves.
- *Lachesis.* For children who cannot help stretching the truth - they always tend to exaggerate and over-dramatize.

Children Who Stammer

Different remedies may be administered in these cases:
- *Ambrea grisea, Argentum nitricum, Causticum* (for children who start stammering after an unpleasant or threatening event), *Gelsemium, Kali bromatum.*

Problem Children

It would be impossible in the context of this book to cover all the problems children have adapting to the world as they grow from infancy to adolescence. Here are just a few examples of remedies you can use:
- *Hepar sulph.* For aggressive, belligerent children, who may turn to pyromania as a way of expressing their frustration.
- *Lycopodium.* For children who are selfish, very reserved, seemingly inaccessible.
- *Natrum muriaticum.* These children are extremely taciturn and clearly have trouble communicating.
- *Mercurius.* These types of children are impulsive and can be bullies - they always have to be the leader of their gang; they may also exhibit sadistic tendencies.
- *Staphysagria.* For children who are short-tempered and vengeful.

Angry Children

- *Anacardium.* Their mood seems to improve after eating. When hungry, these children can become unbelievably angry.
- *Chamomilla.* For children with a nervous temperament, who are very demanding.
- *Stramonium.* Intentionally naughty, these children can throw tantrums and become violent to the point of delirium.

Tired Children

(For chronic fatigue, more psychological than physical, and which seems to intensify towards the end of the school term.)

- *Argentum nitricum*. Children are emotional and feverish, and are always afraid of not being good enough.
- *Calcarea phosphoricum*. Children are stubborn; they need approval and security.
- *Natrum carbonicum*. For children who have guilt complexes.

Unstable (Moody) Children

- *Mercurius*. These children are impulsive and unable to accept discipline - they become talkative, disruptive and aggressive when they have to submit to authority.
- *Natrum muriaticum*. For children who refuse to talk, to the point of having a nervous breakdown.
- *Thuja*. These children are traumatized by school; their attitude leads them from one failure to another.

Lazy Children

- *Baryta carbonicum*. Children make slow progress and hesitate because of worry or fear of the future; they are often excessively meticulous.
- *Graphites*. Children are apathetic, can't make up their minds and don't like work.
- *Sulphur*. Despite their laziness and messiness, these children are ambitious.

Passive Children

- *Opium 15 C*. These children are slow, seem to live in a daydream and are not in touch with reality.

Children Who Lack Self-Confidence

- *Lycopodium*. They seem to be lacking strength and reject others to the point of becoming aggressive.
- *Natrum muriaticum*. Children who always blame others for their own failures.
- *Petroleum*. For children who are extremely over-sensitive.
- *Pulsatilla*. These children always need someone to hang onto, without

whom they don't seem to be able to function.

Sleepwalking
- *Kali bromatum*. Children are anxious, and the only way they can get rid of their anxiety is to become agitated; they talk a lot in their sleep.
- *Phosphorus*. Children who get over-excited.
- *Silicea*. These children blush easily and often have wet, clammy hands.

Shy Children
- *Ambra grisea*. These children are always keyed up and nervous.
- *Coca*. For children who fluctuate between two extremes: either they can't stop talking or they are prostrate with fatigue.
- *Kali phosphoricum*. Whatever the situation (pleasant or difficult) these children are always upset.

Chicken-Pox

This mild childhood disease usually poses no problems, apart from diagnosing it correctly.

After an incubation period that lasts about two weeks, little blisters (vesicles) appear on the face, usually bordering the hairline. They become very itchy, and are accompanied by headaches and fever around 100°F (38°C). The fact that eruptions appear on the mucous membranes in the mouth, and on the scalp, distinguishes chicken-pox from a simple skin rash.

3 granules, three times a day:
- *Antimonium crudum 5 C*. For children who are susceptible to digestive problems. Itching is intense. The tongue is white and coated, skin blisters contain a thick white liquid which forms a yellowish crust.
- *Belladonna 4 C*. For children who develop high fever (see the section on Fever).
- *Mercurius solubilis 4 C*. Children are extremely thirsty; the tongue is coated yellow; they are constipated and sweat profusely, especially at night.
- *Mezereum 4 C*. The crusts last too long or each vesicle is surrounded by a white ring and covered with a thick white crust, under which yellow pus forms.
- *Pulsatilla 4 C*. Children exhibit a state similar to tuberculosis - they are

moody and their temperature fluctuates irregularly.

Convulsions (Infant)

Medical name: *infant eclampsia*. This disorder, which is relatively common, is distressing to watch and a sure remedy has still not been found.

You can, however, use chickweed to relieve the symptoms. This weed, which is also a heart tonic, grows wild in fields throughout summer, right up to the first frost. Administer it as an infusion or as a tincture.

3 granules, three times per day:

- *Chamomilla 9 C*. When a toothache causes convulsions (also see Teeth).
- *Cina 9 C*. For children with worms (see the section on Parasites).
- *Ethyllicum 9 C*. If you suspect that hereditary alcoholism is the cause of the convulsions.

Diarrhoea (In Infants)

Certain forms of diarrhoea are particular to infants and as such require specific remedies.

3 granules, every three hours:

- *Aconitum 5 C*. Diarrhoea is green like cooked spinach and is brought on quite suddenly by exposure to cold; infants are agitated, cry and don't like to be held; fever can be high.
- *Argentum nitricum 5 C*. This diarrhoea is more serious than the *Aconitum* type, although it has the same spinach green colour; it may last for several days; the stomach is bloated, and the child emits a lot of gas. A characteristic sign is that these infants seem to crave sugar.
- *Magnesia carbonica 7 C*. Stool is greenish in colour and foamy; infants suffer from continual colic, which is very painful - they are doubled over and vomit all the milk they drink.

Diarrhoea Due to Teething

- *Chamomilla 5 C*. Stool is hot and burning, smells like rotten eggs, but retains this consistency only during teething; one cheek is hot, the other cold. These infants are often agitated and dissatisfied, but calm down in a car or when being held and rocked.
- *Podophyllum 5 C*. Stool comes out in spurts, preceded by copious gas,

and yellow in colour; the liver is painful and infants rub the right side of their stomach; the rectum is swollen during defaecation.

Directions for Use
(Infants and Children)

Homeopathic remedies are actually more effective in young children and infants because of the relative purity of their bodies, which are free of toxins: this makes it easier for an appropriate therapy to take effect.

In fact, there's really no difference in dosage instructions for adults and children. In all cases, homeopaths will tend to use higher dilutions, the more certain they are of the similitude between the symptoms exhibited by patients and the effects produced in experiments ("provings") with the medication, i.e. the resemblance between problems experienced by patients and the effects of experimental dilutions on healthy people.

Infants

Dissolve 5 granules in 50 grams of mineral water and administer the mixture by feeding with a teaspoon. You can also mix granules with milk or water, and feed with a bottle. The solution must be used within 24 hours.

As is generally true for homeopathic medications, dosages are increased depending on the seriousness of the case and the intensity of the symptoms.

Older Children

Administer granules orally and ask children to let them melt on their tongue as much as possible. Swallowing the granules doesn't really matter, since the medication will penetrate the mucous membranes of the oesophagus as well as those of the mouth.

If possible, try to administer medication (two or three granules at a time) at least 20 to 30 minutes after a meal (or a snack) or after ingestion of any liquid (juice, milk, etc.)

Frequency of Taking the Medication

You are in the best position to judge how frequently to administer the homeopathic remedies you use. You just have to follow a few simple rules:

- The principle of administering homeopathic remedies is as follows: as soon as an improvement in the patient's condition is observed, you increase the time period between dosages, until you can finally stop them altogether.

- For conditions which have stabilized, administer the medication more often, the more intense and acute the symptoms are. This could be every five minutes in cases where symptoms are very acute.

Ears (Problems With)

Ear-ache appears suddenly, during the course of a throat infection, and obviously in cases of otitis, i.e. ear infection (see the section on Otitis).

- Administer a few drops of *Plantago tincture* directly into the affected ear.
- *Chamomilla 4 C.* For cases where the pain is unbearable, causing children to become extremely agitated.

Fever (In Infants)

Fever is one disorder that homeopathy can fight very effectively. Whether it is caused by measles or whooping cough, a throat infection or scarlet fever, the condition is part of the normal process of a child's growth.

Fever - An Ally or An Enemy?

We must not forget that childhood illnesses often play an appreciable positive role. The fever which usually accompanies them burns up harmful microbes and toxic substances which, if not eliminated, could eventually lead to more serious problems. In this sense, fever is an internal defence mechanism of the body.

In fact, it has been observed that adults who did not experience fever during childhood are more susceptible to all kinds of disorders, including cancer. In addition, skin rashes also help to eliminate toxins. That is why trying to prevent rashes from appearing at all can result in much worse problems, like heart trouble, nervous conditions or lung disorders.

Also, it's not a good idea hastily to get rid of an illness with a few pills made from chemicals - they do nothing to eliminate the real toxins which are the cause of the problem.

Help Nature Do Its Work

Infusions made with horsetail *(Equisetum arvense)* help stimulate kidney function. Also note that infectious diseases become established much more easily in bodies suffering from nutritional or vitamin deficiencies.

You can also prescribe warm baths in water with an initial temperature of 102° to 104°F (39 - 40°C) which is then cooled gradually to 98.6°F (37°C), then to 95°F (35°C). Keep patients in the water for about a quarter of an hour; then rub their body before dressing them and putting them to bed.

Also look at the symptoms described in the section on Children's Flu.

When To Worry

Don't worry needlessly; it will do nothing for your health or the child's spirits. But watch out for the following symptoms: the child is too calm; when you observe stiffness in the nape of the neck (a sign of meningitis) or when the child is unusually drowsy, which is a common symptom of a cerebral disorder.

3 granules, about every two hours:

- *Aconitum 4 C*. When the skin is dry and burning - this remedy helps patients eliminate toxic substances through the skin. *Aconitum* is also effective in combating sudden fevers, which are accompanied by anxiety, agitation and palpitations.
- *Apis mellifica 5 C*. Children are rather drowsy, their sleep is punctuated by cries; they can't stand heat, they are never thirsty, and the face is puffy.
- *Belladonna 5 C*. Children are agitated, sometimes even delirious. They seem to be burning up, their eyes are unusually brilliant and they suffer from headaches. They shiver and are very thirsty, but can only drink a few drops at a time.
- *Bryonia 5 C*. Children don't want to get out of bed; the slightest movement is uncomfortable or painful; they drink large quantities of water.
- *Chamomilla 5 C*. Children are agitated and irritable. Fever is stronger in the morning; one cheek is often redder than the other.
- *Dulcamara 5 C*. To combat fevers resulting from a cold. Children do not perspire, but sleep badly.
- *Ferrum phosphoricum 12 C*. Helps the body burn up toxic substances.
- *Ferrum phosphoricum 5 C*. For slight fever; the face is sometimes flushed, sometimes pale. Children do not perspire, but sometimes have nosebleeds.
- *Gelsemium 5 C*. Fever is intense. Children are drowsy and can hardly keep their eyes open; they remain inert in bed, are not thirsty, but suffer

from violent headaches.

- *Mercurius solubilis 5 C.* Children sweat a lot, especially at night.
- *Nux vomica 5 C.* When they move, children shiver and/or tremble; they're often in a bad mood, don't like to have their covers removed and complain of stomach-aches.
- *Opium 5 C.* For cases where a profound drowsiness is accompanied by slight delirium; the face is congested, and the child mutters and moves only when removing his or her covers.

While Waiting for a Doctor

- *Pulsatilla 5 C.* Children are moody and complain about everything; they want to be held, throw off their covers constantly, sweat profusely when they are covered, are always too hot and refuse to drink.
- *Rhus tox 5 C.* Children are physically agitated, and often catch cold in damp weather. Fever stays high, stomach-aches develop, as well as pain in the limbs.

Also consult the sections on Childhood Flu and Teething.

Flu (Childhood)

The following advice pertains to flu as well as all other infectious diseases:

1. When fever appears, stop giving solid food, and maintain the fast as long as the fever persists. In any case, sick children probably won't want to eat anything.
2. Orange, grapefruit or grape juice help eliminate toxins and quench thirst. Carrot juice is effective when the liver is affected.
3. Kidney function can be stimulated to a great degree by infusions of *Solidago;* elder-flower infusions help perspiration.
4. To wash patients, use solutions containing thyme or juniper needles - these help reduce traces of even slight perspiration.
5. Cabbage leaves applied to the liver area help liver function.
6. Maintain proper oral hygiene, getting rid of deposits on the tongue by regular brushing (use an antiseptic gargle regularly).
7. Keep the sick child's room well ventilated.
8. Break the fast first with fruits, then with light vegetarian meals.
9. *Chelidonium 2 C* and *Podophyllus 3 C. 5* granules every three hours if the flu is intense.

Viral Flu

If not cared for properly, viral flu can have serious consequences: rheumatic pains, eczema, pneumonia, chronic abdominal lesions, lesions of the liver, kidneys or stomach.

Wrapping children in warm bedding or immersing them in hot baths will be necessary to induce sweating. As for all cures involving sweating, check to make sure the heart isn't under too much stress.

The medicinal plant *Nephrosolid* stimulates elimination through the kidneys and liver. *Echinaforce* (Echinacea remedy) prevents inflammation and irritations.

Maintain a liquid-based diet (grapefruit juice, diluted myrtle juice, black cherry or diluted beetroot juice). If children absolutely must ingest solid food, make sure it contains no fat or albumin.

Finally, don't try to speed up the recovery time unnecessarily. Children need time to regain their strength after a viral infection.

3 granules, three times a day:

- *Aconitum 5 C*. Children are very agitated - they won't stop crying and complaining. They are very hot and need to be comforted constantly.
- *Arnica 5 C*. For cases where muscular pains are accompanied by intense sensitivity to touch; children cannot stand cold, and shiver for no reason.
- *Arsenicum album 4 C*. These cases are worrying - children are alternately agitated and prostrate; they have diarrhoea and vomit; when they do drink, it is only in small amounts.
- *Bryonia 5 C*. These children are dissatisfied and grumpy, no matter what you do for them; they want to drink very often and suffer from painful joints; they cannot stand cold.
- *Eupatorium perfoliatum 5 C*. Children have pains in their legs, right to the marrow of their bones; they also suffer from headaches and are generally very weak.
- *Gelsemium 5 C*. Children are very passive and hardly move; they suffer from painful headaches, and seem exhausted.
- *Nux vomica 5 C*. Susceptible to cold, these children prefer to remain under the covers, and suffer from pains throughout their body. They also feel nauseous.
- *Pyrogenium 5 C*. Children are agitated and cannot sleep; their pulse is irregular - sometimes rapid, sometimes slow.
- *Rhus tox 5 C*. Children develop herpes sores on the lips; the tongue is coated, the tip of the tongue is red; they are fairly agitated.

Growing (Problems)

Various remedies can help children overcome growing problems, depending on their type.

You can also do a lot to help the growth of children by administering remedies indicated for various types of intoxication which are transmitted or acquired - consult the section on Pregnancy and Childbirth.

3 granules every three hours:

- *Calcarea carbonica 5 C*. For children whose head is large in proportion to the rest of the body, who are late in learning to walk, whose teeth are late in growing and painful when they do appear. These children are very sensitive to cold, rather slow, quiet, even apathetic. They catch cold often, develop eczema easily and can't bear to drink milk.

- *Calcarea phosphorica 5 C*. These children are more lively and nervous than the *Calcarea carbonica* type. They get over-excited easily and also get tired quickly. They are usually too tall for their age and suffer from growing pains like stiffness in the neck and nape. They are often hungry between meals and have a predilection for smoked and salted meat. They get tired very quickly, especially if they have to make some physical or mental effort. They tend to cough in cold weather, and their chest becomes painful to the touch.

- *Calcarea fluorica 5 C*. For children whose bones don't grow normally; joints are lax, and bones tend to be deformed. Visible veins in the centre of the forehead and at the base of the nose, are characteristic signs of the *Calcarea fluorica* type. These children never seem to stand up straight. They also seem to have problems thinking in an orderly and coherent way.

- *Natrum muriaticum 7 C*. The effect of this remedy is to help the body retain lime salts, which are necessary to ensure calcification of bones. *Natrum muriaticum* can be used for the three *Calcarea* types described above - these often develop herpes sores on the lips, and eczema in areas where skin is folded (armpits, backs of the knees, etc.).

Measles

(See Also Rubella - German measles)

Although not dangerous in itself, this viral disease should always be taken seriously because of possible complications.

The illness starts about two weeks after contamination. First the eyes start to run. Children try to avoid light, they develop a cold (inflammation of the nasal passages) and a hoarse cough. Then the characteristic Koplik's spots appear (they can be observed only if the teeth are already formed) - small bright white points in a red area, on the inside of the cheek.

Next come the skin eruptions and fever - small reddish spots separated by areas of healthy skin, which cover the face, neck, chest, stomach, then legs (if there's no fever then the child probably has German measles). Eruptions start disappearing in the same order they appeared.

Fever, which starts shortly before the skin eruptions, usually rises to about 102°F (39°C), then falls, only to rise again to 104°F (40°C), where it remains. If fever persists for more than three or four days after the skin eruptions, then steps should be taken so that the homeopathic treatment can intervene in a decisive way.

A Good Illness

Once again, homeopathy tries, above all, to make sure that the illness proceeds properly, so that the body eliminates the greatest possible amount of viral material and toxic bacteria through the skin. Of course the children suffer for a while, but if they are robust they will easily fight off the disease, and develop a greater immunity.

Preventive Measure

In case of an epidemic, *Belladonna 4 C,* 2 granules every 24 hours, and *Arsenicum album 5 C,* 2 granules every two days, around supper time.

Once the Disease Is Contracted

2 granules, twice a day:

- *Aconitum 5 C.* A remedy which is often prescribed at the outset of the illness. Fever is high, pulse is rapid, skin is dry. Children are nervous, irritated, anxious, suffer from insomnia, and their nasal passages are irritated and often bleed.
- *Belladonna 5 C.* An initial remedy. Fever is high, skin is hot and moist, the tongue is coated. Children are weak, but have trouble sleeping.
- *Bryonia 5 C.* Children are very thirsty, congested, often constipated, and the skin eruption has difficulty breaking out. Bryonia can be alternated with *Aconitum.*

- *Euphrasia 5 C*. Eyes are irritated, and there is abundant discharge from the nose.
- *Ipecac. 5 C*. Children suffer from nausea and vomiting. Also administer towards the end of the skin eruption when the tongue is no longer coated and the cough is phlegmy.
- *Mercurius solubilis 5 C*. The nose is irritated by a constant discharge of clear mucus.
- *Pulsatilla 5 C*. Prescribe towards the end of the illness, or if you suspect the onset of a cold with yellowish nasal discharge and abundant flow of tears.
- *Sulphur 30 C*. 5 granules at night. Administer this medication once, at the outset of the illness - it helps eliminate toxins rapidly by speeding up formation of the skin eruption.

  Note that Sulphur should only be administered to children of the *Aconite* type. In *Belladonna* types (nervous and agitated) it may slow down the process.

Mumps

This common illness is harmless in children. It attacks the salivary glands situated behind the ears and is very easy to identify because of the characteristic hamster-like appearance of the face due to swelling of one or both sides of the neck.

In exceptional cases, it also causes inflammation of the testicles (orchitis) when it occurs during boys' puberty, which can result in reproductive problems. In these cases it is imperative to consult a doctor.

Mumps, which is contagious and can reach epidemic proportions, is caused by a virus. The incubation period lasts between one and three weeks. It is passed on through the saliva - the illness usually lasts seven days from the day before the appearance of the inflammation. It is during that time that the risk of spreading the disease is greatest, either by talking to other children, or through objects that have been in contact with the affected child's saliva.

Mumps epidemics usually occur towards the end of winter. It is of some comfort to know that, in 95 percent of cases, children become immune to further infection once they have had the illness.

Initial symptoms include general discomfort, shivering, pain in the ears and headaches.

Hot sitz baths are soothing: increase the temperature gradually from 96.8°F

(36°C) to 104°F (40°C) and then wrap the child in dry towels. Arabic vegetable essence helps stimulate digestive functions; in some cases you may have to flush out the digestive tract (enema, colonic irrigation).

Hot compresses of water to which you add a few drops of *Arnica* or *Calendula tincture* help soothe the pain.

3 granules, every three hours:

- *Apis mellifica 5 C*. Fever is intense, children feel stiffness in the nape of the neck and suffer from headaches.
- *Belladonna 4 C*. Inflammation of the glands occurs suddenly; these become very sensitive to the touch and cause shooting pains. Children are feverish and agitated.
- *Mercurius solubilis 4 C*. The most general remedy. Children are feverish, sometimes cold and shivering, sometimes hot; at night they are thirsty and sweat profusely. The tongue is coated with a yellowish substance, breath smells bad, and patients experience difficulty opening their jaws.
- *Rhus toxicodendron 5 C*. The area around the glands is red and swollen; children hurt all over and are very agitated, especially at night. Fever is high, and accompanied by shivering and a dry cough.

  A particular symptom of *Rhus toxicodendron* cases is the development of cold sores, usually on the lips, as well as a red triangle on the tip of the tongue.

Night Terrors
(See Also Behaviour Problems)

Some children are terrified of sleeping in a dark room and insist on having a night light on all night long. Also, once they finally fall asleep, they tend to be very agitated.

2 granules before going to bed, or if the child cannot sleep:

- *Kali bromatum 4 C*. For children who sleepwalk, or who suffer from nightmares.
- *Stramonium 4 C*. For children who grind their teeth in their sleep.

Otitis

In most cases of otitis a doctor should be consulted. However, if it is a recurring condition and if no fever develops, you can treat the disorder yourself.

Otitis can be diagnosed by the inflammation of the ear, the colour of the tympanum (ear drum) and, in some cases, by the pus which flows from the affected ear. Penicillin, which you should not hesitate to use under the right circumstances, prevents the disorder from developing complications, especially mastoiditis. Otitis can cause partial deafness (which may not be immediately detected) and is therefore certainly not an illness to be taken lightly.

In cases where pus is emitted, clean the ear with a cotton bud, but do not probe too deeply. To ease the pain, place a hot, moist compress over the affected ear, and wrap the head in a soft cloth or towel.

Also, onion compresses help displace the infection down into the neck. Avoid foods which are spicy or hard to digest - stick to a diet based on fruit.

3 granules every three hours:

- *Aconitum 5 C.* If the otitis is probably caused by exposure to cold, or if it appears very suddenly.
- *Calcarea carbonica 5 C.* A basic remedy, applicable in all chronic cases.
- *Capsicum 5 C.* Otitis is accompanied by burning in the throat, and the ears are sensitive to the touch.
- *Capsicum annuum 5 C.* If the otitis is related to a sore throat or a head cold (which are frequent causes).

This is also an additional precaution against mastoiditis.

- *Belladonna 5 C.* In cases where the condition is accompanied by general aches and pains and fever, and congestion of the facial area.
- *Mercurius solubilis 4 C.* Suppuration appears after the ear drum is unblocked (which can occur spontaneously, or through surgical intervention).

Rubella (German Measles)

German measles produce many of the same symptoms as measles and scarlet fever.

Despite popular belief, this illness does not strike only children; women between the ages of 15 and 35 can contract the disease with its characteristic skin rash which, in their case, is usually found in the folded skin areas behind and around joints, especially ankles, wrists, hands and knees.

Danger to Babies

If contracted in the second or third month of pregnancy, women should consult a doctor immediately: in four out of five cases, the disease will cause malformations or other major problems in the foetus.

This is why an accurate diagnosis of the illness is essential. A host of complications can be avoided once the virus (and its virulence) has been identified. The disease is passed on via nasal secretions.

Differences Between Measles and German Measles

An absence of inflammation of the eyes and throat, as well as an absence of fever when the skin eruption appears, are the characteristic signs that you're dealing with a case of German measles (Rubella) and not ordinary measles. Another important sign is the appearance of ganglions behind the ears, on the nape of the neck, in the armpits and in the folds around the groin area. Also, in German measles there are no spots (Koplik's spots), even if the mucus is red.

Eruptions usually disappear after about three days. You may want to quarantine a child for a week or so, which is the usual period of isolation, depending on who the child is likely to come in contact with.

Choose from among the following three remedies (2 granules every 24 hours):

- Dulcamara 4 C.
- Mercurius solubilis 5 C - the most common remedy.
- Pulsatilla 5 C. For children who can't sleep without a light on.

Scarlet Fever

Scarlet fever is one of the more serious childhood illnesses. In fact, it is a streptococcal infection accompanied by a sore throat and a typical rash. You are bound by law to report any cases of the disease to the medical authorities. If not immediately treated with antibiotics, affected children - as well as their brothers and sisters - must remain absent from school for a sufficient period of time. The disease is most common between the ages of two and eight years. Boys are more likely to contract it than girls. Complications arising from scarlet fever can have a harmful effect on the kidneys for the rest of a child's life.

The incubation period of scarlet fever, which lasts about eight days, produces no tangible signs whatsoever. Then the first symptoms appear: shivering, aches, fever rising to 104°F (40°C), very rapid pulse (between 140 and 150 beats per minute), abdominal pains made worse by vomiting.

Another characteristic sign is the colour of the tonsils, which become unusually bright red. The tongue has a white coating, except around the edges and at the tip which are also bright red. During the following week, this red colour will gradually move towards the centre of the tongue.

The rash appears on the mucous membranes of the mouth, 48 hours after the initial symptoms. It then spreads, mainly affecting folded areas around the joints, especially the elbows. Skin starts peeling (desquamation) around the fifth or sixth day.

Of course, as soon as the first symptoms appear, you should consult a doctor as soon as possible. What makes scarlet fever difficult to identify is the fact that it does not always produce the rash or initial fever. In some acute cases, homoeopathic doctors will even prescribe allopathic antibiotics (rendering unto Caesar the things which are Caesar's!).

If possible, hang red curtains on the walls around the sickbed. Maintain room temperature at about 65°F (18°C) and give patients stewed fruit and fruit juice as long as the fever is above 104°F (40°C).

Preventive Treatment in Case of Epidemic

- *Belladonna 4 C.* 2 granules morning and night.
- *Arsenicum album 5 C.* 2 granules every 48 hours.

Once the Disease Is Contracted

- *Ailanthus 4 C.* 2 granules per day. This is the most common remedy. It should be started early and can sometimes halt the development of the disease completely. Administer with *Gelsemium sempervirens* 5 C, 2 granules every 12 hours, and *Belladonna 4 C,* 2 granules every 12 hours.

Teething
(See Also Teeth and Infant Diarrhoea)

Teething is often accompanied by fever and sometimes complicated by diarrhoea, colds, bronchitis or even otitis (see sections concerning these disorders).

Typically, one cheek is burning hot, while the other is pale and cold. Infants are agitated, cry a lot and only calm down when held. Teething is a difficult period, both for children and for their parents.

In cases where children calm down if they are given something to bite on (a piece of sugar, a rattle, a biscuit, etc.) you can rub the gums with *Plantago tincture* to ease the discomfort.

3 granules, every three hours:

- *Belladonna 9 C*. Infants are exhausted and suffer from spasms or even convulsions; especially recommended when canine (eye) teeth are coming through.
- *Borax 5 C*. For nervous infants with viscous, mushy, yellowish or greenish diarrhoea; when rocked these infants become nervous and pale.
- *Chamomilla 5 C*. The most general remedy, usually effective when administered every five hours; also use when teething troubles are accompanied by a head cold, intestinal colic, flatulence or diarrhoea. These infants are hypersensitive, grumpy and bent double - they cry, salivate profusely, are agitated and sometimes convulsed.
- *Ferrum phosphoricum 5 C*. 2 granules every hour while waiting to see a doctor. In cases where there is fever and the condition is complicated by sore throat, bronchitis, otitis or colic.
- *Kreosotum 5 C*. Infants are skinny and wrinkled; they develop painful gingivitis and diarrhoea; their breath and stool have a particularly unpleasant odour; skin on the bottom is irritated.
- *Magnesia carbonica 5 C*. Infants are hypersensitive and nervous (although less so than in Chamomilla cases); they develop intestinal colic, which is eased when they are able to pass wind.
- *Podophyllum 5 C*. Diarrhoea, although smelling bad, is not painful; infants are not grumpy, agitated or hypersensitive (as in *Chamomilla* cases).

Tonsils

The tonsils are part of the lymphatic network - a collection of vessels through which a colourless or amber-coloured liquid flows. This liquid has a composition similar to blood plasma. The function of the lymphatic system is to defend us against microbes - it acts as a kind of filter.

This is why tonsils, far from being a useless encumbrance, are important organs which should be preserved if they are in good health. In case of illness, everything should be done to try and cure the problem before resorting to surgical removal.

Tonsillitis

Tonsillitis refers to inflammation limited to the tonsils and surrounding tissue, inflammation which appears when patients suffer from a throat infection. Allopathic medicine routinely prescribes antibiotics to treat the problem, in order to avoid any possible complications, which do not often occur but can be serious: cardiac problems, pericarditis, and nephritis for example.

Emergencies

If the fever is very high, call a doctor. Also call in a physician if the inflammation is severe or if the child cannot swallow anything.

Consult the section on sore throats for an appropriate remedy.

Don't forget that "painting" or spraying the throat with a powerful antiseptic solution is useful. Gargling with lemon juice is also helpful. Also apply compresses as soon as symptoms appear, alternating between cabbage leaves and clay. An infusion made from *Solidago* leaves helps eliminate toxins in case of a throat infection. *Santasapina,* a syrup made from pine buds, helps fight coughing.

Abscess of the Tonsils

- *Hepar sulph. 7 C. 5* granules every 48 hours, with *Pyrogenium 7 C, 5* granules every 24 hours. If the abscess seems to be going down, administer *Hepar sulph.* first. If not, administer *Pyrogenium.*

Vaccination

Simple vaccination can sometimes be dangerous, so it's better to take precautions if you decide to have your children vaccinated.

Get Well Informed

For more information on the subject, consult the book *The War on Microbes Has Started* by Dr. Chavanon. The doctor shows how immunization can be achieved using homeopathic remedies obtained from various microbe and bacteria cultures. This kind of immunization has been shown to be more active and without danger.

- *Vaccinotoxinum 9 C.* 10 granules the morning after the vaccination.
- *Diphtherotoxinum 9 C.* 10 granules in the morning, two or three days after the injection, and *Formol 9 C,* in the morning, four or five days after the injection. Indicated for diphtheria and tetanus vaccinations using so-called anatoxins (inactivated bacterial toxins).

Homeopathic Vaccinations

In addition, there are a series of homeopathic vaccines (called *Nosodes)* which can arm children against various hereditary illnesses. Administer one every ten days, one after the other.

- *Ethyllicum 9 C* will protect children against possible toxic accidents.
- *Luesinum 9 C* cleans out the mother's body, neutralizing the toxic effects of chronic hereditary disorders, like syphilis for example.
- *Psorinum 9 C* is effective against problems like psoriasis, rheumatism and eczema.
- *Medorrhinum 9 C* fights hereditary gonorrhoea; to be used especially in cases where the disease has been detected in the mother or father of the child.
- *Nux vomica 9 C* protects children against chronic nervous disorders.
- *Syphilinum 7 C*. 2 granules, every 20 days as a simple precaution against long-term effects of possible hereditary syphilis, even if only a potential threat.
- *Tuberculinum 9 C*. As its name indicates, this is an antidote for hereditary tuberculosis. This doesn't mean that the disease is transmitted at birth - what can be transmitted is a homeopathically constructed resistance if children are born into an environment where they are likely to be exposed to this infectious disease.

Weakness (General)

A child may show signs of weakening, look generally sick and suffer from loss of appetite. If one of the following remedies does not provide prompt relief, do not hesitate to consult a doctor.

3 granules, once a day:

- *Abrotanum 4 C*. For infants who are losing weight, especially in the lower limbs. They have trouble standing or sitting up; the face is wrinkled, their eyes are dull and circled with dark rings. Follow up the treatment with *Natrum muriaticum 5 C*. This type of case, in particular, requires the intervention of a doctor.
- *Calcarea phosphorica 5 C*. For children who are growing rapidly, and who often suffer from headaches, especially when making some mental effort (studying). They show signs of sexual arousal. They tend to eat a lot between meals, and sleep is agitated.

- *Iodum 5 C*. Although they eat a lot and can't seem to satisfy their appetite, these cases continue losing weight. They are constantly agitated (hyperactive) and they seem to exhaust themselves.
- *Natrum muriaticum 7 C*. One dosage of 3 granules. Repeat 15 days later if necessary. Combine with another medication. For cases where children continue losing weight, despite the fact that they eat a lot; they are depressed, and have trouble making the least physical or mental effort; they seem to be permanently moody; they are often thirsty.
- *Silicea 5 C*. For children who are so thin that they have trouble staying out in cold weather and develop colds and bronchitis far too easily.

Chapter 3

The Nervous System

> *Homeopathy has had considerable success treating disorders of the mind. You will notice that, in general, dilutions are higher than for other kinds of problems. This is simply because the best experimental results were obtained with these concentrations.*

Abulia

This disorder is characterized by a total, or partial, lack of will-power, which places subjects in a highly contradictory position. They know they have to do things but never seem to get around to actually doing them. These cases generally need to be treated by a psychotherapist or psychoanalyst.

- Baryta carbonica 7 C. 5 granules per week, in conjunction with Opium 7 C and Aethusa cynapium 7 C, 2 granules in the morning, on alternate days.

Alcoholism

Homeopathy can, in certain cases, provide relief for people who fall prey to alcoholism, either by helping them overcome the desire for alcohol, or by combating the symptoms produced by intoxication.

In most cases, however, people will need specialized help to break the harmful habit completely.

Moderate Compulsive Drinkers

People who drink moderate amounts, but who do so constantly in order to get stimulation, can use the following treatment: *Hyoscyamus niger 4 C,* 2 granules twice a day; *Lachesis 5 C,* 2 granules once a day; *Nux vomica 9 C,* once after ten days.

Inveterate Drinkers

We recommend trying *Lachesis 30 C* and *Nux vomica 30 C* without the patient's knowing (you can put them in the patient's soup once a week, for example). To neutralize aggressiveness due to alcohol privation, add *Hyoscyamus 9 C* and *Staphysagria 9 C,* 3 granules of each. Other remedies include:

- *Arsenicum album 5 C. 3* granules three times per day. These people suffer from constant gastric and intestinal problems, vomit when they eat or drink anything.

- *Asarum 7 C. 3* granules twice a day. For alcoholics who are susceptible to cold and who abuse strong alcoholic drinks. They are often nauseous and doubled over with feelings of heaviness and anxiety in their stomach. They get up very early and feel a need to drink right away. They are hypersensitive and cannot stand noise.
- *Aurum 9 C.* 3 granules once a week. These people are susceptible to cold, congested, often hyperactive and fluctuate between states of anger and depression, with frequent thoughts of suicide.
- *Capsicum Mother Tincture.* Two or three drops added to a litre of wine will put the drinker off alcohol.
- *Hyoscyamus 5 C.* 3 granules every three hours. For people who hallucinate, thinking they're surrounded by mice or rats which they try to fend off with convulsive movements of their arms. In addition, these people are agitated and aggressive, and often try to provoke people around them by exposing their genitals.
- *Lachesis 7 C.* 2 granules three times a day. Subjects are over-excited and can't stop talking, then they fall into states of nervous depression. They can also be aggressive. They are worse just after waking up; when they manage to get to sleep, they'll often wake up suddenly with the sensation of someone trying to strangle them.
- *Nux vomica 5 C.* 2 granules every 2 hours. This is the remedy for a hangover, when subjects suffer from nausea, trembling and dizziness. Chronic alcoholics usually wake up in a bad mood, suffer from digestive problems, headaches and haemorrhoids. Their sleep is often troubled by nightmares populated with monsters and other fantastic apparitions.

Anorexia
(See Also Appetite, Nervous Breakdown)

This disorder usually affects adolescent girls who sometimes starve themselves to the point of wasting away in order to attain some inaccessible aesthetic ideal. Of course, this only explains their behaviour on a superficial level - various underlying motivations, which differ depending on the case, are the real causes of this bizarre behaviour.

It's useless and even harmful to try and force an anorexic child or adolescent to eat - doing so will probably only strengthen their resolve not to eat. In most cases, the help of a specialist is required.

Try as often as possible to offer the anorexic person a varied and balanced diet. Serve a cup of camomile tea half an hour before meals and a teaspoon of Lehning's Vegetable Tonic after meals. Also *Alfalfa 1X* and *Avena sativa 1X*. However, the best way to stimulate appetite is still movement - exercise, walks in the fresh air, gardening, for example - while avoiding excessive drinking.

- *Cina 9 C.* 3 granules twice a day. Lack of appetite alternates with voracious eating.
- *Lachesis 5 C.* 3 granules three times per day. People who get very excited during the course of an evening, and prefer to drink alcohol rather than eat the delicious food on their plates.
- *Lycopodium 4 C.* 3 granules three times a day. These people are full soon after they start eating or, conversely, seem to gain more appetite as the meal goes on. Also for people who are very picky about what they will and will not eat.
- *Mica 9 C.* 3 granules three times a day. These people are depressed, even desperate. ("Life is uninteresting, so why should I eat?") They are often cold and irritable. Their pulse is slow and weak.
- *Sepia 9 C.* 2 granules three times per day. For anorexics who are indifferent to everything and everyone, and who say they just want to be alone.
- *Sulphur 7 C.* 3 granules twice a day. For anorexics who say they are full as soon as they start eating.

Anxiety (Anguish)

This is another so-called "modern affliction". It seems to have become a normal part of life in today's society, if you look at the reports of the number of barbiturates and tranquillizers people consume every year.

Of course, anxiety is nothing new. But it is true that our world is changing more rapidly than ever before, while our belief systems (religion, family, traditions, personal relationships etc.) are becoming ever more fragile (see the Introduction for more comments about the changing nature of the quality of life in modern society). More than ever, people need to find ways of staying calm. Modern solutions (like drugs) leave a lot to be desired, since all they do is help us forget and avoid reality.

A good first step consists of simply cutting out coffee, tea, chocolate and alcoholic drinks, whenever possible. If you smoke, try to confine your smoking to after meals.

Physical activity is also an excellent antidote for anxiety. It's no surprise that millions of people around the world are jogging, or are passionately engaged in some other form of sport. And it's true that half an hour of jogging releases a substantial number of endorphins into the body (a substance similar to morphine, which is thought to be secreted by the brain during sessions of strenuous exercise) which do a lot to curb the effects of stress or depression.

Sometimes, however, our worries are of a more metaphysical nature, and watching TV or doing exercise cannot help us unless we have decided to ignore the problem. This is why so many people are turning to meditation or spend hours in sensory deprivation tanks, to find some measure of tranquillity.

The following remedies deal with some of the multiple forms of anxiety common in today's society.

- *Aconite 5 C.* 2 granules every three hours. Against feelings of fear or imminent death. Also for people who have palpitations due to anxiety.
- *Argentum nitricum 7 C.* 3 granules twice a day. When anxiety is caused by anticipation about some forthcoming event. Also for people who always act precipitately and for whom time always seems to pass too slowly.
- *Arsenicum album 5 C.* 2 granules every eight hours. Anxiety is accompanied by agitation; subjects are desperate, lack self-confidence, believe they are incurable and can't stay still. Their depression comes in cycles: they are unable to function for a couple of days, after which they feel better for a couple of days, then fall back into anxiety and depression, and so on. Also for cases where anxiety is intensified as night falls or for people who are alone.
- *Calcarea carbonica 9 C.* 3 granules once a week. Fear of the future causes intense anxiety.
- *Cocculus 9 C.* 3 granules once a week. Time always passes too quickly for these hypersensitive people - they find themselves slow, ineffective.
- *Gelsemium 9 C.* 3 granules once a day. For anxiety which produces trembling.
- *Glonoinum 9 C.* 3 granules once a week. Too much blood flowing to the brain disturbs these people - they think too fast and too intensely.
- *Ignatia 5 C.* 3 granules once a day. Subjects are nervous and sad, and have trouble breathing, as if something were blocking their throat. Also

for rapid and radical mood swings, changing from optimism to high anxiety in a few seconds. Sudden mood changes are a characteristic of this type, as well as *Arsenicum album*.

- *Kali carbonicum 9 C*. 3 granules every three hours. Anxiety is lodged in the stomach.
- *Medorrhinum 9 C*. 3 granules twice a day. These people seem to have no notion of time; they are night owls, preferring to live at night rather than during the day. They are absent-minded and act hastily, but less so at night.
- *Phosphorus 4 C*. 2 granules once a day. For people who suffer from periodic depression due to vague, rather philosophical fears, especially when they are alone; they are sometimes very sensitive to changes in the weather - an imminent storm will affect their mood, for example.
- *Staphysagria 5 C*. 3 granules per day. Anxiety is characterized by brooding, bearing grudges against others, etc. Subjects tend to become obsessed with bad memories and feel an intense desire for revenge.
- *Stramonium 9 C*. 3 granules per day. For cases of anxiety which cause people to stammer or to break out in a cold sweat. Also against fear of the dark.

Apathy
(See Also Nervous Breakdown)

Indifference, lack of interest in anything, stale emotions - sounds like a pretty minor problem, you may say. Yet suffering from a total lack of interest and energy can be like a living death, even though a person may be in the best of physical health.

Apathetic people soon lose their will to live because they can't find or create any sources of joy or pleasure (which are rare enough unless people make any effort). For some this effort comes naturally, whereas others have to work at it.

Note: the symptoms described for the following remedies characterize acute cases of apathy and are therefore more pronounced than in cases of temporary or relatively mild apathy.

- *Ambra grisea 5 C*. 2 granules per day. Subjects seem to be lost in a cloud and do not react to anything; they may spend entire days dreaming about the past.
- *Anacardium orientale 9 C*. 2 granules twice a day. These people seem to

remain in a state of reverie; they can be irritable and incapable of making decisions. Their perceptions (hearing, touch, etc.) seem to be affected, and in acute cases they will experience hallucinations, mostly auditory.

- *Helleborus niger 7 C*. 3 granules per day. A particular kind of depression sets in, where people hardly seem to perceive what is going on around them; they are apathetic and in a kind of stupor. They become physically weak - the more you try to console them, the further they withdraw into their own world.

- *Muriaticum acidum 5 C*. 2 granules per day. People are sad, taciturn and irritable. They sometimes suffer from headaches and dizziness; symptoms are aggravated in damp weather.

Apprehension
(See Also Stage Fright)

People sometimes get very apprehensive about forthcoming events (whether they're certain to happen or not) to the point of suffering from uncontrolled fits of trembling. Most of these fears can be overcome through individual or group therapy. The most effective therapy consists of helping apprehensive people confront their real or imagined danger, which they usually think is worse than it really is.

- *Argentum nitricum 9 C*. 3 granules three times a day. Anxiety arises when these people are faced with the idea of doing something they're not accustomed to doing, or with some forthcoming event.

Bulimia

It takes about twenty minutes for our brain to receive a message from our stomach telling us we're full. Twenty minutes, during which time we often continue eating, twenty minutes when we literally stuff ourselves. That's why some people say that the moment to stop eating is when you're enjoying your meal the most.

When we completely lose control of our appetite, we are often trying to avoid dealing with problems that are going to get worse in any case. Also, diabetes can cause some people to become bulimic. And in the early stages of pregnancy, bulimia is perfectly normal.

- *Iodum 9 C*. 5 granules once a week. Subjects are voracious eaters, never satisfied, and are constantly agitated as they try to get rid of their obsessions. They are often irritable and abrupt.

- *Natrum muriaticum, 7 C.* 3 granules every two days. Subjects crave an unlimited amount of fruit.
- *Sulphur 9 C.* 5 granules once a week. These people are generally good-natured and jolly, but at the same time highly egotistical and proud. Their joviality is often a façade, as they try to hide their profound distress.

Claustrophobia

Claustrophobia is a fear of enclosed spaces and can be more or less acute, depending on the case. For really distressing cases, take *Argentum nitricum 5 C,* 2 granules every two hours, while waiting to see a doctor.

Cold (Hypersensitivity to)

Being hypersensitive to cold can be an important symptom of some larger disorder, in the same way as an extreme intolerance of noise is a sign of a more serious problem.

- *Asarum 9 C.* 3 granules every two days. These people are weak and constantly on edge, and cannot tolerate noise as well as cold.
- *Calcarea silicata 9 C.* 5 granules once a week. These people are thin and pale, mentally fatigued, hypersensitive, irritable, and seek solitude. They cannot tolerate extreme heat and humidity as well as cold, and all of these aggravate the symptoms.
- *Petroleum 12 C.* 5 granules once a week. These people are thin and fear winter and cold weather in general; their skin is dry, thick and dull, and cracks easily; they don't perspire enough and often suffer from depression and an inability to make decisions.

Concentration

There are exercises which can help us develop our powers of concentration, but here, too, we sometimes lack the necessary motivation to overcome problems of this kind.

- *Aethusa 9 C.* 5 granules once a week. For students who have trouble concentrating; the condition may be aggravated by summer heat and sometimes in the morning; they may suffer from headaches and may often be in a bad mood.

- *Anacardium 9 C.* 5 granules once a week. For people who are exhausted by intellectual work; they are indecisive and may suffer from memory loss.
- *Natrum muriaticum 9 C. 5* granules once a week. For students who are dehydrated and skinny, who drink a lot of liquids and have an enormous appetite.
- *Oleander 9 C.* 5 granules once a week. Memory is weak, mental effort produces a general sensation of heat.
- *Silicea 9 C.* 5 granules once a week. For students who are timid, nervous and fearful.

Discouragement
(See Also Nervous Breakdown)

Although they are not stimulants, certain homeopathic remedies can sometimes help people overcome their own inertia.

- *Ambra grisea 9 C.* 5 granules every two days. After a difficult period, a personal loss or some other stressful event, subjects are depressed and lack energy.
- *Kali phosphoricum 9 C.* 3 granules twice a day. Subjects feel intellectually exhausted, are sad, anxious and indecisive; they tire rapidly and are further weakened by any effort; they have a low tolerance of cold or noise. On the other hand, their energy seems to revive to some extent after meals.

Exhaustion
(See Also Convalescence, Nervous Breakdown, Mental Fatigue)

Although less dramatic than nervous breakdown, nervous exhaustion is nevertheless a serious disorder. Subjects are more conscious of their day-to-day reality than are people suffering from a nervous breakdown, but they still don't see things as they normally would when in good health. This is why, whenever possible, they shouldn't be left alone to fall into a state of more severe depression.

- *Agaricus 15 C.* 10 granules once a week. Subjects are weak, both mentally and physically; they can't tolerate cold, tremble a lot and lack co-ordination in their movements. They are sad and discouraged, suffer from memory loss and sometimes feel dizzy for no reason. Symptoms are worse in the morning, after sexual intercourse or after making a mental effort.

- *Carbo vegetabilis 9 C.* 10 granules once a week. Subjects seem to have no energy; they can't tolerate cold, they're pale and look anaemic; the tip of their nose is sometimes bluish (cyanosis); symptoms are aggravated in the morning and at night, or in confined spaces which are too hot or too cold.
- *Phosphoricum acidum 9 C.* 3 granules per day. For students who are exhausted and whose mental faculties fall into a state of torpor; they may suffer from loss of memory; they develop an aversion to studying and conversation, and seem melancholic and discouraged. Symptoms are aggravated by mental or physical exertion but are eased by calm and solitude.
- *Phosphoricum acidum 15 C.* 10 granules once a week. Mental faculties are sluggish; these people suffer from memory loss, seem indifferent to everything, avoid conversation and mental effort.

Hallucinations

The term hallucination refers to any distortion of our sensory functions (sight, hearing, taste, touch and smell) inasmuch as these are the vehicles through which we interpret the outside world. Hallucinations concerning sensations outside our own bodies are called cenesthesic hallucinations.

These cases require the intervention of a trained specialist. If subjects are willing to drink, give them an infusion *of Santane No. 9* ,* which will help calm them down. A simple lime-blossom infusion, sweetened with honey, is also effective for this purpose.

While waiting to consult a physician, you can try one of the following remedies:

- *Absinthium 5 C.* 2 granules every two hours. For alcoholics who become over-excited, suffer from spasms, irritability and dizziness.
- *Absinthium 12 C.* 10 granules once a week. As for the 5 C dilution, but use for chronic cases.
- *Antipyrine 5 C.* 2 granules three times per day. These people are mentally over-excited and suffer from visual or auditory hallucinations. They are

---

* Santane No. 9: Tilia flowers, Crataegus, rose, peppermint, melissa, bitter-orange, origanum, lupulus, lavenders; produced by Iphym, France.

often feverish and prostrate.
- *Cannabis Indica 9 C.* 3 granules twice a day. Subjects have visual or auditory hallucinations, and/or visions of grandeur; they are often mentally over-excited - they have a lively mind, but alternate between states of hilarity and anxiety.
- *Hyoscyamus niger 7 C.* 2 granules per day. For visual hallucinations.
- *Stramonium 9 C.* The face is flushed and congested during a crisis; subjects are mentally over-excited and physically agitated; they are afraid to be alone or in the dark. During states of delirium, they are terrified by visual hallucinations.

Hypersensitivity
(See Also Cold, Personality Problems)
- *Brucea 9 C.* 5 granules every three days. Subjects cannot stand being touched.
- *Colchicum 9 C.* 5 granules every three days. Subjects are hypersensitive to smell, with a strong aversion to cooking odours in particular - they suffer from nausea and are therefore unable to enjoy food. The simple thought of food can make them sick.
- *Hydrophobinum 9 C.* 3 granules every two days. This is a general remedy for hypersensitivity to noise, smells, light, touch, etc. For example, the sight, sound or even the idea of running water is enough to provoke various problems: irritability, headaches, urge to urinate, etc.
- *Platina 7 C.* 3 granules every day. For women whose vulva is very sensitive to touch, rubbing clothes, etc.
- *Coffea 12 C.* 10 granules per week. For generally hypersensitive people - they are nervous and mentally overactive.

Hypochondria
Hypochondria is a well-known disorder - all you have to do is sit down and read a medical dictionary for a few hours and you'll find symptoms that correspond to about a dozen diseases. People convince themselves they are seriously ill. They become obsessed and are sure that the symptoms they're feeling prove they're sick. (Yet there is nothing physically wrong with them!)
- *Aurum metallicum 9 C.* 5 granules every two days. These people are

melancholy and seem to want to die.

- *Natrum muriaticum 9 C.* 2 granules every two days. Subjects are reserved and uncommunicative about their (mostly digestive) problems, and tend to brood constantly.
- *Phosphorus 7 C.* 3 granules every three days. Subjects are anxious and fret about the least sign that could be a symptom of disease. They are generally friendly and enjoy the company of other people.

Insomnia
(See Also Sleep)

People who suffer from chronic insomnia should re-examine the way they live. Of course, you can't get rid of all your worries with a magic wand. We must learn to stay calm even under difficult circumstances.

We could also try to change our frame of mind, so that we would be less vulnerable to stress. A good walk is a great way to clear your mind. Also, avoiding crowded shopping areas in the evening before going to bed sometimes helps you get to sleep more easily.

Cut Out Stimulants

You should cut out a stimulant such as coffee, at least gradually, by cutting out those cups in the late afternoon. Morning coffee is the hardest to cut out completely.

As with many other health problems, insomnia can be an indication that something is wrong with a person's lifestyle. Whatever you do, try not to fall into the habit of relying on sleeping pills - the body becomes dependent on them, and you soon won't be able to do without them. In addition, two hours of natural sleep is worth five hours of drug-induced sleep.

- *Lemon balm tea,* to which you add a little hops, is an excellent sedative. There's also the traditional *Valerian tea,* however its effect is more temporary. *Kuhne Baths* (see section) also help in overcoming insomnia.
- Also very effective: *Passiflora 1 X*, five drops in a little water, whenever you wake up.

Three granules of one of the following remedies, an hour before going to bed (repeated if necessary), in 5 C dilution if the condition is temporary, and 9 C if it is a long-term problem:

- *Aquilegia 5 C.* For nervous women whose sleep is short and agitated and who sometimes experience spasms and trembling.

- *Argentum nitricum 7 C*. Insomnia is caused by apprehension about some event.
- *Arnica 7 C*. People are agitated and find their bed too hard. Administer after prolonged worries or mental strain.
- *Avena sativa 1 C*. For general insomnia.
- *Belladonna 5 C*. Insomnia persists, despite a person's fatigue.
- *Chamomilla 7 C*. For nervous people who have nightmares and perspire a lot in their sleep.
- *Cora 5 C*. Insomnia due to altitude.
- *Coffea 7 C*. An overactive mind (the inability to stop thinking) prevents these people from sleeping.
- *Gelsemium 7 C*. Insomnia due to mental fatigue; even when exhausted, these people just can't get to sleep. Also for cases of insomnia due to the shock of a tragedy or loss.
- *Ignatia 7 C*. Depressed, tormented by grief, these people are constantly yawning and sighing, yet they can't get to sleep. They are sometimes awakened by itching sensations.
- *Kali phosphoricum 5 C*. For insomnia linked to mental strain.
- *Nux vomica 5 C*. Late hours, too much work, coffee and prolonged discussions before bed are routine for these people.
- *Passiflora 5 C*. These people are agitated, nervous, weak and exhausted, sometimes tormented by grief.
- *Stramonium 7 C*. For cases of night terrors, or fear of the dark that prevents children from sleeping.
- *Sulphur 5 C*. People who are very light sleepers and wake up at the slightest noise; they also have troubling dreams.
- *Valeriana*. This form of insomnia is characterized by excessive mental activity, a feeling of pins and needles in their legs and changing moods.

Melancholy

Melancholy, even when it is understandable, can sometimes last longer than necessary. This indicates that there is some other, underlying cause, or that a person is susceptible to depression. Homeopathy can be of some help in combating these negative influences.

3 granules of one of the following remedies every two days:

- *Ignatia 9 C.* People are very sensitive and start crying for no reason; they are introspective and tend to brood. Children are brilliant, but are pushed too hard by parents and/or teachers to perform well at school.
- *Gelsemium 9 C.* Subjects are fearful, try to avoid contact with others, and demonstrate an inordinate fear of exams or speaking in public. They sometimes seem to be in a daze.
- *Kali phosphoricum 9 C.* Subjects are timid, fearful, over-emotional, discouraged and lack self-confidence; they are indecisive, lack will-power and are very sensitive to pain and noise. They become even weaker when they have to make any kind of effort, but seem to revive somewhat during meals.
- *Lachesis 9 C.* These people are characterized by a total lack of joy - they keep brooding about the same old negative thoughts; they suffer from insomnia, are saddened by their own life and unfortunate events seem to leave an indelible trace in their mind.
- *Lycopodium 12 C.* People are depressed and lack self-confidence to the point of thinking that they are good for nothing; they tend to be morose and taciturn; they suffer from memory loss, and can be irritable and authoritarian; they often lose their train of thought when talking.

Memory

There's a saying that "memory is the faculty that forgets". In fact, its function consists of selecting and filing information, in the form of facts and important names. Interestingly enough, our mental health depends on our ability to forget a certain amount of that information.

It's not hard to comprehend how important remembering and forgetting are. If we were to remember everything - every little detail of everyday life, our least little problems and all our pains - life would become hell.

We all suffer from emotional shocks at some time in our lives. Isn't it something of a blessing that the memory of those events fades in time, becoming less acute and less painful. . . in the present?

Memory can be compared to a blackboard in a classroom: students could not read anything if someone didn't wipe off the previous day's lessons every night.

A problem arises if the student who cleans the blackboard does so a little too zealously, erasing information which is useful for the next day's class. Even the most brilliant mind is severely handicapped by a faulty memory. None of us can completely control our memory. Sometimes we'd like to forget, at other times we just can't remember things.

- *Anacardium orientale 9 C.* 3 granules three times a day. For students who have studied to the point where they can't assimilate information any more, and start forgetting what they've already learned. Also for people who forget recent facts and names and, as a result, begin to lose self-confidence; they may also be touchy and indecisive.
- *Baryta carbonica 9 C.* 10 granules once a week. These people are slow learners, or unable to keep their mind from wandering.
- *Caladium 9 C.* 3 granules three times a day. For those who suffer from temporary amnesia and often lose their train of thought.
- *Kali bromatum 9 C. 3* granules three times a day. These people forget or jumble their words; they are sad and indifferent, and tend to have nightmares
- *Kali phosphoricum 9 C.* 3 granules three times a day. People have trouble concentrating on a single idea; they are depressed and overworked.
- *Luesinum 9 C.* 3 granules three times a day. For those who tend to forget names of people and places.
- *Medorrhinum 9 C.* 3 granules three times a day. For memory that hardly functions at all.
- *Nux vomica 9 C.* 3 granules three times a day. These people suffer from memory lapses and have trouble working.
- *Phosphoricum acidum 9 C.* 3 granules three times a day. These people are forgetful, especially in the morning.
- *Silicea 9 C.* 3 granules three times a day. Subjects lack self-confidence, have trouble concentrating and spend a lot of time day-dreaming.
- *Sulphur 9 C.* 3 granules three times a day. Subjects forget proper names and recent events.

Mental Confusion
(See Also Nervous Breakdown)

People can sometimes fall into states of depression and develop fever to the point of becoming delirious. These people are prey to a general disorder known as mental confusion, and require the help of a doctor or therapist. While waiting to consult a specialist, you can use one of the following remedies to alleviate the symptoms:

- *Baotisia 9 C. 3* granules three times per day. Subjects are incapable of concentrating, and sometimes suffer from a split personality or feel that one part of their body is detached from the rest. They are indifferent to everything and everyone, and believe they have no hope of recovering.
- *Hyoscyamus 9 C.* 3 granules three times per day. Subjects alternate between states of delirium and stupor; they are jealous, suspicious and mistrustful, and constantly blame the people around them; they tend to be exhibitionists and talk a lot about their work.
- *Opium 9 C. 3* granules three times per day. Subjects are so slow intellectually that they seem retarded; they appear indolent and hardly react to sensory stimulation, as if they can't see or hear anything. They are allergic to heat, revive somewhat in the open air or after a cold drink.

Mental Fatigue
(See Also Nervous Breakdown, Exhaustion)

This type of fatigue is characterized by memory loss, lack of self-confidence and irrational fears. Subjects have no interest in anything.

- *Arnica 9 C.* 5 granules every two days. People are prostrate and inert, as if suffering from shock. Conversation seems to depress them even more.
- *Gelsemium 9 C.* 5 granules every two days. Subjects are afraid of everything, tremble and seem to be in a daze.
- *Ignatia 9 C.* 5 granules every two days. Subjects are nervous; they yawn, sigh and cry a lot and often feel as if there's a ball of tension in their throat or stomach.
- *Lachesis 9 C.* 5 granules every two days. After some profound tragedy or emotional shock, people become alternately over-excited and depressed; they talk a lot and their sleep is disturbed by nightmares.

Nervous Agitation
(For Children, See Behaviour Problems)

Can't keep still? It's not easy to overcome nervous agitation or restlessness, once it becomes a part of your personality. We usually don't have the time or the inclination to take the necessary steps: relaxation, travel (in order to get far away from the source of our worries - something we all dream of doing, but which, strangely enough, few people actually manage to do, even if they have the means).

On the other hand, we are sometimes unaware of just how nervous we are, which doesn't mean that our state of agitation has no effect. The physical consequences to ourselves are often long-term and it's the people close to us who pay the price.

Here are a few homeopathic remedies which are likely to help you regain your serenity and peace of mind. This does not mean that you should necessarily limit your treatment to taking a homeopathic remedy - there are many relaxation techniques (yoga, deep breathing, visualization, etc.) which can help ease the tensions you experience in your life.

However, we should point out that taking tranquillizers (except under very special circumstances) does nothing to re-establish lasting mental balance.

Take the most appropriate remedy at a dosage of 3 granules once a week:

- *Arsenicum album 9 C.* For those who are meticulous to the point of being obsessed; they are touchy, they are in constant movement (both mentally and physically), are impatient and show signs of avarice.

- *Iodum 9 C.* These agitated people are thin and anxious; their state worsens when they're hungry; they have trouble coping with heat. They tend to calm down a bit in fresh air or when engaged in some physical activity. They are impulsive, cannot stand noise, and are often in a bad mood.

- *Kali bromatum 9 C.* These people constantly need to move around - their hands or feet are always beating out some mental rhythm. They seem to have memory problems and become more agitated when they have to make some kind of mental effort; physical exertion, on the other hand, seems to calm them down. They often have nightmares.

- *Lillium tigrinum 9 C.* Subjects are always in a hurry, always in a bad mood, gruff. Their ideas are jumbled and lack coherence; they have a hard time concentrating, and seem to lack judgement, harbouring false ideas and opinions indiscriminately. They start to suffocate in rooms that are overheated. Women menstruate early and are sexually over-excited.

- *Mephitis putorium 7 C.* Subjects are nervous, their legs will not stop shaking; they often suffer from insomnia.

- *Tarentula Hispana 9 C.* Excited, agitated and hypersensitive, subjects can't stay in one place; their minds are often wildly over-excited and this is intensified by noise or throbbing music. They calm down in a quiet, tranquil room.

- *Zincum metallicum 9 C.* People have to move their legs constantly.

Nervous Breakdown
(See Also Apathy, Discouragement)

We do not have enough space here to cover all the different types of nervous breakdown. Most cases require the help of a specialist who is familiar with the patient's history.

- *Agaricus muscarius 12 C.* 10 granules once a week. For patients who are in a state of general nervous ruin, due to excessive mental exertion. They are sad, discouraged and unable to tolerate cold; their hands tremble, and symptoms are aggravated by any mental effort and by cold. They have trouble expressing themselves - they lose their train of thought and can't find their words.
- *Ambra grisea 9 C.* 5 granules every two days. Subjects are depressed and apathetic after an emotionally trying or unsettling event. They cry a lot and their condition makes them worry, so they become even more depressed. They are noticeably weak physically, have a failing memory and are very uncomfortable with strangers.
- *Anacardium orientale 12 C.* 10 granules once a week. For people who are irritable, sometimes angry or rude; they have trouble understanding what others tell them, and can't concentrate; they also suffer from memory loss. They lack energy and self-confidence. Symptoms are aggravated when they're hungry or when they have to make a mental effort.
- *Antimonium crudum 12 C.* 5 granules once a week. Subjects are sad and cry all the time, and display suicidal tendencies.
- *Aurum metallicum 12 C.* 5 granules once a week. People cannot tolerate cold and sometimes explode in violent bouts of anger. They are disgusted with life and fearful of their own suicidal thoughts.
- *Caladium 12 C.* 5 granules every three days. For depression that sets in after sexual excesses. These people have trouble concentrating, are irritable and hypersensitive to noise. They sometimes feel dizzy when they close their eyes. Symptoms are aggravated in hot rooms and improve in fresh air and after a good sleep.
- *Causticum 15 C.* 5 granules once a week. Against depression which is often associated with old age. People are weak, stiff, sometimes mildly

paralysed in certain parts of their bodies; they are thin and emaciated, sad, seem anxious, especially at night and in the dark, and don't talk much. Symptoms are eased by warmth in bed.

- *Cocculus 9 C.* 5 granules once a week. For cases where depression is characterized by a slowdown in mental faculties, accompanied by irritability, bouts of anger and hypersensitivity to emotions and to noise. Subjects frequently suffer from recent memory loss and are often in a bad mood.

- *Fluoricum acidum 15 C.* 10 granules once a week. Thin and withdrawn into themselves, these people seem to have lost their memory - they hardly respond to questions that are put to them and cannot sustain any mental effort, which gives them a headache.

- *Hyoscyamus niger 9 C.* 3 granules three times per day. Physical exhaustion is punctuated by temporary fits of excitability, followed by even more marked prostration. Possible origins of this state: extended periods of worry, disappointments in love.

- *Ignatia 30 C.* 10 granules every two weeks. After some kind of tragedy, subjects often cut themselves off from everyone and become silent; they sigh and yawn. Any effort to get them to open up sends them deeper into their shell. Subjects often feel like there's a ball of tension in their throat or stomach.

- *Kali bromatum 9 C.* 3 granules three times a day. The condition is due to money worries or mental exhaustion. These people cannot tolerate cold, they're agitated and constantly shifting, especially their hands. They sometimes have spasms, and may suffer from nightmares.

- *Kali phosphoricum 9 C.* 3 granules three times a day. After excessive mental work, people fall into a state of mental exhaustion, melancholy and discouragement. They are indecisive, hypersensitive, anxious and lack will-power. They find any physical effort exhausting.

- *Lillium tigrinum 12 C.* 5 granules once a week. Subjects are melancholy and anxious, irritable, have trouble concentrating and lack clarity. Trying to console them only aggravates their state; walking in the fresh air eases symptoms.

- *Lycopodium 12 C.* 5 granules once a week. People have absolutely no self-confidence; their mental capabilities and memory seem to deteriorate along with their lack of interest in work and any kind of activity - all they want is peace and quiet - they find any physical effort exhausting.

- *Mercurius 9 C*. 10 granules once a week. Subjects are self-centred, and have problems with comprehension and concentration. They suffer from memory loss and are slow to respond. They are agitated, always want to go out and meet people and are very sensitive to changes in temperature.
- *Natrum carbonicum 12 C*. once a week. Subjects are weak and tired, cannot tolerate cold, extreme heat or stormy weather, which causes headaches and exhaustion.
- *Natrum muriaticum 15 C*. 10 granules once a week. Subjects are sad and discouraged, they cry a lot, brood about things, are indifferent to everything except their own sorrow. They often resist being consoled.
- *Nux vomica 9 C*. 10 granules once a week. Overwork leads to burnout. Subjects are sad and discouraged, disgusted with their job, and have trouble making any kind of mental effort or concentrating; they are irritable and extremely tense.
- *Phosphoricum acidum 9 C*. 5 granules once a week. Physical, nervous and mental exhaustion, intellectual slowness and torpor resulting from overwork, or worries; subjects find they have trouble remembering things and are uninterested in facing any intellectual challenge; symptoms are aggravated by any kind of effort.
- *Sepia 12 C*. 10 granules once a week. Subjects are totally lacking in energy; they are melancholic and apathetic; they cannot tolerate cold and are indifferent to everything; they avoid conversation and seek solitude; they're often irritable and grouchy, but seem to feel better after a good night's sleep.

Nervousness
(See Also Anxiety, Noise, Hypersensitivity, Insomnia, Stress, Trembling)

We're all nervous to some extent, but that doesn't mean we're all sick. In proper doses, nervousness acts as a stimulus, as in the case of athletes whose nerves make them more aware, thus improving their performance.

But nervousness can become excessive, cause people to tremble, say things they don't mean, drop objects and do exactly what they don't want to do - in short, it can make life miserable.

At that point, people generally try to change their habits or living conditions, in order to give their body more rest - they take a holiday in the country, for example. But people who can't afford to get away whenever they need a break must look for other solutions, unless they succeed in mastering one or more relaxation techniques.

If you are excessively nervous, you should, once again, take a close look at your diet. The first thing you should do is restrict your intake of coffee and alcohol. The recommended diet, which is the same as for Gastritis (see section), is designed to eliminate substances likely to produce exaggerated excitation of the nervous system.

On the other hand, vitamin C is an excellent natural source of nourishment for the nerves. Yeast, which contains vitamins B_1 and B_2, also acts as a fortifier for the nervous system. Use brewer's yeast extract if you have digestive problems. Avoid places and situations that are likely to cause stress, try to find peace and quiet and get more sleep.

- *Agaricus 9 C.* 10 granules once a week. Constant trembling of the hands results in pronounced clumsiness. These people are often sad, have trouble expressing themselves and finding their words.
- *Aquilegia 6 C.* 3 granules three times per day. For women whose sleep is agitated and too short and who sometimes get muscle spasms.
- *Asarum Europum 9 C.* 10 granules once a week. Subjects are hypersensitive, their nerves are on edge; they cannot tolerate even slight noise and are especially disturbed by grating or squeaking noises.
- *Asafoetida 9 C.* 3 granules per day. Irritable and moody, these people have a low pain threshold; they sometimes get spasms; symptoms improve in the fresh air.
- *Borax 9 C,* three times per day. Both children and adults are pale and skinny; they are nervous, anxious, upset for no reason, frequently in a bad mood, and jump at the slightest noise. Symptoms seem to be aggravated when they lean forward.
- *Chamomilla 9 C.* 10 granules every two weeks. These people only calm down when surrounded by vibrations: in a train, at the cinema, or working with the radio on.
- *China 9 C.* 3 granules three times a day. Nervousness is accompanied by hypersensitivity to smells and to touch.
- *Chloralum 4 C.* 3 granules three times per day. For nervous people who suffer from frequent headaches, which are aggravated by alcohol.
- *Kali bromatum 9 C.* 3 granules three times per day. Subjects are nervous, somewhat depressed, agitated, with hands and fingers that are incessantly

moving. Any mental effort makes them even more nervous.

- *Kali phosphoricum 9 C. 3* granules three times per day. Subjects' legs are constantly agitated.
- *Nitricum acidum 9 C. 3* granules three times per day. People are nervous, weak and tend to lose weight. They are often gloomy and prostrate, indifferent, irritable or weary. Their condition gets worse if they lack sleep.
- *Nux vomica 9 C. 3* granules three times per day. Subjects are both nervous and irritable.
- *Valeriana 9 C. 3* granules three times per day. Subjects are very excitable, moody, and alternate between states of euphoria and irritability; the tendency is more marked when they are hungry.
- *Zincum 9 C. 3* granules three times per day. For people whose legs are constantly agitated, even when they sleep.

Nightmares
(See Also Night Terrors in Children)

It's normal to have a nightmare now and then, but when they occur on a regular or even daily basis, they become a source of unpleasant tension which can destroy a person's sleep. Note that intestinal worms can be a cause of nightmares in children.

An infusion made with orange flower syrup, taken before going to bed, is effective. Also 2 grams of *P.C. Sedative** , if needed. A lime-blossom bath just before going to bed can also help.

2 granules the morning after a nightmare:

- *Kali bromatum 9 C.* Subjects are generally weak and very sensitive; children tremble at the slightest contact or noise; nightmares are recurring; adults often feel insecure, sometimes have difficulty expressing themselves and suffer from mental exhaustion.
- *Stramonium 9 C.* Children are afraid of the dark, very agitated, almost wild, sometimes cruel; they are afraid of water. Adults talk incessantly, suffer from feelings of guilt and, in extreme cases, from hallucinations.

---

* Sédatif P.C.: Abrus precatorius, Aconitum napellus, Atropa belladonna, Calendula officinalis, Chelidonium majur, Viburnum opulus; produced by Boiron, France.

Noise (Hypersensitivity to)

Hypersensitivity to noise is most often accompanied by headaches; we are edgy, we may suffer from dizzy spells, and the slightest noise makes us jump or tremble.

A single disorder rarely occurs on its own - it's as if we sometimes become veritable magnets for all kinds of problems. And a sorrowful or ill-tempered disposition seems to make us even more vulnerable. Research on people's tolerance of noise has only begun to discover the numerous problems that it can engender.

Urban environments place our nerves under severe stress, all the more so since we are genetically unprepared for coping with a milieu that is so radically different from anything mankind has had to face before: in its present form, the urban environment is less than a hundred years old, which represents only a fraction of a second of human existence as a whole.

Of course, being hypersensitive to noise is only one of a group of symptoms which are part of a larger problem, and it is precisely on this larger, more global scale that homeopathic remedies are most effective.

Practising some kind of relaxation technique should become an integral part of everyone's life - relaxation should be taught at school! - so that we learn to maintain a degree of inner calm, which will help us deal with the day-to-day problems we all have to face.

5 granules once a week:

- *Asarum 9 C.* For nervous people who are hypersensitive, susceptible to cold and "allergic" to even the slightest noise (especially squeaking). They often get headaches and can hardly stand the feel of their own clothes.
- *Cantharis 9 C.* Subjects are anxious, agitated and sometimes nasty; their irritability is aggravated by noise and by the sight of water.
- *Iodum 9 C.* Subjects are agitated, thin and anxious; they feel worse when they haven't eaten, and cannot tolerate heat; they tend to calm down out in the fresh air or when engaged in some physical activity. They are impulsive, can't stand noise and are often in a bad mood.
- *Kali phosphoricum 9 C.* Subjects are timid, fearful, excessively emotional, easily discouraged and completely lacking in self-confidence; they are indecisive, lack will-power and are very sensitive to touch and to pain, as well as to noise; they are quickly exhausted by any kind of effort,

but revive somewhat after meals.

- *Nux vomica 9 C.* These people are hyperactive, nervous, congested, impatient and always tense; in many cases they are heavily addicted to coffee and/or alcohol. Symptoms improve after a good night's sleep.
- *Theridion 7 C.* 10 granules once every two weeks. People are agitated and constantly feel the need to be doing something; they are also hypersensitive to touch and sometimes feel as if the noise around them is penetrating their entire body, right into their teeth.
- *Strychninum 9 C.* Subjects are very excited, both physically and mentally; they are irritable and explosive; they have exaggerated physical reflexes and are sometimes susceptible to cold draughts.

Oppression
(See Also Asthma, Shortness of Breath)

The sensation of not being able to breathe, as if there were a weight on your chest, is sometimes of nervous origin. This "oppression" is usually accompanied by psychological discomfort.

- *Ignatia 9 C.* 3 granules three times per day. The most general remedy.
- *Opium 7 C.* 3 granules three times per day. People feel oppressed, as if they are suffocating the moment they try to sleep; they tend to be drowsy all day long.

Personality Problems

Included under this heading are a number of "personality disorders" that can be treated with homeopathic remedies, often to the great relief of the sufferer and the people around them.

Problems are presented in their so-called pathological state, i.e. when they become serious. You don't have to identify all the symptoms to choose a given remedy. Also, you don't have to wait for a case to become pathological before trying a remedy.

Whenever possible, try to combine the homeopathic treatment with some kind of personal intervention - therapies and therapists exist for almost any kind of problem. If you think the problem is a minor one and does not require therapeutic intervention, then you may want to look at the situation from the point of view of personal development: the aim is not just to get rid of a problem, but also to enrich your life and your personal relations.

That's why it's always a good idea to define in concrete terms the changes you wish to make. You can do this through communication, either with people close to you or in the more formal setting of group or individual therapy sessions. It's always harder, and sometimes discouraging, to try and do this kind of "work" all on your own.

Aggressiveness
(See Also Anger)
- *Mercurius solubilis 9 C.* 5 granules once a week. Subjects always have to be the leader, the centre of attention; they tend to be violent (sometimes directing their aggression at animals) and quarrelsome.
- *Nux vomica 9 C.* 10 granules once a week. People are impatient and irritable - they don't ask, they demand!
- *Staphysagria 9 C.* 10 granules once a week. Subjects are often in a bad mood; they get angry easily and are prone to throwing and breaking things when upset.

Anger
(See Also Aggressiveness)
Note: After a bout of anger, you can administer 3 granules of *Colocynthis 9 C* to help calm people down.
- *Cereus serpentinus 9 C.* 10 granules once a week. For people who are prone to terrible fits of rage; they can be disgustingly rude and profane; when not angry they tend to be depressed.
- *Cimex 12 C.* 5 granules once a week. People are subject to violent anger and want to break things.
- *Colocynthis 5 C.* 2 granules every half an hour. These people are very short-tempered and tend to fall sick after a bout of anger.
- *Ignatia 5 C.* 2 granules every half an hour. Especially for women with unstable personalities who get upset easily and who develop various other problems because of their anger.
- *Nux vomica 9 C.* 5 granules every week. For business people who are intolerant and uncompromising.
- *Stramonium 12 C.* 10 granules per week. Face is congested, eyes are shining, people become violent and nasty.
- *Veratrum album 9 C.* 5 granules per week. Subjects are anxious and

constantly critical of others. Once angry, they become furious, start screaming and want to bite or scratch.

Arrogance
(also see Overbearing Pride)
- *Lycopodium 9 C*. 5 granules once a week. These people criticize others all the time and are torn between their desire for solitude and their inability to be alone. They cry easily and cannot stand being contradicted. They are bitter and suffer because of their dark, brooding thoughts, which they cannot get rid of.
- *Platina 9 C*. 5 granules once a week. These people are proud but also melancholic; they have a pronounced attachment to beauty; they feel they are not appreciated and misunderstood. Subjects often have a very high opinion of themselves and are in conflict with people around them, suffering as they are from fear and insecurity. Symptoms are aggravated by emotional stress, nervous fatigue, frustration and touch.
- *Veratrum album 9 C*. 5 granules once a week. Subjects are anxious, exceedingly critical of others and quick to lose their temper.

Authoritarianism
For this condition, as well as for many other personality disorders, it must be understood that administering a homeopathic remedy cannot completely resolve the problem. In most cases, treatment should include therapeutic intervention by a professional, and a change in location and/or living conditions, so that the problem does not continue to arise at the slightest provocation.
- *Aurum metallicum 9 C*. 5 granules once a week. These people are prone to violent anger and have trouble controlling their instinctive reactions; however, they seem to be able to regain their good humour quickly enough; they have problems living with other people.
- *Nux vomica 9 C*. 5 granules once a week. People tend to be touchy and get very angry over insignificant things; they are resistant to any new ideas, and are often sad, worried and shut themselves off from the rest of the world.

Bigotry
Here, it's the people around the subject who suffer most; bigots cling to rigid (and often contradictory) views and tend to judge everyone around them severely.

"Live and let live!' you say, over and over again, but without effect. But don't forget that bigoted people need warmth perhaps more than anyone.

- *Stramonium 7 C.* 3 granules twice a day.

Brooding

- *Natrum muriaticum 7 C.* 5 granules. Subjects are introverted, seldom communicate, and seek solitude in order to brood about their past.
- *Sepia 7 C.* 5 granules every two days. For subjects who punish the people around them by refusing to speak for long periods of time.

Capriciousness

- *Chamomilla 9 C.* 5 granules once a week. Never content, never satisfied, these people are often rude and vengeful; they don't like to be approached or touched; children often throw tantrums towards nightfall.
- *Cina 9 C.* 5 granules once a week. Subjects are stubborn and grumpy; they don't like to be looked at or approached; they do an about-face and reject something they wanted a moment before. Children are timid and fearful, they don't like being touched or held, and yawn a lot.
- *Staphysagria 9 C.* 5 granules once a week. These individuals are hypersensitive and short-tempered. They are often in a bad mood and tend to brood about past sorrows.

Clumsiness
(See Also Nervousness)

- *Natrum muriaticum 9 C.* 3 granules per day. The more edgy these people become, the clumsier they are - their movements become even more abrupt and imprecise than usual.

Crying

- *Ignatia amara 9 C.* 10 granules once a week. Tears are interspersed with heavy sighing.
- *Natrum muriaticum 9 C.* 10 granules once a week. Subjects are sad and always about to burst into tears.
- *Pulsatilla 9 C.* 10 granules once a week. For emotional types who start crying for no apparent reason; they seek the company of others.
- *Sepia 9 C.* 10 granules once a week. Here, too, people cry for no apparent reason, but seek solitude instead of company; when you try to

console them, the crying gets worse.

Fears

Administer the appropriate remedy at a dosage of 3 granules of a low dilution (5 C) every hour for people suffering from acute fear. If the fear is debilitating or continual - in which case you're dealing with a phobia - the dosage would be 10 granules of a higher dilution (9 or 12 C) once a week.

To help people recover after a crisis, administer 3 granules *of Aconite 9 C.*

- *Aconite* for fear of dying.
- *Actaea racemosa* to combat the fear of giving birth or the fear of going insane.
- *Argentum nitricum.* Subjects are afraid of solitude, crowds, open spaces, heights, and suffer from general anxiety.
- *Belladonna* fights fear of animals.
- *Brucea* alleviates the fear of being touched.
- *Calcarea carbonica* can be effective against fears concerning the future.
- *Causticum* for fear of the dark.
- *Hydrocyanic acid,* also for fear of the dark.
- *Hyoscyamus* against fear of water and infection.
- *Lycopodium* to treat fear of responsibilities.
- *Phosphorus* alleviates fear of ghosts and disease.
- *Pulsatilla* reduces apprehension about the opposite sex.
- *Radium bromide* for fear of solitude and of the dark.
- *Rhododendron* fights fear of storms.
- *Stramonium* prevents fear of darkness and of tunnels.

Guilt (Excessive Feelings of)

- *Lachesis 9 C.* 5 granules once a week. Subjects tend to complain about their fate; they can become violently angry and then regret what they do or say; they are sometimes jealous for no reason.
- *Lillium tigrinum 9 C.* 5 granules once a week. These people are melancholic and despairing and often depressed and meticulous.
- *Pulsatilla 9 C.* 5 granules once a week. These individuals are gentle, likeable, affectionate, but can become rather resigned - they seek other people's sympathy; they can often be sad and taciturn.

Impatience
- *Argentum nitricum 9 C.* 5 granules once a week. These people do everything in a hurry.
- *Nux vomica 9 C.* 5 granules once a week. Individuals are nervous and irascible; they enjoy working and being active; in a negative sense they are always tense, often overworked and irritable, and impatient to get a reaction or a result.

Intolerance
- *Nux vomica 7 C.* 5 granules every two days. Individuals have trouble assimilating new ideas, and can't stand being contradicted.
- *Staphysagria 9 C.* 5 granules once a week. For short-tempered people who don't hold anything back and who cope with tragedies or setbacks.

Intolerance of Being Contradicted
- *Aloe 9 C.* 5 granules once a week. Individuals are sad; their moodiness is aggravated by hot, damp or foggy weather.
- *Aurum metallicum 9 C.* 5 granules once a week. These people are anxious, rather unstable, incapable of adopting a "live and let live" attitude; they are limited by their background - severe restrictions during childhood, very strict parents, etc.
- *Bryonia 5 C.* 5 granules once a week. People are anxious, confused, irritable and timid; they seek solitude and almost always talk about their work.
- *Lycopodium 9 C.* 5 granules once a week. Subjects are depressive, anxious and very sensitive; they are very critical, can be intelligent, but are narrow-minded.
- *Nux vomica 12 C.* 5 granules once a week. For those who are active and make good workers, but who are always tense; they have trouble accepting new ideas; they can be irritable, quarrelsome and short-tempered.
- *Sepia 9 C.* 5 granules once a week. People are melancholic and tend always to see the dark side of things; they have trouble getting organized, and tend to spend time alone and brood over problems, even though they fear solitude; a restoring sleep usually alleviates the symptoms.

Irritability

- *Arsenicum album 7 C.* For people who are agitated.
- *Chamomilla 9 C. 5* granules every three days. Subjects are nervous, irritable, capricious, and don't like to be touched. Children, however, seem to regain their good humour when held or rocked.
- *Cina 9 C. 5* granules every two days. Adults are nervous, irritable and short-tempered; children complain all the time.
- *Hyoscyamus 7 C.* 5 granules once a week. Subjects are suspicious, short-tempered, hypersensitive, aggressive and ramble on when they talk.
- *Lycopodium 5 C.* 3 granules three times per day. These people suffer from liver and digestive problems, and become irritable, annoyed and nervy. They can sometimes explode in anger.
- *Moschus 5 C.* 5 granules every half an hour. For nervous breakdowns and intense irritability bordering on hysteria.

Jealousy

- *Apis 12 C.* 5 granules once a week. For jealousy that turns to rage.
- *Hyoscyamus 15 C.* 10 granules once a week. For people who are fearful and jealous, irritable and suspicious.
- *Lachesis 12 C.* 10 granules once a week. For cases of unfounded jealousy, where subjects are insecure, and fear being discarded.

Laziness

- *Carbo vegetabilis 9 C.* 10 granules once a week. These people seem to be asleep on their feet; they are incapable of collecting their thoughts; they become more active out in the fresh air.
- *Gelsemium 9 C.* 10 granules once a week. People seem stunned (in a daze); their senses are dull.

Lethargy
(See Also Apathy)

- *Hydrocyanic acid 9 C.* 3 granules twice a day. These people are prostrate, seem completely absorbed in their thoughts; their eyes hardly react to light.

Moodiness

- *Actaea racemosa 9 C.* 5 granules once a week. People are hypersensitive and talkative, and are deeply affected by any emotional problems (especially during the menopause and pregnancy in women) and exposure to damp cold. They fall into melancholy, sigh a lot, are tearful and unresponsive.

- *Ambra grisea 5 C.* 3 granules three times a day. People become hypersensitive after a prolonged period of worry.
- *Crocus 9 C.* 5 granules once a week. Women arc unstable and moody, and are especially affected by heat. Fresh air relieves the symptoms.
- *Ignatia 9 C.* 5 granules once a week. These moody individuals often have real problems and setbacks to deal with; nervous fatigue goes hand in hand with sadness; setbacks result in feelings of insecurity. This remedy is especially effective in these changing and turbulent times.
- *Lachesis 9 C.* 5 granules every two days. After some tragedy, emotional shock or personal setback, these people alternate between being excitable and talkative (especially in the morning), prostrate and depressed (usually at night). Sleep is disturbed by nightmares.
- *Nux moschata 5 C.* 5 granules once a day. Bordering on nervous breakdown, these hypersensitive people fluctuate between states of exhilaration and melancholic apathy.
- *Pulsatilla 9 C.* 5 granules once a week. For those who are laughing one minute and crying the next; they can be distracted, indecisive and short-tempered. Young women are fearful of the opposite sex.
- *Veratrum album 12 C.* 5 granules once a week. People are sad, anxious and tend to be inactive and even prostrate, moaning and groaning. But their moods can undergo sudden changes, and they can quickly become agitated, over-excited and violent.

Nastiness
(See Also Aggressiveness)
- *Chamomilla 9 C.* 10 granules once a week. Despite the fact that these people are usually aware of the wrong they are doing to others, they seem unable to control their behaviour; they are also generally irritable and nervous.

Overbearing Pride
- *Lycopodium 9 C.* 5 granules once a week. Failure, for these people, is unbearable.
- *Platina 9 C.* 5 granules once a week. Excessively proud and rather

aggressive, these people think they are superior to others, when in truth they are timid and insecure.

- *Veratrum album 9 C.* 5 granules once a week. People who always criticize others about their defects and mistakes.

Self-Confidence (Lack of)
(See Also Stage Fright and Behaviour Problems
in the Chapter Childhood)

- *Lycopodium 12 C.* 10 granules once a week. For people who are depressed, and who have lost their desire to be active and to work; they tend to suffer from abulia; they feel worthless, yet continue to be irritable; they cannot tolerate being contradicted and are sexually weak.

Slow-Wittedness

- *Baryta carbonica 12 C.* 5 granules every three days. For people who have trouble understanding things.
- *Calcarea phosphorica 15 C.* 5 granules once a week. For adolescents who grow too quickly, become nervous and agitated; as soon as they start something they give it up; they have trouble concentrating and deciding what is and is not a priority; they tend to suffer from migraines.
- *Mercurius 9 C.* 5 granules every two days. People have trouble expressing themselves.
- *Onosmodium 12 C.* 3 granules every two days. People have trouble understanding things and concentrating; they give in to a kind of cerebral depression (torpor) which is aggravated by hot, humid weather and alleviated by rest and sleep.

Suicidal Tendencies

- *Alumina 15 C.* 10 granules once a week. At the sight of blood or a knife, these people are overcome by the impulse to kill themselves. In general they have problems organizing their thoughts, they are indecisive and never satisfied.
- *Aurum metallicum 12 C.* 10 granules once a week. Individuals are anxious and never satisfied with themselves; they cannot control their impulses, which are passionate and aggressive; although unstable, they are basically happy people.
- *Naja 15 C.* 10 granules once a week. These people have sudden impulses

to put an end to their lives; they are more likely to experience these impulses after a storm, after a meal, or after drinking alcohol.

- *Natrum sulphuricum 15 C.* 10 granules once a week. Subjects want to commit suicide because they are disgusted with life (a feeling which they find very difficult to fight) when in a state of nervous depression. They generally avoid other people.

Suspicion

- *Anacardium 9 C.* 5 granules once a week. These people are excessively suspicious.

Violence

- *Hepar sulph. 12 C.* 5 granules once a week. For people who have violent thoughts, talk rapidly and aggressively. In general this type of person is sad and gets depressed at night.
- *Hyoscyamus 9 C.* 10 granules once a week. During childhood these people like to fight and tend to come to blows. As adults they are suspicious, jealous, and often find themselves in conflict with the people around them.
- *Veratrum album 9 C.* 5 granules once a week. When angry these people become agitated to the point where they shout and try to bite; in general they are anxious and always blaming others for their faults.

Schizophrenia
(See Also Nervous Breakdown, Moodiness)

This serious disorder requires treatment by a doctor. It is usually characterized by a split in personality. Absorbed in a different reality, subjects lose contact with the world around them, become delirious and generally cannot take care of their own basic needs.

They often have to be placed in an institution, since family and friends are rapidly exhausted by the constant attention and supervision schizophrenics require.

In certain cases, at an early stage in the development of the disease, it is possible to administer homeopathic remedies for nervous breakdown. The following instructions may prove useful.

- *Anacardium 12 C.* 10 granules once a week. For chronic cases of split personality. Patients get the feeling their mind is separated from their body, and have trouble perceiving external reality; they are often irritable, and their indecisiveness about contradictory impulses makes them very unstable.

- *Baptisia 12 C.* 10 granules once a week. Patients are calm but in a state of mental confusion; they cannot concentrate; they think they are two people, and that one part of their body is detached from the rest. They feel incapable of ever getting better.
- *Cannabis Indica 10 C.* 10 granules once a week. Patients are hyperactive, euphoric and ramble on incessantly. Their mind seems not to be affected, but they experience sudden mood changes, becoming anxious for no reason, for example. They sometimes suffer from delusions of grandeur or are afraid of going insane.
- *Stramonium 12 C.* Once a week. Patients are very agitated, they have anxieties and sometimes have hallucinations. They tend to be violent.

Sleep-walking

As you probably know, you should never wake up a sleep-walker.

- *Artemisia vulgaris 9 C.* 5 granules once a week. For very nervous people.
- *Kali bromatum 9 C.* 3 granules three times per day. Sleep is agitated, people moan, groan and cry out, and often have nightmares.
- *Kali phosphoricum 9 C.* 3 granules up to five times per day. For grouchy people whose sleep is agitated.

Stammering

Charlie Chaplin, Winston Churchill, Demosthenes, Paul Valéry - they all stammered. So there's no reason to get discouraged if you have a child who stammers. Try to avoid situations where she/he may be made fun of; if the treatment below is not effective, you may want to consult a psychotherapist or psychologist (or both) for help.

- *Stramonium 9 C.* 3 granules per day.

Tics

Nervous tics are involuntary movements which occur for no apparent reason.

In the case of children, you can't expect them to get rid of a tic through an effort of will - it is therefore useless and even harmful to try to force them to stop. It's better to find ways to calm them down, distract them and reduce sources of stress.

- *Mygale lasiodora 7 C* and *Thuja occidentalis 7 C*. 5 granules per week on alternate weeks.

Trembling
(See Also Nervousness)

- *Gelsemium sempervirens 5 C*. 2 granules immediately. For trembling caused by emotions, the onset of fever or by abuse of coffee, alcohol or tobacco.

Chapter 4

Circulatory System

Apoplexy (Stroke)

The attack: a person appears healthy one second, then suddenly collapses and loses consciousness. The face is congested and bloated, breathing is laboured, the sphincter opens uncontrollably. People may also remain conscious and be aware of the paralysis that strikes one side of their body, without being able to do anything about it.

Apoplexy is, in fact, a kind of coma, induced by the rupture of a cerebral artery which then floods a part of the brain.

Warning Signs

Slight or partial paralysis, blurred vision or even total blindness, falling for no reason, intense headaches, dizziness and vomiting; these are all alarm signals and are worrying enough symptoms in themselves.

Precautionary Measures

Stroke is more common after the age of fifty. If you are in that age group, you should make lavish meals the exception rather than the rule. In addition, avoid unusually strenuous physical exertion (especially if you're not used to it) and don't overwork. Make sure you get out in the fresh air and do a moderate amount of daily physical exercise (walking, gardening, etc.)

In Case of a Crisis

Get the stroke victim to a doctor as quickly as possible. While waiting, slip two granules of *China 4 C* under the patient's tongue, followed ten minutes later by two granules of *Opium 5 C*. If you can't get to a doctor right away, continue the treatment with *Glonoinum 4 C, Arnica montana 5 C* and *Ethyllicum 5 C*.

3 granules every hour:

- *Aconite 5 C*. The face, as well as the whole head, is flushed and hot. Patients go pale as soon as they try to get up. They are intensely thirsty and anxious, agitated and afraid of dying. Symptoms are aggravated by heat or closed confined spaces and soothed by fresh air.
- *Arnica 5 C*. Patients are numb and in a state of stupor. They feel exhausted, as if their body has been battered. They are in such a stupor that they can hardly respond to questions. At night they become more agitated and find their bed is too hard.
- *Glonoinum 5 C*. Eyes are bloodshot, patients suffer from headaches

accompanied by dizziness; they clench their teeth, and breathing is laboured; they cannot raise their head, which seems much too heavy; their condition is aggravated - and sometimes caused - by heat or exposure to the sun. They have palpitations and orientation problems (they don't know where they are), their pulse is rapid and strong.

- *Helleborus 5 C*. Patients remain in a daze, as if stunned; they are calm and silent; pulse is slow, the face is pale and deeply lined, eyebrows furrowed, and urine is a dark colour. Patients respond slowly to questions, as if they cannot understand what is being said - they groan and emit incomprehensible sounds, accompanied by repeated movements of the head, arms or hands - they may keep lifting their right hand to their head, for example.

- *Lachesis 5 C*. During an attack the face turns purple, the head is hot while the feet are cold. Patients are incoherent and babble incessantly; they have pains around the eyes or in the nape of the neck and cannot stand the least pressure around the neck or waist; symptoms are aggravated after sleeping, even for a short time, and are alleviated after bleeding from the nose.

- *Opium*. The face is dark red; eyes are staring and half-closed, pupils are dilated. Patients are inert, unresponsive and oblivious to everything around them; breathing is slow and deep; the face and chest are wet with perspiration, the pulse is slow; every now and then a gurgling puffs out the cheek; limbs are cold and the face becomes gradually paler.

- *Phosphoricum acidum*. Totally apathetic and oblivious to their surroundings, patients cannot understand what is being said to them; they are sometimes delirious, suffer from memory loss and mental confusion, and cannot find their words.

Treating the After-Effects

5 granules once a week:

- *Baryta carbonica 7 C*. A long-term remedy; ruddiness has disappeared and patients are pale. They are very sensitive to cold, have frequent palpitations which are aggravated by movement or when they are lying on their left side. Even a minimum of effort is exhausting, and makes them want to sleep. Some mental confusion remains - forgetting familiar places, names, etc. People will often rub their face with their hands, a sign of hypertension.

Arteriosclerosis

This disease results from premature ageing of blood vessels and especially arteries. They become hard and thick inside and, in turn, force the heart to work a lot harder to get blood through the circulatory system to various parts of the body.

An essential aspect in the development of this disorder is the amount of fatty substances people consume: it seems that animal fat in particular tends to leave fatty deposits in the arteries. Arteriosclerosis starts with a kind of flat tumour that causes calcium deposits to build up. The artery loses its elasticity, which increases blood pressure and can result in a stroke or a heart attack.

Three Factors

Foods rich in animal fats produce cholesterol in the blood. Eating too much meat, eggs or cheese, or foods which contain a lot of albumin, are responsible. Alcohol and tobacco abuse are also a direct cause of cardiovascular disorders.

It appears that ageing of the blood vessel walls is due to a lack of unsaturated fatty acids. Unsaturated fatty acids are found in natural oils and fats, but are destroyed by high temperatures, refining processes and oxygenation, for example.

On the other hand, saturated fatty acids contain little oxygen, which makes them difficult to digest - which is why reason people feel so heavy after eating a meal rich in saturated acids, which would contain a large amount of refined oil or fat (the kind most commonly used).

Hydrogenation of fats and oils through electrolysis, which uses metallic salts for the process, also destroys much of the nutritional value of the natural product.

There are other factors which must also be taken into consideration: lifestyle (sedentary or active), obesity, stress (work-related or personal), sex (women are usually affected about twenty years later than men), age (even though the disease can occur in young people).

Precautionary Measures

Try to use non-hydrogenated oils and fats (like vegetable oils) whenever possible - these contain more unsaturated fatty acids because they are cold-pressed. Sunflower oil, poppy seed oil, linseed oil, sesame seed oil (which contains up to 43 percent unsaturated fatty acids) are some of the products you should buy instead of processed oils produced by modern industry.

Among foods rich in unsaturated fatty acids are nuts like almonds, pine kernels, sesame seeds and linseed.

Vitamin E has a beneficial effect on disorders like heart disease, diabetes, arthritis, varicose veins and arteriosclerosis.

Finally, certain foods help food drainage: onions, raw grated carrots, brewer's yeast, leeks, prunes, tomatoes, lemons, garlic and watercress.

Apart from these recommendations, consult the section on Gastritis for a more detailed description of what constitutes a healthy diet.

While waiting for a complete medical examination:

- *Sulphur 9 C.* 5 granules once a week.
- *Baryta carbonica 7 C* and *Aurum metallicum 7 C,* two granules in the morning on alternate days.
- *Cupressus 7 C* and *Kali iodatum 7 C,* 2 granules around supper-time (six in the evening), on alternate days.

Arteritis (Arterial Thrombosis)

This is a problem which begins suddenly. Related to the contraction or dilation of blood vessels, it arises after an obstruction of one or a number of arteries by a blood clot.

Pulse is irregular, affected arteries are painful to the touch, red and thick. A doctor should be consulted immediately. A more general treatment is in order, since arteritis is not a disease per se, but rather a group of symptoms which indicate a state of intoxication.

The body is reacting to a lifestyle which is incompatible with its needs and puts it out of balance. A basic remedy of *Lachesis, Lycopodium* or *Thuja* should be accompanied by a change in lifestyle (stopping smoking, sleeping in a calm place, special exercises for the lower limbs, frequent walks, etc.).

Temporal Arteritis

As its name indicates, the disorder appears around the temples. Patients have a slight fever. Since ocular complications are a possibility, a doctor should be consulted immediately. While waiting to see a doctor: *Glonoinum 5 C, Secale cornutum 5 C, Aurum metallicum 5 C,* one after the other, 2 granules every 24 hours.

Arteritis of the Lower Limbs

This disorder is very common. Legs feel heavy, people tire rapidly from any physical exertion. Blood pressure is normal in the arms, but above normal in the legs.

If the correct treatment is administered early enough (i.e. if the disorder was correctly identified right from the start) then the chances of a full recovery are good.

3 granules once a day:

- *Aurum 5 C*. Patients are susceptible to cold and feel intoxicated. Pulse is irregular and patients feel as if they had weights attached to their feet. They wake up at night and sit up suddenly, leaning forward so as not to suffocate. They feel as if their heart stops beating for a moment, then starts again.
- *Secale cornutum*. Subjects have pains in their arms and legs, and suffer from anxiety; they have palpitations and hot flushes; symptoms improve when walking in the fresh air.
- *Cactus 5 C*. In addition to palpitations, these people have severe cramps which oblige them to stop whatever they're doing - for example, it is impossible for them to continue walking or climbing a flight of stairs. A feeling of oppression and a tightening in the chest (constriction) resemble angina. Lying on the left side aggravates the symptoms, which improve in the fresh air.
- *Nux vomica 5 C*. Subjects are often in a bad mood, get angry easily, are impatient and irritable. They can't stand light or noise. Their extremities are numb, while their heels are very sensitive. They drag their feet when they walk, and affected limbs feel numb. They suffer from low blood pressure in the lower limbs, which may be caused by various factors such as tobacco addiction, taking too much medication, etc.
- *Sulphur 5 C*. Patients are always moving around in bed, trying to find a cool place, since they feel as if their feet are burning up. They get cramps at night, are tired when they wake up in the morning and find that just standing up is exhausting; they also have a constant desire for fresh air.

Asystole (Cardiac Standstill)

This state of intense crisis generally occurs in people who have already shown signs of a weak heart. Symptoms include difficulty in breathing, shortness of breath (dyspnoea), abnormal pulse (either too slow or too fast), purplish skin colour, decreased amount of urine and swollen ankles.

Asystole requires emergency treatment. Contact a doctor. Keep patients immobile, except for the legs which you should move from time to time to prevent complications like thrombosis (clotting in a vein).

- *Crataegus oxyacantha 4 C*. 2 granules every half an hour. For cases where the pulse is rapid and weak.
- *Digitalis purpurea 4 C*. 2 granules every half an hour. If the pulse is weak, irregular and slow, and breathing stops when patients fall asleep.

Follow-up

Once the crisis is over, patients should adopt a suitable diet: no salt, lots of potatoes, rice, fruit, honey.

2 granules every 24 hours:

- *Apocynum cannabinum 5 C*. This functional remedy helps calm the feeling of oppression and normalizes the strength and rhythm of the heartbeat. Patients still urinate very little, are intensely thirsty and have a queasy feeling in the pit of the stomach. They may suffer from occasional blackouts.
- *Crataegus*. This is a heart tonic. Pulse is weak, irregular and accelerated (more than 90 beats per minute). These people have high blood pressure; physical exertion as well as excessive heat aggravate the symptoms, while rest and fresh air soothe them.

  Pain is felt under the left clavicle. Patients sometimes experience mental confusion and/or depressive melancholy.
- *Digitalis*. A heart tonic: in homeopathy, as in orthodox medicine, the weakness of the heart muscle needs to be compensated in order to treat asystole, a condition of mechanical origin.

  The pulse is weak, irregular and slow (less than 60 beats per minute); respiration becomes laboured when patients fall asleep; they suffer from frequent dizziness, and feel as if they're going to black out every time they stand up; extremities are cold and numb.

Basic Remedies

These remedies aim to treat the person's disposition, making the body less susceptible to the disorder.

2 granules once a day:

- *Arsenicum album 5 C*. Palpitations are worse at night and after defaecating. Patients are thin and weak, usually elderly, and suffer from oedema. *Arsenicum album* is effective for asystole of both the left and right sides of the heart.

- *Carbo vegetabilis 5 C.* For very acute cases, characterized by a bluish colour in the face and extremities (cyanosis); patients are anxious, constantly short of breath; the heart beats furiously, veins are swollen; the body is pale, they have cold sweats, especially on the face, and experience a burning sensation around the area of the heart.
- *Phosphorus 5 C.* The liver is sensitive to the touch; you will notice stasis (stagnation) of the veins, especially the hepatic veins, and a weakened myocardial state, especially on the right side; the slightest effort causes shortness of breath. Patients' condition is aggravated by any physical effort, including walking, and by cold. Pain in the liver is also more intense when patients lie on their left side. Extremities are cold, and there are yellow spots on the abdomen.

Cardiac Problems

Palpitations

Palpitations can be caused by a number of factors: nervousness, emotional trauma (like fear or worry), tobacco addiction, diphtheria, high blood pressure, acute articular rheumatism, pulmonary tuberculosis, as well as a host of other possible causes.

In any case, when palpitations occur, you should try to get out in the fresh air and lead a calm life, with as few sources of stress as possible. Avoid stimulants like tea, coffee, tobacco and even Coca-Cola, which contains caffeine.

See also Palpitations in the section on Emergencies.

Paroxysmal Tachycardia

In these cases, people experience repeated bouts of tachycardia which start and end suddenly, and last from a few minutes to a few hours. Heartbeat may go as high as 180 to 220 beats per minute. If this happens to you and you haven't already consulted a doctor, do not hesitate to do so.

As usual, lack of exercise and fresh air may be the cause of various problems like dizziness, headaches and even cardiac failure.

In Case of Crisis

Deep breathing and lying flat with the arms crossed can help soothe symptoms during a crisis. Also try and get the patient to drink a little water or swallow a piece of bread.

3 granules once a day, or 2 granules every half an hour in case of a crisis:

- *Aconitum 5 C*. 2 granules. When palpitations are caused by violent fear or by cardiac irregularity; for patients who are anxious and afraid of dying, who have chest pains and feel numbness in their left arm and pins and needles in their fingers.

  Patients should remain in a prone position, with the head raised on a pillow. Pulse is rapid and hard; the face, which is flushed, goes pale when patients try to stand up.

- *Cactus grandiflorus 5 C*. These people feel as if their heart is being squeezed in a steel vice; the sensation is aggravated when they lie on their left side; palpitations are violent, cardiac rhythm is accelerated, while the pulse is weak.

  Patients experience heaviness on the chest; palpitations are more pronounced on the right side and are aggravated by movement.

- *Crataegus 5 C*. This is the basic remedy for cardiac fatigue and disturbances of cardiac rhythm. Patients often feel as if their heart were increasing in volume, and sometimes have pains under the left clavicle.

  They are often irritable and in a bad mood, and may fall into a state of depression. Symptoms are aggravated by physical exertion and overheated rooms, and soothed by rest and fresh air.

- *Digitalis 5 C*. Patients try to remain immobile, fearing that their heart will stop beating if they make the slightest movement; pulse is weak and slow; symptoms improve with rest.

- *Gelsemium 5 C*. Unlike the *Digitalis* type, these people fear that their heart will stop beating if they do not move; they feel like they're about to faint at any moment; pulse is slow, and patients appear to be in a daze.

  Symptoms are the same for palpitations due to emotional shock, tobacco addiction or stage fright.

- *Glonoinum 5 C*. Violent palpitations accompanied by anxiety; patients have the sensation of blood suddenly flooding into their heart; palpitations are felt in all parts of the body; pulse is slow, the face is flushed, and people feel as if the congestion spreads upwards from the heart to the head, which feels like it's going to explode.

  Veins in the temples and neck are swollen; in serious cases they have a fixed stare, as if the person were disoriented. Alcohol, tilting the head forward and heat aggravate symptoms, which improve in the fresh air.

- *Ignatia 5 C*. After a serious setback or emotional shock, people may become very nervous, their pulse accelerates, and they feel like there's a ball in their throat which is strangling them. These palpitations may also be caused by tobacco smoke - palpitations get worse in smoky, stuffy rooms or when near a lot of perfume.
- *Spigelia anthelma 5 C*. Palpitations can be seen even through clothes, and patients can hear them as well; they feel pains in the left arm and chest, especially the left side; palpitations are aggravated when they drink coffee or when they are lying down, especially on the left side.
- *Naja 5C*. Patients cannot speak; they cough, their left arm is sometimes numb, their legs are weak, especially at night. Palpitations are worse just after waking up and when they are lying on their right side.
- *Lillium tigrinum 5 C*. Subjects feel as if their heart were being squeezed in a vice; the left arm is painful and numb; they are often awakened by hot flushes in the middle of the night; they constantly have to urinate, and palpitations radiate outwards from the genital area, from left to right, up to the back and arms.
  Patients are feverish, and suffer psychologically as well - they feel desperate and overwhelmed with anxiety.
- *Lycopus virginicus 5 C*. The heart beats rapidly and violently; people are agitated and nervous, and tend to suffer from high blood pressure; their hands tremble and they can distinctly hear their heart beating. Palpitations are aggravated by heat, when they move and when they concentrate on the problem.
- *Spigelia 5 C*. Here again, palpitations are so strong that patients can feel them distinctly or see them through their clothes; pains radiate from the heart region towards the shoulders and left arm. Movement causes patients to become more anxious and oppressed.
  Symptoms are aggravated when lying on the left side or leaning forward; lying on the right side or raising the head on a pillow eases the condition.

Cerebral Haemorrhage

Cerebral congestion is caused by high blood pressure. It occurs under varying circumstances, which are generally easy to identify.

People may get very angry, experience some intense emotion, spend too much time in an overheated room, eat too much or drink. . . whatever the circumstances, the face goes red, veins in the temples start vibrating, and people feel a trembling sensation in their heart and pain around the scalp.

They have palpitations and feel dizzy, their vision becomes blurred or they may go completely blind (temporarily); they are overcome by waves of anxiety, they start suffocating and lose their balance.

A doctor must be called immediately; loosen clothes which are too tight (shirt collar, belt, underwear, etc.) and apply cold compresses to the forehead. While waiting for the doctor, slip 2 granules of *China 4 C* under the tongue, and then a quarter of an hour later 2 granules of *Opium 5 C*.

- *Aconite 5 C*. The head is burning hot; patients have a headache and become pale if they try to stand up; they are agitated, have a fear of impending death; the left arm is numb, they experience itching sensations and pains in the fingers; pulse is strong and full; heat aggravates symptoms, while fresh air soothes them.

- *Belladonna 5 C*. For cases of sudden congestion occurring after exposure to cold; the face is so red it looks like all the blood is concentrated in it; people complain of an excruciating headache; eyes are bloodshot, pupils are dilated.

  Patients are very sensitive to noise and light, and seek solitude; drinking liquid causes spasms in the throat; symptoms have the particular characteristic of appearing and disappearing very suddenly; patients feel better when they are immobile and quiet, with their head tilted back.

- *Gelsemium 5 C*. Patients are weak and slightly paralysed; they feel heavy and numb, both physically and mentally; they are not thirsty, and tremble slightly; they should be made to move around whenever they feel their heart weaken. Sunshine, tobacco and hot weather seem to aggravate symptoms.

- *Glonoinum 5 C*. This congestion is due to intense heat. The face becomes flushed and hot; eyes are bloodshot; patients lose their sense of orientation and suffer from such severe headaches that they think they're going to die; pulse is rapid and strong; jaws are clenched together, pupils are dilated; symptoms are aggravated by the sun and by alcohol, and are soothed by fresh air.

- *Lachesis 5 C*. The face is red and swollen; during a crisis patients become delirious and dizzy; they feel pain above the eyes and in the nape of the neck, and tightness in the chest; they are very sensitive to touch, especially around the throat; fresh air and bleeding from the nose (or menstrual bleeding in women) alleviates the symptoms.

- *Opium 5 C.* For cases where patients fall into a coma or comatose sleep (see the section on Coma); pupils are small, eyes half-closed and glassy; the face is dark red; patients are hot and sweat profusely, and seem oblivious to everything around them; limbs are stiff.

  In less critical cases, patients feel numb and indolent; they cannot tolerate heat and feel better out in the fresh air or while drinking or eating.

- *Veratrum viride 5 C.* The face is red but goes pale as soon as the patient tries to stand up; eyes are bloodshot, and people suffer from headache at the back of the head; pulse is slow, and a red stripe is visible in the centre of the tongue.

Cyanosis

Cyanosis is characterized by the bluish colour of the skin and mucous membranes. There are a number of possible causes, among them a weak heart, intoxication and emphysema.

3 granules once a day:

- *Antimonium tartaricum 5 C.* People tend to be short of breath and tire easily; they are sometimes very weak and tremble excessively; they have a strong aversion to milk, preferring acidic foods like citrus fruits which, in fact, aggravate the symptoms.

- *Carbo vegetabilis 5 C.* For cases of chronic and persistent cyanosis; extremities (and sometimes the whole body) are very cold, yet patients experience burning sensations.

  Dairy products, fat, and hot, humid weather aggravate the symptoms, which also get worse towards nightfall. Cold weather in winter seems to soothe symptoms.

- *Pulsatilla 5 C.* People are rarely thirsty, and symptoms (which are psychological as well as physical) vary greatly. The skin may be covered with very noticeable little blue veins (varicosity); people feel better lying down with their legs raised; also for girls or young women with irregular periods, whose legs are red and swollen and who feel uncomfortable in hot rooms.

Embolism

A clot or fatty deposit is obstructing a coronary, cerebral or pulmonary artery. In the first case, see the section on Infarction. For cerebral embolism, see Apoplexy. For pulmonary embolism:

- *Arnica 4 C*. 2 granules every two hours while waiting for a doctor, who should be called as a matter of urgency. Patients experience excruciating pain in the chest; they suffocate, and expectorate phlegm tainted black with blood.

Haemorrhage

(See Also Haemorrhage in the section on
Accidents and Emergency Disorders)

2 granules every 24 hours:

- *Cactus 5 C*. For general haemorrhaging; blood is a dark colour and coagulates rapidly into large clots. Patients feel a pulsing sensation in the area of the blood flow, as well as a constriction if an organ is affected; liver (haematemesis), kidneys or bladder (haematuria), chest (haemoptysis), uterus, ovaries or vagina (metrorrhagia).
- *China 5 C*. For cases of severe haemorrhage after a blow or injury. Patients are very pale, weak, their pulse is rapid; they are dizzy and may black out if they try to stand up.
- *Crotalus 5 C*. Blood is a dark colour but fluid, and it does not form clots; this type of haemorrhage usually occurs in serious infections, hepatic or toxic conditions; it is irritating, and usually has an unpleasant odour; people have palpitations, blackouts, and their body is cold; they are more prostrate than is necessary, even if the case is serious and requires the presence of a doctor.
- *Ipecac. 5 C*. Blood is bright red and flows abundantly; the haemorrhage is clearly aggravated by movement; patients who are nauseous do not feel any relief after vomiting and tend to have fainting spells; the tongue remains uncoated; the possibility of intestinal haemorrhage should not be overlooked.
- *Lachesis 5 C*. Flow of small dark clots which smell unpleasantly; sensation of constriction around the affected organ (see Coccus cacti) which is painful, especially if it concerns the liver; lips turn purple. For

haemorrhage that occurs during menopause or for acute cases of infection which produce blood clots in the faeces.

- *Phosphorus 5 C.* Cases are characterized by an abundant and regular flow of bright red blood, occurring during the course of an acute illness, e.g. acute congestion, circulatory erethism (irritability), weakness of the heart or hepatic degeneration. When lying on the left side, people feel a frequent need to defaecate.

Haemorrhoids

This very common disorder is due to the formation of varicose veins in the rectum and anus. There may be a number of causes: Irritation during defaecation, especially when faeces are dry and hard; fragile veins in some people; weakness of the liver.

Haemorrhoids can also act as a safety valve for people who suffer from hypertension. A doctor should decide which basic remedy is most appropriate.

For temporary problems, *Aesculus compound* ointment and suppositories will ease the symptoms. An appropriate diet can help to avoid constipation, which does nothing but aggravate the problem. Avoid remaining in a sitting position for long periods, take lukewarm or cool baths and lubricate the anus with olive oil before defaecating. *Collinsonia tincture* applied as an ointment can also soothe the condition.

2 granules once a day:

- *Aesculus hippocastanum 5 C.* Burning, prickly pains in the rectum, accompanied by itching; haemorrhoids don't bleed much, if at all; they are purple in colour, and may be aggravated during women's menstruation.

  Subjects are generally constipated. Discomfort is aggravated after defaecation, after long walks or standing up for long periods of time.
- *Aloe 5 C.* The stomach is swollen, haemorrhoids are in clusters, also swollen, burning and sensitive to the touch; people tend to have diarrhoea; a secretion of gelatinous mucus may be observed about an hour after defaecation, which can sometimes be involuntary; subjects often get headaches.
- *Collinsonia 5 C.* For chronic haemorrhoids which are painful and bleed profusely; people feel as if their anus is being pierced with needles, and they are generally constipated; they find it difficult to remain lying down,

and experience intense itching and hot flushes.

- Palpitations are a characteristic symptom of the *Collinsonia* type - these are soothed by hot compresses. You can also use *Collinsonia tincture* as an ointment.
- *Hamamelis 5 C*. Bleeding is abundant, the blood is dark and coagulated; people feel as if their swollen veins arc bruised; the rectum is painful and haemorrhoids, which are a bluish colour, are very sensitive to the touch.

  This disorder frequently appears in people who have varicose veins; it may be accompanied by backaches and headaches; applying cold compresses helps somewhat.
- *Ratanhia 5 C*. Haemorrhoids are accompanied by fissures in and around the anus, and a persistent burning sensation, which is aggravated during defaecation (usually not abundant since people are constipated). Pain is temporarily soothed by applying cold compresses.
- *Nux vomica 5 C*. This type of haemorrhoid isn't very painful and doesn't bleed much; it is characterized by intense itching, by a constant desire to defaecate and by constipation. In addition, the liver is sensitive, and wine and spirits aggravate the condition.
- *Paeonia 5 C*. Haemorrhoids are inflamed, accompanied by fissures, painful ulcers in the anus, constant oozing and itching. Patients suffer a lot while defaecating, and complain of aggravated pain while walking.

Heart

If any organ can be called central, it's the heart. Unfortunately, the heart is subject to a number of disorders which are always harder to cure than to avoid.

One important aspect for keeping the heart healthy should not be overlooked, and that is balanced effort. It's just as harmful to avoid physical exertion altogether as it is to put a strain on the heart from excessive activity.

Fortunately, the body is wise enough to warn us of any imbalance we may be creating. Rather than awkward phenomena which should be got rid of, signs like high blood pressure, cramps and cardiac spasms, as well as other disorders, should be regarded as "our body's language" which we must interpret in order to apply the required basic remedies.

People who suffer from mild cardiac problems should always keep some raisins on them which they can chew if they experience any unease.

- *Arnica, Crataegus 5 C, Cactus grandiflorus 5 C, Calcarea carbonica 5 C*

- these are all tonics which can help patients get back to normal (3 granules per day).

Athlete's Heart

People who do a lot of sports, especially when they're young, tend to push themselves to the limit, encouraged by a system of ruthless competition which some coaches and athletes have now had the courage to denounce.

Certain demanding activities should not be engaged in unless you are suitably prepared, trained and informed of the long-term dangers which they may present. Often, it's twenty or thirty years later that the price must be paid.

3 granules every 24 hours:

- *Arnica 5 C*. If the damage is done and the heart is already overworked.
- *Cactus 5 C*. Physical effort causes dizziness; people feel local constriction and a sensation of weight on the chest; they also have palpitations.
- *Crataegus 5 C*. For cases of overwork and hypertrophy of the heart.
- *Rhus tox 5 C*. For athletes who have pushed themselves too hard; they experience palpitations, causing anxiety; symptoms are aggravated when at rest and improve when they wake up; there may be numbness in the left arm and shoulder.

Hypertension (High Blood Pressure)

A special device is used to measure blood pressure at the moment the cardiac muscle contracts (systolic or maximum pressure) and between two contractions (diastolic or minimum pressure).

In adults, the normal systolic reading is somewhere between 95 and 140, and the diastolic reading between 60 and 90. The World Health Organization (W.H.O.) estimates that hypertension in an average adult can be diagnosed when the blood pressure reading is greater than 140/90.

After a certain age, you have to pay careful attention to the signs your body sends you: headaches, vision problems, buzzing in the ears, insomnia, dizziness etc. If you don't, you may develop more serious disorders: partial or complete blindness, nosebleeds, memory loss, temporary partial paralysis, and so on.

3 granules once a day:

- *Aurum 5 C*. Patients are very sensitive to cold; they are overweight and congested, often wake up suddenly in the middle of the night with their heart beating so hard that they have to stay seated and lean forward.

Cool air and cool baths soothe the condition; the face is often red, patients feel constriction and heaviness in their chest, hot flushes and anxiety.

- *Aconitum 5 C*. The heart suddenly starts palpitating violently, and subjects are overcome with anxiety; they suffer from a headache, their face is flushed and they get dizzy if they try to stand up.
- *Baryta carbonica 5 C*. Dizziness and buzzing in the ears are characteristic signs; these are accompanied by memory loss (people may be old and suffering from arteriosclerosis); subjects distinctly feel their heart beating; the least effort makes them want to sleep and palpitations get worse when they are lying on their left side; pulse is slow and regular. 3 granules every 2 days:
- *Glonoinum 5 C*. People experience sudden congestion and severe headaches, and can no longer find their way round their familiar surroundings (mental confusion); the condition is aggravated by heat.
- *Strontiana carbonica 5 C*. The face is flushed and becomes even more so when patients make the slightest effort; a headache develops, especially at night when patients are in bed with their head down; they cannot tolerate cold which aggravates the condition, as does any physical or mental effort.

  Patients are often in a bad mood; they have a normal appetite - except for meat; they feel pressure on the chest and stomach; feet are cold, with cramps in the ankles and/or soles of the feet; they sometimes suffer from haemorrhoids and diarrhoea; the condition improves while eating and gets worse while walking.
- *Sulphur 4 C*. For chronic arterial congestion: subjects are nervous, have little appetite, their head is hot, they feel their pulse beating, as well as sudden rushes of blood to the head; symptoms are aggravated by heat, after meals, standing up for long periods and by rest. The condition can be improved by mild exercise and dry fresh air.
- *Viscum album 5 C*. For cases where cardiac weakness is accompanied by renal impairment and when there is albumin in the urine. Pulse is irregular, and even minimal effort causes palpitations and shortness of breath (dyspnoea); symptoms are aggravated when subjects lie on their right side.

Hypotension (Low Blood Pressure)

Within certain limits, low blood pressure is not dangerous (consult the section on Hypertension). A consistently low reading of 110 systolic and 70 diastolic usually presents no problem. But if pressure drops below 95 systolic and 60 diastolic, a number of problems may arise: dizziness, syncope, fatigue. For cases of average low blood pressure, people may lack energy and vitality.

To combat low blood pressure, drink an occasional glass of red wine. Also pollen and carrot juice (which does not have the same properties as raw carrots) can help.

2 granules every 24 hours:

- *Crataegus 5 C.* People feel as if their heart is increasing in volume; pulse is irregular, rapid and weak; subjects often feel pain at the base of the heart, they are grumpy and suffer from insomnia; the condition is aggravated by remaining in overheated rooms and improved by exercise.
- *Rauwolfia 5 C.* Symptoms include dizziness, especially at high altitudes, diminished sexual desire in men, loss of energy and motivation, shortness of breath and palpitations. The condition is aggravated by effort, and eased by fresh air. Subjects appear to be almost completely apathetic.
  A characteristic symptom is a decrease or total loss of sexual desire in men; they feel their condition is aggravated by confinement in overheated stuffy rooms, and eased by fresh air.

Infarction (Heart Attack)

An infarction results from the complete occlusion (blockage) of a coronary artery by a clot; attacks occur while people are resting, and especially at night.

Acute pains shoot down the left arm, right to the fingers, as well as to the back and neck. Blood pressure falls very low, pulse is rapid and sometimes irregular; patients go pale, feel nauseous and vomit, and collapse.

A doctor should be called as a matter of urgency. While waiting, administer 2 granules *of Arnica 5 C* then 2 granules *of Naja 4 C* half an hour later. Keep the person lying down, with the upper part of the body raised on pillows. In cases of mild infarction, patients will only have to stay in bed for a few days. Diet should be examined and adjusted to prevent further attacks. These cases should be treated by a cardiologist.

- Cactus grandiflorus 5 C and Calcarea muriatica 5 C. 2 granules twice a day.

Nosebleed

If bleeding is profuse, or if it lasts for more than half an hour, consult a doctor.

Slip 2 granules of *China 4 C* under the tongue if the nosebleed was caused by a blow. Get the person to take slow, deep breaths, and firmly pinch the nostrils.

Use a wet cloth to cool the skin, especially the forehead. If patients are congested after eating a lavish meal or if they're in an overheated room, get them out into the cool fresh air.

If caused by a blow, administer 2 granules each of *China 5 C* and *Arnica 5 C,* alternating them every fifteen minutes.

Be careful about stopping a nosebleed that happens infrequently and lasts only a few minutes, especially in people suffering from high blood pressure. In fact, a nosebleed can act as a "safety valve" for the body - a way of eliminating surplus pressure: in these cases, administering 2 granules of *Melilotus 5 C,* followed by 2 granules of *Crotalus 5 C* half an hour later, is enough to stem the flow gradually.

3 granules one a day:

- *Aconitum 5 C.* When the nosebleed has the effect of relieving a headache or when the patient is congested and anxious. Afterwards, blood pressure should be checked.
- *Hamamelis 5 C.* Dark-coloured blood flows slowly, sometimes abundantly. This kind of nosebleed is triggered by exertion or blows. People feel a throbbing headache around the temples, with a feeling of constriction at the root of the nose.
- *Melilotus 5 C.* The blood which flows is very red, the face is red, the person has a headache, mainly in the forehead. The condition worsens if the weather is stormy, if it is hot and heavy, or variable. The condition is improved when the person lies down, in fresh air. Large amounts of urine are passed.

Pericarditis

Inflammation of the pericardium - the membrane which surrounds the heart, and the origin of the major blood vessels - is characterized by a sharp pain spreading over the chest, which is aggravated by the slightest movement (even breathing).

3 granules every twenty-four hours:

- *Aconitum 5 C.* For cases where pericarditis develops suddenly; pulse is accelerated, strong and sometimes irregular; in addition to pains in the chest, patients feel constricted, as if they were going to faint; they are agitated and cannot lie on their side; they should be kept in bed, with their head raised.

- *Bryonia 5 C.* Patients feel better when immobile, lying on their left side; they feel on the verge of blacking out (syncope), are very thirsty and get dizzy when they try to sit or stand up.
- *Spigelia 5 C.* Pains in the heart region spread to the left arm. Violent palpitations can be observed, even through clothes; patients are extremely anxious.

Phlebitis

Phlebitis refers to the inflammation of a vein. It is very painful and can lead to an embolism.

People feel pains in one of their legs (this often occurs a few days after childbirth); the limb swells up, becomes even more painful and turns white. In cases of acute phlebitis of the limbs, patients must stay in bed for between six weeks and two months, so that the clot which is blocking the vein does not detach and travel to the lungs where it can cause death from pulmonary embolism.

Alcohol compresses and clay poultices as well as washing with *Yarrow (Millefolium) tincture* may soothe the pain. Cutting out certain foods and adding others to your diet can also help reduce the inflammation much more rapidly.

3 granules every 24 hours:

- *Arnica montana 5 C.* For phlebitis following injury. Fever is only slightly high, but patients have trouble sleeping. The body is cold, except for the head and face.
- *Lachesis 5 C.* Prevents infection (septicaemia).
- *Pulsatilla 5 C.* Phlebitis is stabilized, but still causes white swelling (oedema), intermittent pains, mild fever and shivering. Symptoms are aggravated in overheated rooms.
- *Vipera 5 C.* Very sensitive red swelling (oedema) accompanies the venous inflammation; pains are like cramps; they are eased when the affected limb is raised, and aggravated when it is lowered.

Syncope (Blackouts)

The famous and frequent fainting spells suffered by women of the eighteenth and nineteenth century are fortunately a thing of the past. Syncope includes blackouts, partial blackouts and temporary giddiness, and is characterized by partial or complete loss of consciousness due to disturbances of the cerebral circulation.

Usually, people simply faint after some emotional shock, or even after being confined for a prolonged period in a poorly ventilated room.

True syncope is caused by arteriosclerosis, arterial hypertension and exhaustion. If the condition persists or recurs, a doctor should be called in. Pulse is weak, face and lips are pale, extremities are cold.

While waiting for a doctor, loosen any tight clothing, bathe the person's face in cold water and place two or three granules of *Nux moschata 4 C* or *Veratrum album 4 C* on the tongue.

You can also administer 3 granules of *Ammonium carbonicum 5 C* every half an hour if you think the syncope is likely to recur. People who are susceptible to blackouts usually catch cold very easily and often lead a very sedentary lifestyle.

Varicose Veins
(See Also Phlebitis)

Varicosity is caused by stasis of the veins due to poor circulation. Letting the feet get cold, standing up for long periods, or not moving for long periods all result in stasis of the veins. Pregnant women often develop varicose veins, and they should not be taken lightly since they can lead to serious complications such as thrombosis and embolisms.

Injections of saline or glucose, which are designed to neutralize the function of a varicose vein, do not solve the problem. On the contrary, this procedure places an excessive burden on the rest of the circulatory system, which is probably not in much better shape than the affected vein!

Horse chestnut extract *(Urticalcin)* which supplies the body with the calcium it needs, combined with *Hyperisan* promotes natural regeneration of veins. This treatment is especially important during pregnancy.

However, this natural treatment does not work overnight. You should beware of methods and products which promise miraculous results, because they often prove to be a double-edged sword - there may be serious side-effects. Although a natural method may take more time, at least you know exactly what to expect.

3 granules once a day:

- *Aesculus hippocastanum 4 C*. People have a feeling of "fullness" in the affected region; varicose veins are painful and produce a sensation of heaviness; symptoms are aggravated by heat and walking, and soothed by cold baths; people often have to stop and rest while climbing stairs and may develop haemorrhoids.
- *Calcarea fluorica 5 C*. For varicose veins caused by poor diet; the skin is covered with tiny burst blood vessels; people often suffer from lumbago and frequent sprains due to excessive suppleness of the joints.
- *Hamamelis 4 C*. This is the most common remedy; the skin is fragile and sensitive; the slightest blow causes bruising, and people haemorrhage frequently; they also suffer from nosebleeds, blood in the urine and heavy menstrual flow in women.
- *Pulsatilla 5 C*. Extremities are bluish red, the skin is covered with tiny burst blood vessels; patients experience pains in their limbs and always feel better lying down, with their legs raised. Also for girls with irregular periods, whose legs are red and swollen and who feel discomfort in overheated rooms.

Chapter 5

The Digestive System

> *You are what you eat, as the saying goes. And to a great extent, it's true.*
> *Every day we have to make important decisions concerning our health:*
> *choosing what we eat, as well as the importance we give to food, the*
> *atmosphere in which we eat it and so on.*

Acidity

Avoid bicarbonate of soda, which provides only temporary relief and in the long run promotes chronic hyperacidity. Possible causes of acidity are diverse: liver troubles, alcoholism, constipation, overwork and even chronic appendicitis.

Maintain a healthy and simple diet. Eat less bread and sugar and try to eat slowly. Take half an hour rest after meals. You can also drink a glass of freshpressed potato juice in the morning before you have breakfast, at lunch and before going to bed. Also chew on uncooked oat flakes instead of taking bicarbonate of soda to ease symptoms.

- *Arsenicum album 5 C.* Individuals are very thirsty and want to drink small amounts of water repeatedly.
- *Carbo vegetabilis 5 C.* Burning sensations are eased by belching (see Aerophagia).
- *Iris versicolor 5 C.* Burning in the stomach rises up into the mouth, irritating the tongue and teeth, and is not soothed by drinking cold liquids. It can appear at any time. People salivate more than normal, and may vomit up thick viscous mucus. In some cases the liver is very sensitive, people suffer from diarrhoea, vomiting, a burning sensation in the anus, migraines and milder headaches. Symptoms are aggravated at night.
- *Robinia 5 C.* Belches and vomit are acidic; subjects feel a burning sensation right up into their throat, and sometimes even between the shoulder blades; they suffer from headaches around the temples and forehead, which are aggravated by movement.
- *Sulphuric acid 5 C.* As well as burning in the stomach and oesophagus, and a bitter taste in the mouth, subjects are weak; hot drinks seem to improve their condition; they are anxious, agitated, and always thirsty.

Aerophagia

Aerophagia (commonly called belching) is simply expelling gas through the mouth in abnormal quantities, especially after meals. It may be accompanied by various problems, such as palpitations, thoracic pains, respiratory problems, etc.

A good preventive measure is to exercise the abdomen in order to strengthen the abdominal muscles. Also avoid drinking while you eat, try to eat your meals in a calm atmosphere, chew your food well and don't do anything else while you're eating, such as reading or watching television.

3 granules once a day:

- Argentum nitricum 5 C. Belching is very loud, it occurs after meals and lasts for some time. The belching is soothed for a moment, then starts again, accompanied by palpitations, pains in the left side of the chest, and nervousness. For those who eat too quickly and whose stomach is bloated.
- *Asafoetida 5 C*. As in the previous case, subjects are nervous, although somewhat less so; they are more irritable and eat less quickly; their belches have an unpleasant odour and are accompanied by flatulence.
- *Cuprum 5 C*. For those whose stomach rumbles.
- *Carbo vegetabilis 5 C*. For individuals with painful digestion; belches have an unpleasant odour, resembling the food that has been swallowed; also, belching occurs not only after meals, but at any time during the day or night. Subjects suffer from stomach cramps which may spread to the chest; they are short of breath - the expulsion of air provides temporary relief.
- *Ignatia 5 C*. People feel pain in the pit of their stomach, as well as raging hunger around mid-day, which is unusual; they take deep breaths and are constantly yawning; they often feel as if there's a knot in their stomach, which moves up into the throat. *Ignatia* is often prescribed for sensitive, anxious people, whether the anxiety is temporary or a normal facet of their character.
- *Kali carbonicum 5 C*. For those who have trouble digesting; belching is caused by any kind of food, both solid and liquid. Subjects suffer from nausea as soon as they lie down; they often wake up in the middle of the night, overcome with palpitations and anxiety; they have acute chest and back pains, are often depressed and cannot concentrate on their work.
- *Lycopodium 5 C*. For people with liver problems; digestive troubles are

aggravated towards the end of the afternoon, and their belching burns the throat. As soon as they start a meal, they feel bloated, are no longer hungry and are short of breath. Belching produces a burning sensation. *Lycopodium* is often recommended for those who lead a sedentary life and don't do much exercise.

Anal Fissures

Very painful, especially when defaecating, anal fissures are little wounds which take a variety of forms and have a whitish background. They are often accompanied by haemorrhoids.

- Local treatment: ointment made with *Ratanhia T.M., Paeonia T.M.* or *Homeodora cream.* Clean the fissures thoroughly after each defaecation.

3 granules once a day:

- *Graphites 5 C.* Fissures are accompanied by constipation, haemorrhoids and eczema scabs. Stool, when there is any, is large and coated with mucus.
- *Nitricum acidum 5 C.* Patients feel as if there were shards of glass in their anus. Pains persist long after defaecating. Fissures are accompanied by very sensitive haemorrhoids, anal constriction and oozing sores. Patients feel a burning sensation in the anus, and a constant need to go to the toilet (tenesmus).
- *Paeonia 4 C.* Fissures are accompanied by haemorrhoids and ooze constantly. The anus is inflamed and always moist. Pains are intense, occurring both before and after defaecating, and are aggravated by walking.
- *Ratanhia 4 C.* The anus is contracted and dry, and subjects experience shooting pains which are temporarily relieved by applications of cold water or taking cold sitz baths; patients often have worms as well.
- *Silicea 5 C.* When these people try to defaecate, they suffer from contractions and incessant spasms which make evacuating the bowels very difficult - stool comes partially out but then retracts into the anus.

Anal Fistula (Boils)

These very unpleasant oozing ulcers are often developed by people with tuberculosis. It isn't always a good idea to have them treated surgically. Doing so may cause further disorders, since a fistula is often caused by the body's own defence system as a way of eliminating toxic waste material.

- *Berberis vulgaris 5 C.* For anal fistulas that alternate with pulmonary symptoms, such as difficulty in breathing, shortness of breath, etc., or with pains in the ribcage. The anus is ringed with eczema, which is aggravated when subjects scratch, and soothed by cold compresses.
- *Fluoric acid 5 C.* Individuals often develop varicose veins in the lower limbs; they experience itching, especially around orifices like the anus, which is aggravated by heat; fistulas ooze foul-smelling pus which irritates the wound even further.
- *Nitricum acidum 5 C.* This chronic condition tends to demoralize affected people. Needle-like pains are intense, and persist long after defaecating, even if the stool is soft.
- *Silicea 5 C.* The fistula takes on the appearance of an abscess. Spasms of the anal sphincter make evacuation difficult; stool, which may be partially evacuated after straining, is drawn back up into the anus by the spasms.

Appendicitis

The main symptoms of appendicitis are as follows: people are constipated, feel intense pain on the right side of the abdomen below the navel; the region is very sensitive to touch.

When pressure is applied and then released suddenly, pain spreads towards the right; the tongue is coated, patients are nauseous and have fever of between 99°F (37.5°C) and 100°F (38°C).

For people who want to treat their appendicitis, it is generally recommended that they adopt a largely vegetarian diet, cutting out fat, sauces and spices, acidic fruits, fresh bread, processed meats and eggs. They should also stay in bed and go on a juice cure: carrot, myrtle or grape juice mixed with 2/3 spring water.

Apply cold milk compresses to the stomach and drink a laxative tea to help empty the bowels. Complete the treatment with a homeopathic remedy.

Acute Appendicitis

It's not a good idea to refuse surgery in cases of acute appendicitis, which is characterized by high fever, vomiting and shooting pains in the abdomen.

As a last resort, or in situations where you have a few hours to wait before the operation, you can try *Ignatia 9 C,* 3 granules every hour. If symptoms do not radically improve, then there is no choice but to have the operation, which presents no danger to patients (see the section on Surgical Interventions).

3 granules every half an hour:

- *Colocynthis 5 C*. For cases where symptoms are eased if patients lie in a foetal position.
- *Belladonna 5 C*. The abdomen is hot and sensitive, and patients can't bear to be touched in the abdominal region; they also cannot tolerate any movement.

Bladder Problems
(See Also Cystitis)

This hollow organ, made of muscle fibre, can contain up to one and a half pints of liquid. The bladder can also become inflamed. If this happens, people feel a frequent urge to urinate, even though they may only be able to pass a few drops and that with great difficulty. If this happens, drink infusions of juniper berries.

Cholesterol

If the following symptoms are present, it's better to consult a doctor: buzzing in the ears (especially in the morning), dust spots before the eyes, obesity and high blood pressure, pins and needles in the extremities.

In some cases, an increase in cholesterol level is signalled by hardening of one or a number of temporal arteries. However, you should know that research has shown that the presence or absence of lipids and triglycerides are the determining factors in cholesterol problems, rather than the cholesterol itself.

In many cases, cholesterol problems can also be linked to renal or thyroid disorders, to lipoid nephrosis or to hormones found in certain contraceptives.

In any case, it's always a good idea to limit the amount of animal fat you consume, replacing them with a natural rice-based diet, white cheese and salad. Smoking and alcohol abuse should also be avoided.

Consult the section on Arteriosclerosis.

Cirrhosis

For homeopathy to have any effect, it is absolutely necessary for subjects to stop drinking alcohol completely.

To make it easier to do so, add 2 or 3 drops of *Capsicum Mother Tincture* to each litre of wine. Subjects should also eat about 50 grams of lightly cooked calf's liver per day, which should be well-chewed, and 300 to 400 grams of green cabbage, half cooked, half raw.

They should also sleep a lot (12 hours every night), take two naps during the day, one after lunch and one before supper, and abstain from all strenuous activity.

5 granules once a week:

- *Aurum metallicum 7 C*. For those who are melancholic (called Aurum melancholia).
- *Arsenicum album 7 C*. These people are both physically and mentally agitated; they despair of ever recovering and are physically weak; the body is cold, and the condition is aggravated after midnight.
- *Ethyllicum 7 C*. In the morning before eating, people have trembling hands; they lack appetite, are irritable in the morning before eating and expel a slimy white liquid when defaecating; the face is bloated, with abundant varicosity on the nose and cheeks.

  These people have bad breath, suffer from diarrhoea and lots of wind; they sometimes feel slight paralysis of the lower limbs; they can be very talkative at times, to the point of being delirious, and may suffer from anxiety and terrible hallucinations, particularly about animals.

  Symptoms are aggravated by heat, hunger and movement; there is someimprovement in cool fresh air and after resting.
- *Phosphorus triiodatus 7 C*. Subjects are first agitated, then go through a phase of mental and physical depression; they experience nausea and vomiting, abdominal pains and profuse sweating; they are also thirsty.
- *Guercas glandium spiritum 7 C*. In combination with the remedy that most closely resembles the illness (the *simillimum*), this remedy is especially effective against congestion or sclerosis of the liver in agitated or stupefied alcoholics as well as hypertrophy (enlargement) of the spleen.

Colic: Abdominal

Colic is not necessarily accompanied by diarrhoea. Symptoms include cramps, spasms and intestinal irritation and may be an indication of a more serious disorder such as a strangulated hernia, appendicitis, intestinal blockage, etc.

Treating Colic Yourself

Make sure there are no other organic symptoms. Call in a doctor immediately (especially for children) in cases where the stomach is distended, individuals are constipated and cannot release gas, or if the colic attacks occur frequently and are accompanied by nausea, vomiting or fever. If subjects do develop diarrhoea, consult that section for more information.

3 granules every half an hour:

- *Belladonna 5 C*. For intense pain: the stomach is extremely sensitive to the touch - patients can't even stand the contact of their bedclothes. The face is red, the skin is hot; pains may stop suddenly; the condition is eased by lying face down on the stomach; subjects feel totally exhausted.
- *Colocynthis 5 C*. For colic that occurs after exposure to cold. Pains are in the form of intermittent cramps - patients are doubled over and trembling, after which the symptoms ease off for a while. This type of colic can sometimes be caused by a fit of rage.
- *Cuprum 5 C*. During an attack (which is usually severe) patients can't catch their breath and suffer from intermittent spasms and cramps; the face is purple, the lips blue.   Subjects do not defaecate; cold drinks help the condition. The stomach is hypersensitive (as in the *Belladonna* type), but the pain is situated more on the left side.
- *Dulcamara 5 C*. Colic caused by catching cold after exposure to cold, damp weather.
- *Magnesia phosphorica 5 C*. Often prescribed for children. Pain is eased by pressure (people may double up when rubbed) and by heat. The stomach is distended and patients feel better when their clothes are loosened.
- *Nux vomica 5 C*. For colic caused by over-eating or food that is too spicy. The tongue is coated yellow towards the back of the mouth; people feel the need to defaecate, but cannot.
- *Veratrum album 5 C*. As for *Cuprum* types. This remedy is for very severe cases; patients faint from the pain, break out in cold sweats and develop palpitations and cardiac difficulties; the skin of the abdomen is stretched tight and very sensitive.

Colic: Biliary (Hepatic)

Homeopathy cannot dissolve stones (calcium deposits) in the gallbladder. But it can be used to prevent painful recurrences, on condition that patients adhere to a continuous treatment program. The only alternative to prevention is surgery.

3 granules every half an hour:

- *Belladonna 5 C*. Pains come and go suddenly; they are aggravated by noise and sudden movements and when patients are lying on their right side; the stomach is tight and hot.
- *Bryonia 5 C*. Pains are felt on the right side, below the abdomen, are aggravated by movement and soothed by applying firm pressure to the abdomen. These people try to remain immobile, as the least movement is painful. They have a bitter taste in their mouth; they may get dizzy, and suffer from nausea and vomiting; the liver feels inflamed and the tongue has a thick yellow coating.
- *Chelidonium majus 5 C*. Pains come in waves, and may be felt right up to the right scapula (shoulder blade); people feel as if they're being squeezed above the stomach, to the point where they can't stand wearing anything that puts pressure on the area. Subjects also have trouble digesting; their skin and stools are yellowish.
- *China 5 C*. Subjects are hypersensitive; they cannot tolerate noise, touch or movement; firm pressure is more bearable than rubbing; the stomach is swollen, but passing wind provides no relief. Subjects also develop diarrhoea, which gets worse at night or after swallowing food or liquid; they are very thirsty, exhausted, prostrate, and perspire through the night.
- *Colocynthis 5 C*. Pains are intermittent and spasmodic; patients are doubled over, or in a foetal position if lying down. The pain often makes them irritable - an attack may be provoked by a fit of rage.
- *Magnesia phosphorica 5 C*. Patients suffer from violent shooting cramps which come and go rapidly; they are aggravated by cold and cold water, and soothed by heat and applying pressure to the abdomen. They are also hypersensitive and nervous, and are very agitated during attacks.

Colic: Flatulent

Avoid drinking while you eat, and do some daily exercise to strengthen your abdominal muscles. Adjust your diet to cut down on starchy or farinaceous foods

(foods which contain a lot of flour), or at least avoid mixing them with sugar.

3 granules every half an hour:

- *Aloe 5 C*. Characterized by ballooning of the stomach; pains are aggravated before and after defaecating.
- *Allium cepa 5 C*. Usually subjects have got their feet wet or they have eaten watery food such as cucumber or lettuce. Patients are doubled over in pain, which is aggravated when seated and eased by walking; wind is wet and fetid, sometimes accompanied by diarrhoea.
- *Raphanus 5 C*. Pains are eased only if wind is passed; the abdomen is painful to the touch, even of clothing; pain is aggravated by even the slightest movement; the stomach is bloated. The condition sometimes produces respiratory problems - patients feel as if a knot in their stomach is moving up into their throat.

Colic: Renal

Acute attacks are due to the formation of stones (renal lithiasis or kidney stones). Subjects have to urinate frequently; pains are different from those of hepatic colic in that they tend to spread downwards towards the genitals and thighs instead of up into the shoulders. Urinating is painful and may cause bleeding.

Make sure patients drink a lot - if they don't, the urine becomes too concentrated and will eventually form a stone.

3 granules every half an hour:

- *Belladonna 5 C*. Cramps come and go suddenly; patients cannot tolerate contact or movement; the abdomen is hot and swollen; subjects feel a burning sensation when they are able to urinate, which is infrequently.
- *Berberis 5 C*. Subjects experience a burning sensation when urinating; the urine itself is sometimes bloody; pains feel like bubbling and are aggravated by the slightest movement or jolt.
- *Calcarea carbonica 9 C*. The remedy to administer during an attack: 5 granules immediately, along with *Pareira brava* and *Berberis*. For those who catch cold easily and who may suffer from rheumatism. Subjects have a stomach-ache, centred below the navel on the right side; pains ease off when they bend over. This remedy is appropriate for "arthritic" types.
- *Hydrangea 5 C*. The area around the kidneys and bladder is painful; urine contains a thick white discharge.

- *Lycopodium 9 C.* For people who are sedentary and do hardly any exercise. After meals, the skin over the abdomen is stretched; pains in the kidneys are most intense in the late afternoon. Patients shiver right through their body after urinating; the urine is clear but contains reddish sediment, as does the *Calcarea carbonica* type. *Lycopodium* should be taken in high dilutions, with long intervals between doses, with any of the following: *Berberis, Nux vomica, Solidago*.
- *Pareira brava 5 C.* Patients feel pain in their kidneys, lower back, urethra, anus and thighs; they constantly have to urinate, which is so painful that they have to crouch and strain.
- *Ocimum canum 5 C.* Colic is accompanied by vomiting and is situated on the right side; red deposits can be observed in the urine after an attack.

Constipation

Constipation can be caused by nervous disorders, improper diet, psychological problems, stomach or duodenal ulcers, or by cardiac disorders. As far as possible, avoid strong laxatives and purges, which can harm the digestive system.

A simple remedy that works for some people is to eat a few stewed prunes before breakfast in the morning and before going to bed at night, and to drink a glass of warm water before breakfast.

People may also try to improve their psychological condition by getting enough sleep and taking some time off to relax.

Kidney Function: Essential

To stimulate kidney, liver and gallbladder function, take sitz baths with herbal extracts, hot showers, and do aerobic exercise.

Eating Habits

You may want to review your eating habits, especially as far as potatoes and sweets are concerned. Carrot and fruit juices, as well as nuts, can help a lot. Once again, if your lifestyle is sedentary, find the time to exercise.

Constipation Characterized by Frequent but Ineffective Desire To Defaecate

3 granules 3 times per day:
- *Anacardium 5 C.* People feel as if their anus is contracted and stuffed

with a plug. There is some improvement while eating.

- *Lycopodium 5 C*. Constipation due to liver problems, characterized by intensely painful spasmodic constrictions, especially on the right side of the stomach, when patients feel the need to defaecate; accompanied by flatulence.
- *Nux vomica 5 C*. Constipation accompanied by anal spasms and haemorrhoids; often prescribed for sedentary people, who may also be irritable. In the case of infants, they may try very hard to empty their bowels and only manage to pass wind - this makes them cry and they cough.

Constipation Characterized by No Desire To Defaecate

3 granules three times per day:

- *Alumina 5 C*. Patients make a great effort to evacuate; stool comes out in small amounts; they also have trouble urinating; eating potatoes causes flatulence and makes digestion heavy and slow. This form of constipation is often found in sedentary women, older people and children who will not think of going to the toilet themselves.
- *Bryonia 5 C*. Stool is hard, black, dry, slimy and voluminous. People feel as if they have a stone in their stomach as soon as they swallow any food; movement causes them pain, so they end up hardly moving at all; they may be nauseous and dizzy in the morning just after getting up.
- *Graphites 5 C*. Stool is slimy; subjects frequently have pain in the anus, and are often obese and rather drowsy or recovering from a difficult illness.
- *Hydrastis 5 C*. Stool is slimy, sometimes full of mucus, the nausea can happen at any time in the day.
- *Opium 5 C*. For cases of intestinal sluggishness. Stool is dry, hard and black, like marbles. These people have no pain, but remain sleepy for a long time after eating - they are constantly in a state of mental torpor. Children have a tendency to sleep too much. *Opium* is often prescribed for older people.

Constipation Characterized by Stool Which Is Difficult To Evacuate

3 granules three times per week:

- *Alumina 5 C*. Stool is hard and covered with mucus, or soft and sticky with the consistency of clay. Even if the stool is soft, people must make a substantial effort to evacuate.
- *Causticum 5 C*. Stool is long and thin, and passes more easily when standing up.
- *Sanicula 5 C*. Usually for those who are thin; stool is bulky, pale-coloured, hard and dry. Subjects must make a great effort to defaecate; it is painful, and stool which has been partially expelled may be drawn back up into the anus; stool and wind have a fetid odour.
- *Silicea 5 C*. Stool comes out partially, but is then drawn back in by a sudden contraction of the sphincter; especially for teething infants and women during their periods.
- *Sulphur 5 C*. To be taken with *Nux vomica*. People feel as if their bowels are never empty; the anus is red and causes a burning sensation. Sulphur types are usually jovial and stout.

When Travelling

- *Platina 5 C*. 3 granules in the morning and at night before going to bed. Helps adjust to a change of location, habits or lifestyle.

Sea Travel

- *Bryonia 5 C*. 3 granules once a day.

During or After Menstruation

- *Silicea 5 C*. 3 granules per day, before and after periods.
- *Kali carbonicum 5 C*. 3 granules per day during periods.

Diabetes

In 50 percent of cases, diabetes has a hereditary origin. Most of the time, patients develop "full-blown" diabetes characterized by an abundant secretion of urine, excessive thirst and the presence of glucose in the urine. These people are always hungry and never seem able to satisfy their craving for food.

Other symptoms include headaches, loss of sexual desire and skin disorders (boils, intertrigo). The disease is difficult to cope with, both for patients and the people around them. However, there are certain measures that can be taken to make the burden lighter.

The presence of sugar in the blood is not necessarily due to diabetes. It may be a temporary condition, occurring during pregnancy for example. Only a doctor is capable of prescribing proper treatment.

Additional remedies

Prolonged hot showers, especially on the abdomen, stimulate the pancreas. Try to get some acidic milk, and drink at least half a litre per day.

Diet

Proper diet is essential and may re-establish a metabolic balance in mild cases. Abstaining from pastries, sweets, sweet vegetables and fruits is the traditional way to fight the disease. Infusions of myrtle leaves, blackberry leaves and wild walnut leaves, taken once or twice a day, complete the beneficial effects of a proper diet.

You can eat a lot of mushrooms which usually contain a hypoglycaemic substance.

Add as many raw vegetables to your diet as possible: prepare salads garnished with onions and cold-pressed sunflower oil. Nuts are known to have a beneficial effect on the liver, as does carrot juice accompanied by endive salad or other bitter herbs. Chew your food well and swallow slowly. Avoid all foods which contain cooked albumin (egg white) combined with carbohydrates.

Replace strong seasoning with herbs.

What To Prescribe

Once again, we must emphasize the importance of abstaining from pastries, sweets, sweet vegetables and fruits. Of course, these recommendations are very general and **cannot replace treatments prescribed by professionals for individual cases.**

In the case of diabetes during pregnancy, consult a doctor, and make sure you are closely monitored.

2 granules once a day:

- *Acetic acid 5 C*. Patients urinate excessively (polyuria), are very thirsty, pale, thin and weak; they have cold sweats at night, difficulty digesting, abundant saliva, and tend to develop oedema.
- *Amanita phalloides 5 C*. Subjects are thin. As in *Acetic acid* types, they have cold sweats and their body is cold; however, they are less anaemic, less thirsty, and do not crave food as much.

- *Glycerinum 5 C.* Subjects are thin and wasting away; they urinate frequently, but in small amounts.
- *Hydrangea T.M.:* to alleviate thirst.
- *Lactic acid 5 C.* Compared to *Acetic acid* types, these people urinate more often, and may suffer from gastric pains or pains in the joints.
- *Phosphoric acid 5 C.* People urinate a lot (polyuria); urine is a milky colour, and often contains excessive amounts of calcium phosphates (phosphaturia).
- *Uranium nitricum 5 C.* Despite a hearty appetite, subjects remain thin and are intensely thirsty. The disorder is accompanied by intestinal flatulence; urine may be greenish and smell like fish; patients are moody and seem depressed, especially in the morning after getting up.
- *Uranium arsenicum 5 C.* Patients are thin, often thirsty, and may suffer from bulimia and oedema; they are not anaemic and have no flatulence; they get stomach-ache when eating.
- *Uranium compound 5 C.* While travelling.

Diarrhoea

Diarrhoea frequently occurs after meals that don't agree with you, after sudden changes in diet or temperature, or after catching cold. In cases of acute diarrhoea, stay in bed and keep the abdomen warm.

Diet

The best thing is to stick to a diet based on boiled water - for example, vegetable broth and hot herbal tea. The main objective of homeopathic remedies is to cure the disorder more quickly and to avoid possible complications.

Start by abstaining from foods that tend to cause diarrhoea, such as fruit, sweets, raw vegetables, raw or cooked cabbage. To avoid fermentation in the stomach, don't eat fruit and vegetables at the same meal. Make sure you chew your food and salivate well. Drink plain milk, eat oats, fromage frais, soft cheese.

Infant Diarrhoea

To treat diarrhoea in children and infants, serve finely grated apples or oat flakes, and cut out all other foods for a while. In more serious cases, you can limit the diet to infusions of sage or myrtle leaves.

Also use *kaolin* to neutralize irritating toxic substances that cause diarrhoea.

If diarrhoea is accompanied by fever, it's best to consult a doctor.

3 granules once a day:

- *Aloe 5 C*. This is the most general remedy, and should be administered in all cases of mild diarrhoea without vomiting but accompanied by colic pain before and during defaecation. Subjects need to go to the toilet urgently; they may pass watery stool when they think they are urinating or passing wind.
- *Antimonium crudum 5 C*. Diarrhoea is half solid and half liquid, and occurs after over-eating, especially cakes, pastries and acidic wine. People are very thirsty for cold water, are drowsy and prostrate. The tongue has a thick white coating.
- *Argentum nitricum 5 C*. Stool is greenish, mixed with bits of intestinal mucus; diarrhoea is worse after eating or drinking. This type is especially common among children and infants who have eaten too many sweets.
- *Arsenicum album 5 C*. Diarrhoea due to food poisoning, caused by eating food of doubtful quality or freshness, like tainted meat for example. The stool has a fetid odour, and produces a burning sensation in the rectum and anus, sometimes accompanied by bleeding.

Also see Diarrhoea in the section on Infant Disorders.

If Diarrhoea Is Accompanied by Fever and/or Agitation

- *Arsenicum album 5 C*. For children who seem sick or intoxicated; stool is nauseating, and the extremities - and sometimes the whole body - are cold.
- *Calcarea phosphorica 5 C*. For cases of diarrhoea caused by teething in infants.
- *Chamomilla vulgaris 5 C*. For cases where stool resembles scrambled eggs mixed with spinach; it is hot and viscous, has a fetid odour, irritates the anus and is often accompanied by colic pains. Also recommended for infants who are teething.
- *China 5 C*. Diarrhoea that is not painful; stool is yellowish or greenish, and contains some food that hasn't been digested; accompanied by flatulence. This type of diarrhoea is caused by beer, milk and fruit. The abdomen is swollen, and patients are exhausted; the condition gets worse at night and after meals.
- *China rubra 5 C*. This type of diarrhoea is not painful, but causes swelling of the abdomen and a feeling of weakness after defaecating;

stool contains particles of undigested food and often occurs after eating fruit.

- *Cistus 5 C*. For diarrhoea triggered by coffee.
- *Dulcamara 5 C*. For diarrhoea caused by exposure to cold; preceded by pain around the navel, and accompanied by wind, passing of viscous mucus in the stool, and flatulence. In acute cases subjects are intensely thirsty for cold water and may have shivers down their back.
- *Colocynthis 5 C*. To calm intense abdominal pains, which are only relieved by people doubling over. Subjects are agitated; the condition often occurs after a fit of rage, and is soothed by heat and firm pressure.
- *Gelsemium 5 C*. Stool is abundant and yellowish; this type of diarrhoea may follow an emotional shock, or be due to apprehension about some imminent event, like speaking in front of a large group of people.
- *Mercurius solubilis 5 C*. For diarrhoea due to problems with the biliary tract, the small intestine or large intestine. The tongue is coated yellow and retains teeth marks; stool is greenish and viscous, sometimes bloody; defaecation is accompanied by abdominal pains.
- *Natrum sulphuricum 5 C*. Diarrhoea is painless; bowels are bloated with wind; stool comes out in spurts and is yellowish in colour. In humid weather, people feel a dull pain in the abdomen.
- *Mercurius corrosivus 5 C*. For more serious cases accompanied by intense pain and burning sensations in the urinary tract.
- *Phosphorus 5 C*. For serious cases: stool is nauseating, streaked with blood; defaecation is involuntary - the anus remains distended; accompanied by passing of wind and bleeding; subjects are exhausted and are constantly thirsty.
- *Podophyllum peltatum 5 C*. For diarrhoea which occurs especially in the early morning, around 5 a.m. Stool is watery, yellowish and abundant; it may be odourless or smell extremely bad, depending on the food the person has eaten. This type of diarrhoea is frequently followed by a feeling of weakness in the abdomen and rectum. The rectum has a tendency to prolapse. The condition improves when subjects lie on their stomach.
- *Veratrum album 5 C*. For profuse diarrhoea accompanied by vomiting, general weakness and occasional blackouts. Subjects suffer from severe colic - they are prostrate, the face is pale, cold and covered with perspiration; body temperature is very low (hypothermia), they have

intense spasms and abdominal pains which leave them very weak. In children especially, the vomiting reflex persists even after they have finished vomiting; the complexion is livid and the whole body may be covered with cold sweat.

Digestive Pains

Pain is a signal that should be interpreted, rather than suppressed. We should try to determine the cause of the pain. Stomach and intestinal pains, if not caused by a specific disorder, may correspond to the following remedies.

Note: Medications should be administered at a dosage of 2 granules every half an hour if the pains are intense. Doses should then be spaced out gradually as the condition improves.

Intestinal Pains

- *Cuprum 5 C*. Pains are in the form of bowel spasms, which start and stop suddenly. The abdomen is hard and tight, and very sensitive to the touch. The condition is aggravated by cold and soothed by heat applied to the abdomen, and by cold drinks.   Subjects often feel as if they were being stabbed in the stomach. They suffer from diarrhoea, severe nausea and vomiting, and have trouble urinating.
- *Dioscorea 5 C*. For cases of frequent intestinal inflammation accompanied by abundant flatulence. When pains are at their peak, people feel an intense urge to defaecate and urinate; they may experience exhausting diarrhoea in the morning. If the condition persists or becomes chronic, subjects may develop painful, oozing haemorrhoids; when accompanied by diarrhoea, the pain is intense, as if the intestines were being twisted into a knot; pain is always worse when subjects are leaning forward; stool is yellowish, and after defaecating people feel extremely fatigued.
- *Ipecac. 5 C*. Pains are centred around the navel and travel from left to right; they are accompanied by diarrhoea and constant nausea; vomiting does not provide any relief; the tongue is not coated. These cases occur most frequently in the autumn, when people are more likely to catch cold.
- *Mercurius 5 C*. Abdominal pains are mostly on the right side and are accompanied by kidney problems, diarrhoea or constipation; the stomach

is distended and hard; subjects may get the hiccups, feel nauseous, regurgitate food and suffer from heartburn. The tongue has a yellowish coating, and retains teeth marks.

- *Plumbum 5 C.* People feel is if their intestines were being tied in a knot, and dragged towards their back; the muscles of the intestinal wall are hard and swollen; pain is aggravated by touch, and soothed when subjects lie in a foetal position, or by deep, progressive and prolonged pressure.
- *Veratrum album 5 C.* Violent pains are accompanied by vomiting and abundant diarrhoea, especially at night, and cold sweats (especially on the forehead). Subjects feel weak after attacks; they often experience a sensation of cold around the stomach area; the tongue is dry and discoloured.

Stomach Pains

- *Dioscorea 5 C.* For acute attacks of visceral spasms; people feel heaviness and pain, and have a weak stomach. The pain comes in intense waves and is aggravated when subjects are lying down or leaning forward. Walking, stretching backwards, arching one's back and moving around soothes the pain, as does frequent belching.
- *Belladonna 5 C.* For extremely intense abdominal pains, accompanied by fever. Symptoms appear and disappear suddenly; subjects want to remain immobile, and cannot tolerate physical contact or movement. The stomach is distended, hot and sensitive, and the upper lip is often red and swollen.
- *Chamomilla 5 C.* Like *Belladonna* cases, pains are accompanied by fever; the stomach is distended, but not hot. Subjects are not bothered by movement; they suffer from wind which produces severe stomach pains; the face is flushed and hot; stool is watery and burning, and smells like rotten eggs.
- *Bryonia 5 C.* Subjects feel as if they have a stone in their stomach - the least movement is painful, but pains are soothed by firm pressure on the stomach; coughing also aggravates the pain. The tongue is coated white, patients are intensely thirsty and suffer from nausea and constipation; cold-water compresses ease the condition.
- *Nux vomica 5 C.* The stomach is tight; pains usually start after meals and in the morning after waking up. The stomach swells up about an hour

after eating - it is full of wind, which is difficult to get rid of. *Nux vomica* is often prescribed for those who eat too much, and then vomit. Constipation goes hand in hand with the *Nux vomica* condition - people have weak bowels and are unable to evacuate.

- *Magnesia phosphorica 5 C*. Sudden pains occur at regular intervals - they are intense and spasmodic, causing subjects to lean forward and double over, remain immobile and press their stomach. Expelling wind provides no relief- pains are soothed by heat and friction.

Digestive Problems

Good digestion depends on a number of factors like mood, lifestyle, the kinds of physical activities we participate in and, of course, the kinds of food we eat.

When chronic digestive problems arise, it's always a good idea to examine our habits, or at least those over which we have some kind of control. In many cases, our own ignorance and inertia are the greatest obstacles we have to face in improving our physical and mental condition.

Motivation and a desire to learn are the main tools at our disposal - without them we remain passive consumers of medication, easy prey to recurring disorders which may be quite easy to avoid.

To aid digestion, make sure your diet is suited to your constitution and to your lifestyle. There is no universally correct diet - it's up to each person to study his or her own body and reactions to various foods.

Also consult the sections on Diet, Appetite and Longevity.

Eat Better To Live Better

There are, however, certain constants that should be kept in mind. Good humour, for example, aids digestion and reduces our need to eat a lot. Arguing or discussing contentious issues during meals may often be overlooked as a cause of digestive problems. On the other hand, simply making a meal look attractive can help people digest it well.

Taking the time to savour your food and chew it well is an extremely important factor. After meals, try to relax. Avoid staying seated or leaning forward. In the morning, and before your evening meal, do some abdominal exercises.

Avoid eating too quickly, and don't eat food that is too hot, as this may cause inflammation of the mucous membranes, which is often a precursor to the formation of stomach ulcers (chronic cramps are a characteristic sign). If this happens, drink raw potato juice, diluted with hot water. If you have a digestive problem, you may want to try an oatmeal diet for a while.

Also, whole oat grain can be used to prepare a soothing drink which helps fight inflammation of the mucous membranes. Vitamins A, B_1 and C stimulate digestion, as well as certain herbs like sage, parsley, thyme, bay leaf, chives, celery and chervil. Onions, garlic and shallots also stimulate digestion, but should be used according to personal tolerance.

Regularity Is a Virtue
Eat more acidic foods and proteins at the start of a meal. Eat at the same times every day, as much as possible. Add thyme to your diet, either as a herb or in the form of herbal tea. Also, a glass of tonic sage wine (100 grams of sage soaked in a litre of wine) is an excellent digestive tonic.

Lazy Stomach?
If you have a lazy stomach, feel heavy and drowsy after eating, if meals often don't agree with you (dyspepsia; atony, i.e. lack of stomach tone), if you feel pains, suffer from heartburn, get a bitter taste in your mouth or find that you're still ravenous after eating, then do not drink (even water) during meals - instead drink between meals. Don't eat too much bread during meals, as it bloats the stomach and causes dyspepsia.

2 granules once a day:
- *Abies Canadensis 5 C.* For those with a lazy stomach (atony); they are susceptible to cold, tend to lose weight, and have a constant queasy feeling in the pit of their stomach; although they have a healthy appetite, these people cannot eat big meals or bear to go without food if they're on a diet. They often feel weak, especially if they don't eat on time; they crave meat and other foods, which may be highly nutritious, but they can't digest them properly - they will often suffer from flatulence and palpitations after over-eating.
- *Abrotanum 5 C.* For those who suffer from chronic weight loss, starting with the lower part of the body, despite the fact that they have a voracious appetite; they get stomach-aches while digesting, but can eat relatively large amounts.
- *Arsenicum album 5 C.* For mild food poisoning: people who don't fully recover can benefit from *Arsenicum album,* even long after the food

poisoning. This remedy is also recommended for people who develop pains just after eating or in the middle of the night, as well as for heartburn eased by hot drinks.

- *Bryonia 5 C*. For difficult digestion that is slow and heavy. People feel they are too full, as if there were a stone in the pit of their stomach, which is sensitive.
- *Carbo vegetabilis 5 C*. Foods remain in the stomach and intestines where they ferment, bloating the abdomen and causing pains in the pit of the stomach, shortness of breath and palpitations. Rancid eructation (belching) provides temporary relief.
- *Lycopodium 5 C*. A general remedy for sluggish digestion and also for heavy digestion with heartburn; people lack appetite and suffer from diarrhoea after meals.
- *Natrum muriaticum 5 C*. People feel empty in the pit of their stomach, especially around mid-morning; they are obliged to eat small amounts at frequent intervals, are often thirsty and feel heavy and dehydrated; large meals make them sleepy.
- *Nux vomica 5 C*. Pains or feelings of heaviness start half an hour after meals - pressure on the stomach is painful and people have to loosen their clothing. The back of the tongue is coated white. This remedy is recommended in cases of indigestion due to over-eating.
- *Oleander 5 C*. People constantly feel as if the pit of their stomach were empty - even after meals. They have foul-smelling flatulence, their minds are somewhat groggy, as if numb. Drinking alcohol improves the condition temporarily.
- *Pulsatilla 5 C*. For slow, difficult digestion after eating a heavy meal or because of an inability to digest greasy foods. The mouth is dry, people have a bitter taste and bad breath; the tongue has a thick yellowish-white coating. After meals, people suffer from eructation and regurgitation that tastes of the food they've eaten, and feel a heaviness in the gastric region. The condition is aggravated by heat and hot foods or liquids. Subjects are often nauseous and suffer from diarrhoea; their abdomen is swollen and very sensitive to the touch; they may develop a slight fever and shivers.

Drunkenness

- *Aconitum 5 C*. 10 granules in a glass of water will sober up the person quickly. Take a teaspoon in water every five minutes

It's always better to *prevent rather than cure:* take 4 or 5 granules of *Ethyllicum 5 C* an hour before a meal or party where you think you might drink to excess. Half an hour before, take 4 or 5 granules of *Paullinia sorbilis 5 C* and repeat after the meal.

Flatulence

Work on curing flatulence begins at the dinner table.

Prevention

There are various things you can do if you tend to be particularly flatulent. For example, abstain from drinking while eating, from mixing sugar (especially sugar from fruit) with flour. Also abstain from cooked cabbage. As for other vegetables, season them with savory (herb) while cooking.

Note: these homeopathic remedies should be taken at a dosage of 2 granules every half an hour in cases where pains are intense. Gradually reduce the dose as the condition improves.

- *Abies Canadensis 5 C*. For flatulence accompanied by palpitations.
- *Aloe socotrina 5 C*. When the wind is hot, or occurs during diarrhoea.
- *Arsenicum album 5 C*. When wind has a fetid odour.
- *Butrucum acidum 5 C*. Flatulence is worse at night; pains are so bad that subjects cannot sleep; they sweat profusely through the feet, which smell bad. Lazy digestion and liver function are the causes of the problem.
- *Cajuputum 5 C*. Flatulence with intestinal bloating; the condition gets worse at night; there is, however, no odour.
- *Carbo vegetabilis 5 C*. For simple flatulence.
- *Kali carbonicum 5 C*. Flatulence with abdominal bloating and pains which are worse at around three in the morning.
- *Lycopodium 5 C*. When passing wind seems to ease the flatulence.
- *Sulphur 5 C*. For abdominal pains with fetid-smelling wind which is more abundant in the evening and at night.

Food Poisoning

The body usually responds to food poisoning with diarrhoea, followed by severe abdominal pains and fever. This reaction is beneficial, and if it doesn't occur naturally, the best thing to do is provoke evacuation with a purgative, enema or laxative, in order to eliminate toxic substances by emptying the bowels.

Clean Yourself

Once the purge is complete, go on a fast, which you can ease with cream soups and carrot juice to soothe the liver. There is a positive side to your predicament. You can use the occasion to clean out your system. Your stomach should be able to retain solid food as soon as hunger reappears.

You should always make sure that the meat you eat is fresh and be selective about where you eat out. Also get rid of food in tins that have been even slightly dented.

The more that meats are processed (into sausage, potted meats, salami, etc.), the higher the risk. Boiled meats are less dangerous than roasted meats, where internal temperatures usually don't exceed 45°C.

- *Arsenicum album 5 C.* 2 granules three times a day, if you haven't fully recovered from a bout of food poisoning, even long ago.
- *Calendula T.M.* Add one or two teaspoons to a glass of water, which you swallow as quickly as possible, rinsing it round your mouth as you do so. A quarter of an hour later, take:
- *Botulinum 7 C.* 3 granules, followed a quarter of an hour later by:
- *Pyrogenium 5 C.* 5 granules, and again 15 minutes later by:
- *Arsenicum album 5 C.* 5 granules.

Mushroom Poisoning

If the affected person has eaten mushrooms recently, the following symptoms will be added to those mentioned above: heartburn, sweating and intense thirst.

See a doctor without delay. DO NOT WAIT for the following symptoms to appear: the person seems exhausted and unable to think clearly, and starts getting cold. The situation is dangerous - there is no time to waste.

While waiting for the doctor, make the person drink small amounts of very cold salted water, using one teaspoon of salt (sea salt if possible) per glass of water.

Gallbladder
(See Also Biliary or Hepatic Colic)

The gallbladder is a membranous reservoir situated at the lower surface of the liver. It contains bile. Gallbladder inflammation can be caused by emotional shock, over-eating or unusually strenuous physical exertion. A doctor should be consulted.

In most cases, gallbladder problems indicate the presence of gallstones. While waiting to see a doctor, and in order to soothe the pain, apply cold milk compresses (soak a clean cloth in some cold milk). Compresses should be changed as soon as they warm up from contact with the skin.

Gastritis
(See Also Stomach, Heartburn, Stomach Pains)

The primary symptoms of gastritis are easily recognizable: nausea, belching, difficult digestion (see section) and vomiting that may contain blood (haemorrhage).

Symptoms appear after meals if people over-eat or if certain foods don't agree with them, and are caused by inflammation of the mucous lining of the stomach.

Diet

Set a strict schedule for meals, and force yourself to chew your food well. Also stop smoking and adopt an appropriate diet. The idea is to avoid eating foods that are likely to irritate the mucous membranes in the gastrointestinal system and also to avoid exciting the nervous system excessively.

You should therefore abstain from fatty meat and offal, processed meats (except lean ham), seafood (except oysters, anchovies and sardines), tinned meat, fish, greasy soups, chocolate and cocoa, and strong spices.

Drink wine in moderation, avoiding champagne and burgundy types, as well as strong beer. Cut out strong tea and coffee, strong cheeses, eggs and, to some extent, spinach, beans, lentils, peas and sorrel.

Also avoid sweets and milky coffee, take long walks before and after meals, and try to create an atmosphere that helps you relax in general.

Many cases of chronic gastritis are caused by the excessive consumption of bicarbonate of soda, certain types of mineral water or continuous use of certain laxatives. These only weaken the system, making it more vulnerable, and it is better to do without them because of their harmful side-effects.

3 granules once a day:

- *Argentum nitricum 5 C.* For people who act hastily and who are generally anxious; the condition is aggravated by sweets; they regurgitate and have burning eructation after meals; pains, which radiate all the way up to the left false ribs, are soothed by heat. People belch frequently, especially when upset.
- *Arsenicum album 5 C.* For gastritis caused by food poisoning. Burning pains in the stomach are soothed by heat; people are revolted by the sight of food, and thirst for small quantities of water.
- *Phosphorus 4 C.* Pains in the stomach, accompanied by a feeling of emptiness and faintness, are sometimes soothed by eating and drinking cold liquids (although these may be regurgitated as soon as they are reheated in the stomach). These people suffer from nausea and vomiting, and are hungry immediately after meals.

Hepatitis (Viral)

Viral hepatitis was once known simply as jaundice. As its name indicates, it is caused by the presence of a virus in the body.

People feel as if they have the flu, and develop some fever. They are tired, have no appetite and suffer from headaches and digestive problems. Urine is less abundant and a darker colour. The spleen may become enlarged.

In a second "icteric" phase, the familiar signs of jaundice appear.

A Strict Diet

People who contract hepatitis should stay in bed for two weeks and stop work for at least six weeks. Their entire environment should be thoroughly cleaned (toilet disinfected, dishes kept separately) and they should pay special attention to their personal hygiene, as well as that of the people around them.

For a complete run-down of what to eat and what to avoid, consult the section on Jaundice.

- *Phosphorus triiodatus 7 C.* 5 granules every 10 days.
- *Phosphorus triiodatus 5 C,* and *Lycopodium clavatum 5 C,* 2 granules on alternate days.
- *Nux vomica 5 C, Bryonia alba 5 C, Berberis vulgaris 4 C,* 2 granules per

day of each.

For more information, consult the section on Jaundice.

Hiccups

Hiccups are very common, but can also be very unpleasant. They are caused by the spasmodic contraction of the diaphragm, producing an intake of air which is strong enough to cause the vocal cords to vibrate, producing the characteristic hiccuping sound.

If you can't get rid of your hiccups quickly by holding your breath, take the appropriate remedy every fifteen minutes:

- *Cuprum metallicum 5 C* (for general cases). Place 2 granules on your tongue and suck them slowly. If the hiccups don't stop, try 2 more granules. If they still don't stop, take 5 granules.
- *Hyoscyamus niger 5 C*. 2 granules. When hiccups are accompanied by stomach-ache.
- *Ignatia 5 C*. 2 granules. For hiccups associated with nervous disorders which are aggravated by tobacco and coffee. Also for people who yawn a lot, or who have nausea which gets better when eating. Also recommended for children's hiccups.
- *Moschus 5 C*. 2 granules. For hypersensitive people subject to excessive sexual stimulation, and for hiccups caused by stimulants such as alcohol, coffee, etc.
- *Nux vomica 5 C*. 2 granules. For hiccups due to excessive eating or drinking. *Nux vomica* hiccups may also appear after drinking very cold liquids.
- *Teucrium marum verum 4 C*. 2 granules. For infants who get the hiccups after feeds.
- *Veratrum viride 5 C*. 2 granules. Hiccups are accompanied by a severe headache, usually during the early afternoon. The tongue and lips are dry, the face is flushed.

Indigestion
(See Also Colic, Diarrhoea, Dyspepsia,
Gastro-enteritis, Food Poisoning)

Basically, indigestion is caused by an excess or an incompatibility of foods. The symptoms are general discomfort, hot flushes, cold sweats, hiccups and nausea, cramps, vomiting and sometimes stomach-ache with diarrhoea.

Start treatment by hot showering of the stomach region (if you don't have a shower, use a hot-water bottle, hot towels etc.). Then cover the abdomen, which will appear bright red, with a poultice of raw, finely chopped onions (onions can be replaced by cabbage leaves).

Bear in mind that food poisoning and appendicitis show the same symptoms as indigestion at first.

Every half an hour, depending on the case:

- *Amygdalus 5 C,* 3 granules. For children who throw up everything they eat or drink. There is no diarrhoea, general condition is good, but there is regular morning nausea. Look especially for a tongue that is red at the edges and tip.
- *Antimonium crudum 4 C,* 3 granules. For children who stuff themselves, whose "eyes are bigger than their bellies"! Vomiting is accompanied by belching which smells of the food just eaten. The tongue is coated white.
- *Bismuthum 5 C,* 3 granules. Severe stomach pains accompanied by cramps, occasional vomiting and/or retching. Alleviate pain by drinking cold liquid, or stretching/bending backward.
- *Calcarea muriatica 5 C,* 3 granules. For people who are markedly susceptible to indigestion. Some have slow and difficult digestion, even on a normal diet, vomit after meals and are constipated.
  Others get indigestion when they eat too much. They vomit all liquids and tend to suffer from diarrhoea.
  In both cases, there is a noticeable lack of muscularity and generally weak condition. *Calcarea muriatica 9 C,* 4 granules once a week is recommended for chronic cases.
- *China 5 C* 3 granules. For people who suffer from flatulence and whose stomachs are often bloated and sensitive to the touch. The condition is aggravated after meals and by certain foods such as milk and fruits, containing lots of water.
- *Ipecac. 5 C* 3 granules. To treat vomiting, when the tongue is uncoated. After heavy, fatty meals.
- *Kali muriaticum 5 C* 3 granules. For people who show an intolerance of fatty foods. Vomit is thick and viscous, the tongue is coated white or grey.
- *Nux vomica 5 C* 3 granules. For excessive consumption of wine or other

alcohol. The rear of the tongue has a thick yellow coating, there is nausea after meals, with pains and heaviness appearing about three hours after the meal. Sufferers can't vomit, but there is frequent retching.

- *Pulsatilla 5 C 3* granules. Mainly used for children, after too many sweets or ice-creams. Also for people who can't digest fatty foods like sauces, processed meats, fried foods, etc.
- *Senna 5 C 3* granules. Vomiting accompanied by stomach pains, extreme fatigue, nausea and pale complexion.

Intestinal Sluggishness
(See Also Digestive Atony, Constipation, Difficult Digestion)

One good way to cure intestinal sluggishness is to drink a soup each morning prepared from freshly ground wheat germ. Add a small chopped onion, a crushed clove of garlic and, once cooked, finely chopped parsley and a tablespoon of olive oil.

When laxatives don't appear to work, use the following remedy: prepare an infusion of senna leaves or pods (or some other purgative plant) to which you add a small raw potato with its skin, cut into cubes, a teaspoon of bran and one of linseed. Cook for 15 minutes. Drink this preparation in the morning, and also at night if the case merits.

Intolerance of Certain Foods

This isn't just a question of psychology. Certain foods, whether we like them or not, just don't "fit" our metabolism, especially when we're unwell.

Planning a Heavy Meal?

Before a meal that may be difficult to digest, take *Nux vomica 5 C 2* granules. You can also consult the following list of specific remedies for different foods. Take 2 granules, before or after the meal (if there is no other specific indication).

2 granules every half an hour, when the case merits:

- *Argentum nitricum 5 C.* For sweets, jams, honey, sugar.
- *Calcarea ostrearum 4 C.* For oysters.
- *China 4 C, Bryonia 4 C, Ipecac. 4 C.* 2 granules of each, one hour before eating fruit.
- *Ferrum metallicum 5 C.* For eggs and meat.

- *Ignatia 5 C.* For coffee.
- *Lac vaccinum 4 C.* Intolerance of milk.
- *Lycopodium 4 C.* Carrots, oysters, onions.
- *Nitricum acidum 5 C.* For milk.
- *Nux vomica 5 C.* For alcohol.
- *Egg peptone 4 C.* For eggs.
- *Fish peptone 4 C.* For fish.
- *Ptelea 5 C.* For cheese.
- *Pulsatilla 5 C.* For butter, ice-cream, pastries, fat, pork etc.

Intolerance of Certain Foods in Infants and Children

This section is mainly concerned with digestive problems in infants and young children. Vomiting must be carefully observed to make sure that it isn't a symptom of some other illness, such as gastro-enteritis, appendicitis or food poisoning.

Directions for Infants

Dissolve 5 granules of 5 C in 50 grams of neutral mineral water. The mixture is only good for 24 hours. After that, make a fresh one. Feed to young infants with a teaspoon, as often as required (the more severe the problem, the more frequently).

For very young babies, give 2 granules of 5 C every hour or so. Stop the medication as soon as there are signs of improvement.

- *Aethusia cynapium 5 C.* For babies who immediately vomit their milk in the form of curdled milk.
- *Antimonium tartaricum 5 C.* Infants who can't digest milk, and vomit frequently.
- *Bismuthum 5 C.* Here, too, liquids are rejected immediately, with noisy belching and retching, and a sour odour. The infant cries after eating.
- *Cuprum 5 C.* Violent spurts of vomiting. The infant writhes with pain from stomach spasms. Often accompanied by diarrhoea.
- *Magnesia phosphorica 5 C.* Gastric spasms and facial grimacing, which seem to ease when you hold the infant flat on his/her stomach and apply light pressure to the tummy with your hand.
- *Magnesia carbonica 5 C.* For children who can't tolerate milk. Curdled vomit and various forms of diarrhoea: discoloured and sour-smelling, or greenish, frothy and sour-smelling, or it may contain thick, bloody

lumps.● *Natrum carbonicum 5 C*. For children who can't digest milk. Sour-smelling diarrhoea in noisy spurts, aggravated by hot weather.
- *Natrum phosphoricum 5 C*. Like *Aethusa cynapium,* but for cases of more acidic diarrhoea.
- *Nux vomica 5 C*. For nervous, irritable infants, who have problems after meals and are constipated. Despite their tears and efforts, they cannot pass their stool.
- *Sepia 5 C*. For children who vomit, are sad and morose.
- *Silicea 5 C*. For thin children who feel the cold and vomit often.

Jaundice
(See Also Hepatitis, Viral
for a Description of the Initial Phases)

The causes of jaundice are diverse: catching a cold, suffering some traumatic setback, emotional shock or food poisoning can all bring on the disorder. However, the real cause has to do with blood problems, obstacles in the tracts leading to the liver or problems with the liver itself.

Multiple Causes

Other possible causes are poisoning by industrial or household products, especially chemicals, or food poisoning (especially from mushrooms). Certain pharmaceutical products can also cause the disorder (antibiotics, anaesthetics, anticoagulants, sulphonamides, sedatives, cortisone and its derivatives, etc.)

After the symptoms described in the section on Hepatitis appear (headache, fatigue, loss of appetite, digestive problems, dark urine in small quantities, coated tongue), the person may develop jaundice (icterus) which should be treated as an emergency.

Skin and mucus become yellowish, the temperature rises. Urine becomes even darker and stool is also discoloured. People are often nauseous, refuse to eat, feel ill and develop rashes.

The first thing to do is stay in bed. Treatment for most cases lasts between four to six weeks, and it's better to let the illness take its course instead of trying to curtail it prematurely. Which doesn't mean that no steps should be taken. On the contrary...

What To Do and What To Eat

Drink at least one glass of fresh carrot juice per day. Bathe the region around the liver with hot water, and alternate cabbage compresses and clay wraps. Drink diuretic infusions (horsetail, cough grass, birch, rosehip) and continue doing so even after the illness is cured. Radishes, chicory and artichoke all have a beneficial effect on the liver.

Cut out fatty meat and offal, processed meat (except lean ham), seafood (except oysters), anchovies and sardines, tinned meats, fish, greasy soups, chocolate, cocoa and strong spices.

Also cut out sweets and coffee with milk. Drink wine in moderation, avoiding champagne and burgundy types, as well as strong beer. Abstain from strong tea or coffee, strong cheeses, eggs and, to a lesser extent, spinach, beans, lentils, peas and sorrel.

If jaundice is accompanied by gastrointestinal problems (such as diarrhoea or vomiting), nervous disorders (mental confusion, delirium, exhaustion) or any haemorrhaging, it is absolutely essential to consult a doctor as soon as possible.

3 granules 3 times per day:

- *Berberis 5 C*. Pains are piercing and sharp, like a knife blade, in the region of the liver and kidneys; urinating is difficult, and the urine is a reddish colour. Patients feel intense itching and are constipated despite a frequent urge to go to the toilet.
- *Bryonia alba 5 C*. Shooting pains in the liver are accompanied by a feeling of intense heaviness; the liver area is sensitive to the touch; pains are stronger after meals, or if patients are pushed or have to move; they are also constipated. Some relief is provided by applying firm, sustained pressure, or when patients are lying on their right side. The mouth is dry and has a bitter taste; patients are nauseous, which is aggravated by movement; they have headaches, are often irritable and in a bad mood.
- *Chelidonium 4 C*. The main characteristic of *Chelidonium* cases is constant pain below the right shoulder blade, accompanied by pains in the liver. The tongue is coated yellow and retains teeth marks; patients have a bitter, salty taste in their mouth. The liver is swollen, patients are constipated, and stool is whitish; people crave hot food and liquids and are averse to cold food and liquids.
- *Colocynthis 5 C*. Pains are so intense that patients are often doubled over; they have a bitter taste in their mouth; urinating is difficult; pains are aggravated by cold and soothed by heat.

- *Digitalis 4 C*. The pulse is very slow, weak and irregular. The liver is swollen and painful. Patients' extremities are also swollen (oedema), passing urine is infrequent and difficult, and patients tend to black out easily.   The distinctive characteristic of *Digitalis* cases is nausea, which is aggravated by the smell of food.
- *Nux vomica 5 C*. Like *Bryonia alba, Nux vomica* is characterized by local sensitivity of the liver and constipation (although patients feel as if they need to go to the toilet). Firm pressure eases the pains, which are aggravated after meals; patients also feel very drowsy. The rear part of the tongue has a thick yellow coating.
- *Myrica 4 C*. Pulse is slow (less so than for *Digitalis* cases, however); the skin looks almost tanned; passing urine is infrequent, and urine itself is yellow and frothy, while stool is soft and discoloured. Patients suffer from severe pains in the chest in front of the heart.
- *Phosphorus 5 C*. For severe cases of jaundice. The liver is enlarged and patients are unable to lie on their right side; they may develop diarrhoea (painless but tiring) with greasy particles or constipation with small whitish stools.
- *Podophyllum 5 C*. A characteristic remedy for serious digestive problems. Patients can't keep anything down; they suffer from diarrhoea of a clear yellowish colour, especially in the morning, and sometimes accompanied by anal prolapse; patients tend to rub their abdomen. The condition is aggravated by movement and touch, and soothed by eating hot food and drinking hot liquids; patients feel better in a sitting position, leaning back.. Digestion is slow, accompanied by excessive yawning and drowsiness. Urine is yellowish and the pulse is slow.
- *Juglans cinera 5 C*. Pains in the liver shoot right up to the right shoulder or the left shoulder blade; they are accompanied by headaches above the nape, morning nausea, itching, burning diarrhoea and insomnia, usually after three o'clock in the morning.
- *Lachesis 5 C*. For jaundice affecting alcoholics.
- *Nux vomica 7 C*. For chronic liver congestion. The liver is sensitive to the touch, even to contact of clothes; subjects are constipated and tend to develop haemorrhoids; the back of the tongue is coated yellowish-white. Subjects are often extremely nervous and irritable; the condition is aggravated by eating and especially by rich foods, coffee and alcohol.

Kidneys
(See Also Renal Colic)

Kidneys are filters which can clean close to 60 litres of fluid per day. Their activity is essential to the survival of the body. If they stop working for more than 48 hours, uraemia will result.

An enlarged prostate is the surest sign of this disorder and must be remedied as quickly as possible. If the problem, which occurs mostly in older males, cannot be cured with hot compresses of plants in 24 hours, then catheters will have to be used, which can cause considerable discomfort.

In cases of kidney stones which obstruct the urethra (the canal through which urine passes), hot baths accompanied by light massage can have excellent results. To stimulate kidney activity in a general way, add chopped parsley to soups and sandwiches. Avoid salt, eat less meat, strong spices and refined sugar. When problems arise, take care to eliminate sugar-based foods from your diet.

Infusions like *Solidago* (also known as "golden rod"), couch grass or horsetail also help to activate the kidneys, as well as onion compresses.

On the other hand, certain precautions like drinking cold liquids slowly and protecting the kidneys from cold draughts, can also help to avoid complications.

Kidney Problems

Twice a day:

- *Berberis vulgaris 4 C.* 2 granules. Pains spreading to the hips, thighs or groin, and a burning sensation in the urethra or bladder when urinating are two common symptoms of *Berberis vulgaris*. The kidneys are terribly painful and sensitive to the touch, and the urine (which passes in small amounts) is dark coloured with greyish or brick-red sandy deposits.

Three times a day:

- *Cantharis 5 C.* 2 granules. The symptoms are more or less the same as for *Berberis vulgaris*, but the person seems markedly more agitated and the pain affects the kidneys more strongly.
- *Hydrangea 5 C.* 2 granules. The pain is felt more on the left and at the neck of the bladder. Characteristically, urine contains traces of blood and whitish sediments.
- *Pareira brava 4 C.* 2 granules. In this case, the pain starts from the kidneys and spreads to the thighs. The need to urinate is felt almost constantly, but violent straining then causes the person to crouch when urinating.

Liver
(See Also Hepatic Colic)

The liver is an essential organ that affects both our physical and mental well-being. It plays an important role in digestion, in the transformation of sugars and in the production of red blood cells. The liver is like a central exchange through which our mental attitudes influence our body, and the kinds of food we eat influence our mental state.

Multiple Symptoms

Do you tend to get drowsy between meals? Do you often suffer from nausea, dizziness, migraines, or break out in itching rashes? Are you nauseated by sweets or does fried food give you an upset stomach? Are you always thirsty? Do you find food cooked in grease repulsive? If so, there may well be something wrong with your liver.

The liver can also cause certain types of mental exhaustion. Are you depressed, always tending to see the dark side of things, or do you find the people around you hard to take? Once again, the cause of your problems may be a malfunction of your liver.

Before describing the remedies that can help cure liver disorders, we will discuss a few ways to avoid possible liver problems.

Start by Reviewing Your Diet

For cases of mild liver malfunction, start by reviewing your eating habits. Do you eat fatty foods? Lots of meat? Sauces? Sweets and cream? If so, you may have to make some changes.

If you succeed in modifying your eating habits, you can have a decisive influence on your health. And for those of you who have to undergo basic treatment, eating the proper foods will act as a powerful complement in effecting a cure. And don't forget that a balanced diet provides its own reward in the form of general well-being.

Black Radish

You can start by drinking radish or black radish juice (in capsules which dissolve in water, called *Raphanus sativus*). Of course, you'll have to reduce your cholesterol intake: eat more fish and less meat, and as little vegetable oil as possible.

You can eat as many fresh and dried fruits as you want (prunes, raisins, figs), green vegetables, lean fish, celery, potatoes, rice, salads and yoghurt. Eat oysters with every meal (when in season) and as many artichokes, celery and carrots as you can manage. Carrot juice also has a beneficial effect, as do bitter vegetables like endive and dandelion salad.

Non-Hydrogenated Oils

Opt for cold-pressed sunflower and sesame seed oils. Sesame seed oil is especially beneficial in cases of liver and gallbladder disorders. Sesame seeds also stimulate heart function (among other things) and act as a nerve tonic.

Of course, these recommendations are very general. To attain and remain in good health, you'll have to develop your own routine, based on trial and error depending on how you react to various foods - you can choose the combinations of foods that seem to work best for you.

Good Humour Makes for Good Meals

Making sure you eat proper foods is not the only thing you have to do to ensure good health. It isn't merely what you eat, but also how you eat that affects your body. If you are constantly worried about all kinds of problems and are unable to cope with stress, then don't be surprised if you develop liver problems.

That's why it's important to eat in a pleasant atmosphere. Avoid bringing your problems to the table - the dinner table is not the place to settle accounts. Concentrate on chewing your food well before swallowing it. It's also not a good idea to read or watch TV while eating.

Good Humour

In other words, avoid mulling over problems while eating. Make your meals a time for relaxation and pleasant conversation, and concentrate on the joys of eating wholesome, well-prepared food. You'll find this an excellent and rewarding exercise. Also, it's a good idea to give your digestive system a break now and then by fasting for a day.

After a few years, you'll realize that good health is not a moral issue at all. From a practical point of view, being in good health is simply the best way to take advantage of all the pleasures life has to offer while you're young, and to save time and spare yourself painful strain on your body as you grow older.

Attacks of Queasiness

A chronic liver disorder will be marked by acute attacks in an otherwise healthy person. It has been suggested that nine times out of ten, the attack is of emotional origin - worry, distress, heated discussions, anxiety, etc.

An attack of queasiness (acute hepatic congestion) starts with a migraine headache. Subjects seek darkness and sometimes experience visual problems. They want to be alone, feel constantly nauseous, but do not vomit. As for the area around the liver itself, people feel a kind of heaviness and discomfort rather than real pain.

The best thing to do is drink only water with buttermilk for 24 hours, then stick to vegetable broth and fresh fruit juice for a while.

Acute Attacks

To help patients suffering from acute attacks, administer 5 granules of *Ignatia 7 C* or *Phosphorus triiodatus 5 C,* and *Nux vomica 5 C,* alternated the following day with *Choloformum 5 C* (2 granules of each). To this add *Podophyllum 4 C* and *Berberis 4 C,* 2 granules of each, once a day.

Basic Remedies

These remedies are designed to strengthen the body as a whole, and to modify the way it reacts.

3 granules, once a week:

- *Chelidonium majus 7 C.* The most general remedy. People feel pain radiating from the liver region towards the right scapula (shoulder blade). The skin is yellowish; digestion is difficult, but improves with hot drinks; stool is a golden yellow colour and floats on the surface of the water.
- *Lachesis 7 C.* For liver disorders that are caused by infection. Patients feel ill, vomit bile, suffer from diarrhoea; skin and mucus are slightly yellow in places. Subjects find hot flushes and the contact of clothes or sheets uncomfortable; the condition is always worse after sleeping.
- *Lycopodium 7 C.* People feel heavy on their right side, at the level of the navel, to the point where they can't lie on their right side; their skin is yellowish around the temples; they are very hungry, but feel full after the first few mouthfuls of food, after which they suffer from persistent eructations which burn the throat persistently.

  They develop painful haemorrhoids. Use *Lycopodium* for liver disorders when subjects lose weight, and when secretions (sweat and urine) are extremely acidic. However, it should always be used in combination with another remedy, like *Phosphorus,* in a high dilution (7 to 9 C) or another basic treatment, since the body will be under some stress as it suddenly begins to reject toxins.

- *Phosphorus 7 C.* The liver area is swollen, painful, and sensitive to the touch. Stool is discoloured and difficult to evacuate; sometimes, however, stool is abundant, greasy and comes out in spurts, and has a fetid odour.

- *Podophyllum 7 C.* For chronic liver insufficiency or congestion characterized by problems with biliary secretion, and abundant diarrhoea of a yellow-brown or yellow-green colour, especially early in the morning or after meals. Diarrhoea alternates with constipation; stool is discoloured, and subjects suffer from headaches. Abdominal pains can be soothed with massages and rubbing, and headaches disappear a few minutes after people develop diarrhoea.

- *Sulphur 5 C.* Often prescribed for convalescing patients who experience raging hunger towards the end of the morning, which is soothed somewhat by eating; they are intensely thirsty and have a craving for sweets; flatulence smells like rotten eggs; they are constipated or have morning diarrhoea, are exhausted and suffer from hot flushes. The face is congested, the lips and ears are red. The condition is soothed by skin rashes.

Various Liver Disorders

- *Berberis 5 C.* When the left lobe is affected. Pains start suddenly, are strong enough to force people to double over and are aggravated by any jolts or sudden movements; pains radiate upwards under the left false ribs, and cross the liver region from front to back.

 Also for piercing liver pains which are aggravated by movement and accompanied by pain in the gallbladder, constipation and bad digestion.

- *Chelidonium 5 C.* The liver is painful, especially the right side; people suffer from piercing pains in the back, which shoot up to just under the right shoulder blade. The liver is sen sitive to the touch; the tongue is pasty and coated yellow, with red edges, and retains fingerprints after being pinched.

 Subjects have a bitter taste in their mouth; the condition is aggravated by movement and any kind of physical contact, and soothed by eating and drinking hot drinks, and by staying seated and leaning back. Digestion is slow; people feel drowsy and yawn a lot; urine is yellowish, pulse is slow.

- *Juglans cinerea 7 C.* Pains in the liver shoot up to the right shoulder, or under the left scapula, and are accompanied by headaches situated above the nape, morning nausea, itching, burning diarrhoea and insomnia (usually after three o'clock in the morning).
- *Lachesis 7 C.* For liver pains affecting alcoholics.
- *Nux vomica 7 C.* For chronic liver congestion. The liver is sensitive to the touch, even to contact of clothes; subjects are constipated and tend to develop haemorrhoids; the tongue is coated yellowish-white. Subjects are often extremely nervous and irritable; the condition is aggravated by eating (especially rich foods), coffee and alcohol.

Nausea

2 granules per hour:

- *Antimonium crudum 5 C.* For nausea caused by over-eating. The tongue is coated white. Also recommended for nausea that is relieved by eating.
- *Bryonia 5 C.* For nausea that increases during meals, or nausea which is eased by moving around.
- *Cocculus Indicus 5 C.* For nausea accompanied by dizziness or occurring after exposure to extreme cold or travelling.
- *Colchicum 5 C.* When the mere smell of food causes nausea.
- *Ipecac. 5 C.* If the nausea persists, and becomes permanent, and even vomiting doesn't help. The affected person salivates a lot.
- *Nux vomica 5 C.* When you've eaten too well and too much, take this after the meal. The back of the tongue has a yellowish coating. Also for nausea caused by smoking.
- *Symphoricarpus 4 C.* For nausea which is aggravated by any movement.

Parasites (Intestinal)

It can happen that some people live with intestinal parasites for years, even decades, without being aware of it. They should question themselves about the reasons for their bad health, anaemia and the dark rings around their eyes.

Although homeopathic treatment cannot guarantee total effective elimination of intestinal parasites, or parasites in general, it is still better at least to try and get rid of them first by using natural and homeopathic methods. If it doesn't work, more drastic measures will be required.

It's Sometimes Better To Wait

In infant cases, make a few attempts with homeopathic remedies before turning to allopathic medication. These toxic substances are sometimes worse than the problem they are meant to cure, since infants may not be able to metabolize them, even in the dosage recommended by a doctor.

What homeopathic cures do is first to ease the symptoms caused by the parasites, and then to neutralize the toxic substances produced by the worms, especially those that attack the nervous system.

Above all, however, homeopathic medicine works on the person's susceptibility, making he/she more resistant to invasion. As in most instances, an efficient immune system - which can be seen as a definition of "good health" - is our best protection.

So even if you decide to opt for allopathic treatment in a given situation, you should nevertheless continue with the homeopathic remedies, which will in no way obstruct the allopathic medication, quite the contrary. The following brief descriptions will enable you to identify the most common forms of parasites.

Parasites

Certain parasites, such as *Ascaris lumbricoides,* can travel from the intestines right up into the lungs, where they sometimes cause bronchitis before descending back through the digestive passages (sometimes even appearing in the mouth, in cases of a bad cough). They reach lengths of between 15 and 25 centimetres (6 to 10 inches).

Oxyurids are the most common intestinal parasites. They measure between 2 and 12 millimetres, and the females lay their eggs in the folds of the rectum.
Toxins secreted by worms cause intense anal itching. This can serve to spread contamination, since children will scratch themselves and gather eggs under their nails.

So during treatment, personal hygiene must be especially rigorous. Sheets and other bedclothes, as well as the room in general, must be kept clean to prevent re-contamination.

Taenia or the tapeworm can reach lengths of 5 to 10 metres! Its larvae are found in pork. The affected person loses weight despite a hearty appetite, suffers from dizzy spells, general discomfort and frequent mood changes. The treatment, which is long-term, is based on *Cuprum oxydatum nigrum* (see the list below).

Trichinae are small worms (between 2 and 4 millimetres) transmitted in pork meat. Troubles start with gastro-enteritis, marked by red skin rashes, followed by muscular pains about ten days later.

The signs:

- Face has irregular yellow blotches.
- The person is irritable, gets angry for no reason.
- Restless sleep, frequent waking up, grinding of teeth.
- Pale complexion, marked by bluish rings around the eyes and around the mouth.
- Breath is acidic and tasteless at the same time.
- Painful abdominal cramps.
- Itching of the anus and nose, especially at night.
- Grinding teeth during the night.
- Over-abundant salivation.
- In the case of oxyurids, frequent clearing of the throat.
- Parasites can cause personality problems. Ascarids: impulsiveness, melancholy, anxiety, inability to work or concentrate, tendency to faint. Oxyurids: irritability.
- Eyelids twitch, and sometimes strabismus appears.
- Despite all these symptoms, one or more lab tests are sometimes necessary to detect the presence of parasites, their eggs or cysts.
- Strange as it may seem, these symptoms are usually more pronounced at the time of a full moon.

Precautions

Avoid eating raw meat, which might be contaminated. As for pork, cook it for half an hour. Wash fruit and vegetables carefully: they may be contaminated with fertilizer. Wash lettuce in salt water and rinse thoroughly. Keep your nails short and clean them before every meal.

When cooking food, use a lot of shallots, garlic and wild garlic (wild garlic especially purifies the blood, the liver and bile, and is recommended for people suffering from arteriosclerosis and hypertension).

Papaya: A Natural Preventive

A good way to make your body resistant to parasites is to chew a papaya leaf at the end of each meal or to swallow a teaspoon of the fruit's black seeds. You can also obtain Papayasan granules for children, and papaya pills for adults.

Unfortunately, domestic pets are sometimes the cause. A dog can transmit tapeworms just by licking your hand.

- *Cina 4 C.* 2 granules twice a day. This is the remedy most often recommended to fight parasites, especially for patients who are hypersensitive, easily angered and unbearable. The person shows all the symptoms listed above. Anal and nasal itching cause disturbance throughout the night. Appetite is sporadic, the tongue is clean, and the person might experience involuntary urination at night.
- *Cuprum 4 C.* 2 granules three times a day. Spasms are observed.
- *Cuprum oxydatum nigrum 1 X* (1st decimal dilution), in 0.25 g packets of powder, one packet morning and night for six weeks, to fight the tapeworm: stomach pains, enormous appetite, dizziness and general discomfort, and mood changes are the symptoms used to detect the presence of this most unwelcome creature.

Also to fight trichinae:

- *Granatum 4 C.* 2 granules twice a day. The signs are accompanied by stomach-aches.
- *Granatum 4 C.* 3 granules twice a day. To combat all worms.
- *Helmintochortos T.M.* Take ten drops a day in a little water, for eight days.
- *Indigo 5 C.* 2 granules three times a day. For cases where discomfort is eased when the person moves.
- *Natrum phosphoricum 5 C.* 3 granules three times a day. For cases with stomach pains.
- *Sabadilla 5 C.* 2 granules three times a day. For people who suffer from stomach pains and itching in the ears. Children are nervous and susceptible to cold, but aren't especially moody. Coughing begins as soon as the child lies down.
- *Spigelia 5 C.* 2 granules three times a day. The distinctive symptoms for

this type: palpitations, coupled with coughing, very bad breath, stomach pains and anal itching. *Spigelia* fights ascarids as well as oxyurids.

- *Stannum 4 C.* 2 granules per day for ten days. For cases with convulsions, stiffness, weakness and/or blackouts and melancholy. This remedy fights tapeworms.
- *Teucrium marum 5 C.* 2 granules four times a day. Fights oxyurids and ascarids. Itching of the anus and nasal passages, aggravated by heat (hot beds, rooms etc.). The person is nervous, irritable and agitated throughout the night.
- *Viola odorata 4 C.* 2 granules four times a day. Very effective in building up resistance to parasites, fighting them when they are present and modifying the person's susceptibility to parasites.
- *Viola odorata 5 C.* 2 granules once every two days. Creates unfavourable conditions for parasites, and helps the body to get rid of them in a radical manner.

Poisoning

While waiting for a doctor, try to get the patient to vomit by tickling the back of the throat. A specialist is essential for determining the appropriate treatment.

Also refer to the section on Poisoning in the chapter on Accidents, Emergencies and Disorders.

Stomach

Various disorders may affect the stomach and cause digestive problems.

Note: medications should be administered at a dosage of 2 granules every half an hour if the pains are intense. Doses should then be spaced out gradually as the condition improves.

The Sensation of Having a Foreign Body in the Stomach

- *Abies nigra 5 C.* The sensation arises immediately after meals; subjects often lack appetite in the morning but even more before large meals; however, they suffer from raging hunger pangs in the middle of the night.

Sensation of a Distended Stomach

- *Cajuputum 5 C.* The sensation is accompanied by flatulence, which occurs in almost spontaneous spasms; people may have palpitations and pains in their heart during digestion. Constipation is often a secondary symptom.

- *Bovista 5 C*. When the sensation is stronger in the morning on waking up.

Ulcers

Ulcers are open wounds in the stomach or intestines. To some extent they are a modern disorder, resulting from a lifestyle of stress and hurried meals, which eventually break down our body's natural defences.

That is why trying to solve the problem through surgery is only a superficial approach. If you feel intense, very localized pain about four hours after meals, then you probably have an ulcer. But there are measures you can take to soothe the condition and avoid surgery, which is an extremely radical treatment without being really effective.

Of course, you must watch out for emergency signals: a stomach which is contracted and as hard as wood, sudden pain as if someone had punched you in the stomach, dark stool which would indicate haemorrhage and occasionally vomiting. All these indicate that something is drastically wrong - surgery should be performed within six hours.

But this kind of crisis can be avoided by adopting a lifestyle that is more compatible with the needs of your body. Try to look at a change of lifestyle as a benefit to your body rather than a punishment, and you'll soon realize that making the necessary changes will do a lot more than merely treat your ulcer, since you'll generally feel in much better shape than before. Remember, real health is more than just the absence of disease.

First, take your time when you eat. Don't read or watch TV during meals, since doing so tends to disrupt digestion, just like gobbling down some cake or ice-cream after a meal. Eat slowly, and chew your food well.

Avoid spicy foods, fizzy drinks, very hot soup and other liquids. Also cut down on the amount of salt you eat. Aspirin and cortisone derivatives should be avoided altogether.

Make a habit of drinking a glass of fresh potato or cabbage juice before meals. If you don't like the taste, add them to a bowl of soup, but don't cook them. You can also drink a teaspoon of powdered wood charcoal dissolved in a glass of warm water at the end of meals. A natural way to ease heartburn is to chew on raw oat flakes.

3 granules twice a day:

- *Argentum nitricum 5 C.* Pain is situated below the false ribs, and is aggravated by eating sweets (which people crave almost to the point of obsession). The pain is localized in the back - eating or applying pressure to the stomach makes it worse. People suffer from burning eructation and flatulence, as well as constant nausea. Diarrhoea is greenish in colour.

- *Arsenicum album 5 C.* People are feverish; burning pains occur after eating, which is the characteristic symptom of this type - they are soothed by applying hot compresses.

- *Bismuthum 4 C.* Pains begin immediately after eating, both in the pit of the stomach and at the back of the throat; people have to lean back to ease the pain; they cannot tolerate drinking water, preferring wine instead, and tend to regurgitate food long after it has been swallowed; headaches alternate with pains which cross the stomach at the level of the navel and get worse when walking.

- *Kali bichromicum 5 C.* Dull pains are accompanied by a feeling of pressure and heaviness, and spread right up to the shoulders. As well as suffering from discomfort during meals due to excessive acidity, patients experience sudden bouts of very acidic nausea; they are frequently constipated and feel a burning sensation in the anus and rectum; the tongue is red and dry.

- *Lycopodium 5 C.* People sit down to eat with a ravenous appetite, but feel full after a couple of mouthfuls; they suffer from excessive eructation and a burning sensation in the throat which can last for hours. Passing wind soothes the condition somewhat; stool is hard and difficult to evacuate; the liver is painful and sensitive to the touch.

- *Nux vomica 5 C.* For those who allow themselves to over-eat (especially greasy foods) and drink too much; they are often irritable; pains, in the form of cramps, begin about half an hour after meals. People have to loosen their clothing, especially around the waist; the back part of the tongue is coated.

Vomiting
(See Also Hepatic Colic, Constipation, Difficult Digestion,
Indigestion, Intolerance of Certain Foods,
Lazy Digestion, Nausea)

There are many possible causes of vomiting, from sea-sickness to ulcers to constipation. Vomiting may also be the only sign of an impending heart attack in older people.

Every half an hour:

- *Aethusa cynapium 4 C* (see Directions for Infants). For infants who immediately bring back up curdled milk; they are constantly sleepy and seem to get more and more weak and thin. Administer with *Calcarea carbonica 4 C* to combat acidity of the digestive tract.

- *Antimonium crudum 5 C*. 2 granules. The tongue is always coated with a milky-white substance; vomiting occurs after over-eating or drinking too much alcohol.

- *Bryonia alba 4 C*. People vomit water or bile just after meals; they are anxious and agitated, and drink small amounts of water. This type of vomiting may be the result of eating food which has gone bad.

- *China 4 C*. The tongue is yellow, people have a bitter taste in their mouth and feel weak after vomiting. The condition is caused by eating fruit that is not ripe.

- *Iris versicolor 4 C*. 2 granules after each time a person vomits. For cases of vomiting bile; individual feels a burning sensation in the stomach, throat and the digestive tract right down to the anus; the condition is accompanied by frequent headaches.

- *Ipecac. 4 C*. 2 granules. Vomiting due to improper diet. The tongue is clean, but subjects tend to be drowsy; vomiting does not provide any relief; over-abundance of saliva causes people to swallow constantly.

- *Nux vomica 4 C*. The tongue is coated yellow; people feel a heaviness in their stomach, but their condition improves with sleep. This disorder is due to the abuse of coffee or alcohol.

- *Pulsatilla pratensis 5 C*. The face is pale, the mouth pasty, the tongue yellowish; however, patients do not exhibit excessive thirst. Caused by eating too many pastries or fatty foods.

- *Sulphuricum acidum 5 C*. 2 granules every half an hour. In these cases, vomit is so acidic that patients can feel the deposits on their teeth.

Subjects are most often alcoholic.

Vomiting Blood

- *Ipecac. 4 C.* 2 granules every two hours. Blood is bright red. Patients are constantly nauseous, and tend to become numb.
- *Kreosotum 4 C.* 2 granules every two hours. People feel as if there were ice water in their stomach; drinking water leaves a bitter taste in their mouth.
- *Millefolium 4 C.* 2 granules. When blood is black and coagulates easily; patients are prostrate.

Chapter 6

Genito-Urinary System

Amenorrhoea (Lack of Menstruation)

Menstruation sometimes stops for various reasons other than pregnancy and menopause, for example ovarian malfunction, thyroid disorders, problems of the nervous system or tuberculosis.

In adolescents, the causes may be psychological and are often linked to anorexia. Even travelling by plane can disrupt the menstrual cycle.

Drink infusions of marjoram and mugwort (*Artemisia*) each evening and take a teaspoon of brewer's yeast before main meals. Avoid spices, alcohol, coffee, tea and sauces. Make breathing and physical exercises a regular part of your daily routine.

2 granules three times per day:

- *Aconitum 5 C*. When menstruation stops after catching cold or because of a shock. For women who are agitated and anxious.
- *Bryonia 6 C*. When pains and sensitivity in the lower abdomen are aggravated by movement and soothed by firm, prolonged pressure. Menstruation usually stops after catching a cold; in hot weather, periods are frequently accompanied by nosebleeds and headaches. Also for amenorrhoea which occurs while travelling.
- *Calcarea carbonica 5 C*. This remedy is especially helpful for adolescent girls who are pale, who perspire easily and who suffer from gastric and intestinal acidity; they have a milky discharge when urinating. Also for cases of menstruation which stops after a cold bath.
- *Kali carbonicum 5 C*. For young women who are anaemic and whose menstruation has stopped for some months; they are tired and depressed, suffer from aches and back pains, especially in the middle of the night. Any kind of exertion makes them perspire; they catch cold easily, and their pulse is weak and irregular.
- *Lachesis 5 C*. Periods are difficult and accompanied by circulatory problems; also for cases where menstruation stops after some trauma or emotional shock, or because of premature menopause.
- *Lillium tigrinum 5 C*. Interruption of menstruation is accompanied by dizziness.
- *Opium 5 C*. Interruption of menstruation due to a scare.
- *Pulsatilla 5 C*. 2 granules. For gentle-natured women whose periods are interrupted because of anaemia, nervousness or when they get their feet wet. They cannot tolerate heat and have trouble digesting fatty foods,

pastries and fried food.

- *Sanguinaria 5 C*. Interruption of menstruation is accompanied by hot flushes and headaches which are concentrated around the temples.

Bartholinitis

Infection of Bartholin's glands, which lubricate the vagina, is generally characterized by painful inflammation of the outer lips of the vagina. The inflammation quickly increases in volume, and it is usually necessary to surgically drain the pus which accumulates in the swelling after a few days, unless the homeopathic treatment produces rapid results.

It is best to consult a doctor before the gland bursts and the infection spreads. In any case, continue the homeopathic treatment to prevent the condition from recurring and to accelerate the healing process.

- Take supplements of *vitamins C* and *A*. Also take (sitz) baths in bran water or with a decoction of marshmallow root for three minutes, three times per day. You can also resort to vaginal douches, using the following aromatic solution: 2 granules of *Thuja occidentalis T.M.*, 2 granules of *Hydrastis Canadensis T.M., Sabina 6X* (6th dilution), 2 granules of *Essence of Cedar*, 2 granules of *Essence of Cypress*, and *Alcohol 90°* (q.s.p. 250 cc).
- Also 3 granules three times per day:
- *Hepar sulphuris calcareum 5 C* and *Pyrogenium 5 C*.

Bladder Troubles
(See Also Cystitis)

The bladder is made of muscle fibre, and can hold up to three quarters of a litre of liquid. It is also subject to inflammation, in which case the desire to urinate is frequent, even though only a few drops may be expelled, sometimes with great difficulty and sometimes with a lot of pain. If this happens to you, it can be treated by drinking an extract of juniper berries or infusions of juniper leaves.

Breast-feeding

Studies conducted in Sweden on a number of generations have shown that children who are breast-fed run less risk of becoming diabetic. This fact alone is a good enough reason to feed your child the "natural" way.

Also, mother's milk (and especially milk produced during the three or four days after birth - called "colustrum") provides quantities of mineral salts, vitamins and antibodies which protect infants against disease during the early stages of life.

Breast-feeding also brings mother and child closer together, giving the child its first experience of human contact, which is so essential if the child is to develop in a harmonious and secure fashion.

Soothing music has been shown to have a beneficial effect on breast-feeding.

What To Avoid

Alcohol and allopathic medications are to be avoided (especially drugs like anti-depressants and even aspirin) as much as possible; also tobacco, especially in the first few weeks after giving birth.

Problems With Breast-Feeding

For cases where the nipples are extremely sensitive, whether or not cracks develop, prepare dressing with *Homeodora* cream and apply between feeds. Or you can try *Calendula cream* or *Chamomilla* orally for sore nipples and *Nitric acidum* for cracked nipples.

If Milk Diminishes in Quantity or Quality

Make sure mothers drink enough liquids and eat enough starchy foods (potatoes, beans and lentils, for example), wholemeal bread, honey, fruit, carrots, fennel, brewer's yeast and oranges.

Breast-feeding Diet

Diets of breast-feeding mothers should be rich in protein obtained from lean meat and fish, eggs and hard cheese. They should drink a glass of fresh carrot juice per day and make sure they get enough vitamin A, C, D and E.

Feed more often but for short periods, using both breasts; when the condition improves, spread out the feeds again.

Mother and Child Are Connected

Finally, you should be aware that many emotions are also transmitted through the process of breast-feeding. Strong emotions like anger and fear make mother's milk bad for baby (see *Chamomilla* for this problem). Keep this in mind and work even harder on staying calm and serene at home and with your child.

Homeopathic Remedies During Breast-feeding

Every three hours:

- *Arnica 4 C.* 3 granules. Women have sore nipples for the first few days after birth; they feel exhausted; head and hands are flushed, while the nose and the rest of the body are cold.
- *Bryonia 5 C.* 2 granules. When breasts are excessively swollen.
- *Calcarea carbonica 9 C.* 2 granules. Administer to women who plan to breast-feed, starting right after the birth. Also for cases where breasts are distended and painful, and women (usually blond and slightly overweight types) were often late menstruating.
- *Chamomilla 5 C.* 2 granules. For nervous and agitated mothers; the tip of the breasts is red and very sensitive to touch. Cramps in the uterus felt by the mother as soon she starts to breast-feed are a characteristic sign.
- *Cina rubra 5 C.* 2 granules. For mothers who are fatigued from breast-feeding.
- *Dulcamara 4 C.* 2 granules. When milk suddenly stops flowing after catching a cold; breasts are swollen but not painful.
- *Phellandrum 5 C.* 2 granules. Women suffer from breast pain when feeding.
- *Pulsatilla 5 C.* 2 granules. For mothers who produce too much milk.

Breasts

In cases where lumps appear (mastosis), a doctor should be consulted immediately. You can examine yourself regularly (four or five days before your period). This is especially recommended after the age of forty. Your doctor can provide you with more information on the subject.

The idea is not to make you nervous or afraid once a month, but simply to make sure that you are not hiding anything from yourself. If you do hide the condition for too long, you may make effective treatment impossible.

Appearance

You can use natural methods to firm up your breasts. These methods are not dangerous and only require a certain amount of will-power.

The first thing you can do is use cold hydrotherapy: press a sponge soaked in cold water to your breasts a number of times. Then rub them with eau de cologne (90°). Also doing appropriate exercises (stretching the arms backwards, for example) can help develop a firm chest. However, be careful of sports that may damage the breasts.

Posture also plays an important role. Stand up straight as much as possible, with your shoulders back. This gives a more shapely curve to your chest. Wear an adjustable bra that suits the form of your breasts. It is true that we often don't know how to stand - it's as if our own body were a stranger to us. And it is not necessarily a question of muscles: we sometimes have to modify the balance of our spine before working on the muscles in the back. A course in yoga stretching techniques would be the best way to go about acquiring good posture.

Finally, a healthy diet rich in vitamins will help keep breasts shapely and firm (consult the section on Gastritis for a detailed description of such a diet).

Pains in the Breasts

3 granules once a day:

- *Chimaphila umbellata 4 C.* For breasts which are overdeveloped (hypertrophy), hard and slightly painful to the touch; appropriate for women who are overweight and have trouble urinating.
- *Chimaphila umbellata 7 C.* Breasts are not very developed, hard in places and painful; appropriate for young girls who tend to have skin problems, or for older women who are generally weak.
- *Conium 5 C.* Breasts start to get slightly larger, then diminish in size and become flaccid; also for cases of cysts or benign lumps in the breasts.
- *Conium macula turn 5 C.* If taken early enough, this remedy can prevent breasts from getting soft and flaccid.
- *Belladonna 5 C.* For the onset of abscesses on the breasts; skin is red, and women feel a pulsing, throbbing pain in the affected area.
- *Bellis perennis 5 C.* For pain in the breasts caused by bruises.
- *Bryonia 4 C.* Breasts are swollen, hard and hot, and paler than usual; they feel heavy and any kind of movement, pressure or even touch aggravates the pain; pain is soothed when breasts are firmly bound or supported.

Also for cases of pain in the breasts during each period, particularly when accompanied by intense thirst.

- *Clematis erecta 6 C.* Breasts are swollen and hard, and sensitive to the touch; shooting pain is aggravated at night, but there is no discharge.
- *Phellandrium 5 C.* For breasts which hurt during breast-feeding.

- *Pulsatilla 5 C.* Breasts are blocked and dilated veins can be observed under the skin, especially during periods, which are often late, intermittent, with thick dark blood containing clots.

Cracked breasts

For cracked or chapped breasts, apply an ointment made up of a mixture of 2 grams of *Castor equi* and 20 grams of pure, sterilized vaseline. Prepare a sterilized compress, coated with this substance, and place it on the affected breast.

Childbirth
(See Also Pregnancy, Breast-feeding)

Homeopathic medicine can be very useful for future mothers (see the section on Pregnancy) especially when it comes to reducing the intensity of labour pains.

During Pregnancy

Make sure you take a walk every day and move around enough so that the foetus does not become too large. As for diet, gradually reduce the amount of salt you use during the last two weeks before giving birth, until you have eliminated it completely.

Preparing for Birth

For two months preceding the birth, take *Nux vomica 7 C,* 3 granules per day, to reduce labour pains.

During the last month, take *Caulophyllum 12 C,* 5 granules once a week, to prepare the muscles of the uterus so they will contract as they should.

For the last two weeks preceding birth, take *Arnica 5 C,* 2 granules in the morning and at night. This will make the birthing process more regular, the contractions more efficient, and eliminate risks of infection.

On another level, but one which is also important, mothers who want to get rid of the excess fat that builds up on the thighs and bottom should take *Natrum sulphuricum 9 C* and *Thuja 9 C,* alternating 5 granules of each every two weeks before going to bed, for as many months as possible during the pregnancy.

However, this prescription does not mean mothers should stop doing at least a minimum of exercise and watching their diet closely after giving birth, even though many women find it difficult to stick to a diet during this period.

During Childbirth

- *Actaea racemosa 4 C.* 2 granules every two hours, makes uterine contractions more effective, thereby easing the birthing process. It also calms over-excited nerves which many women experience during the birth (and understandably so).
- *Arnica 5 C.* During labour, 2 granules every hour, alternated with *Cimicifuga 4 C. Arnica* prevents the risk of haemorrhage, helps fight contractions which are too painful and the risk of infection after giving birth. Take two granules every two hours, starting 12 hours before the expected delivery time.
- *Calcarea acetica 4 C.* 2 granules every half an hour if the labour goes on a long time.
- *Caulophyllum 4 C.* When the cervix is rigid and contractions are so short they resemble shivers.
- *Chamomilla 5 C* alternating with *Coffea 4C.* 3 granules every half an hour if labour pains become intolerable.
- *Cimicifuga 4 C. 3* granules every hour. Speeds up dilation of the cervix if it is slow in opening (which makes labour pains ineffective).
- *China 4 C.* 3 granules every half an hour, or even every quarter of an hour, in case of abundant or prolonged blood flow before birth.
- *Coffea 5 C.* 2 granules every hour. For women who complain incessantly during labour. Their eyes are glassy, their face is flushed and swollen; the cervix is hardly dilated at all.
- *Kali carbonicum 5 C.* 2 granules every half an hour. Pains spread to the thighs and buttocks, and labour does not progress as it should.
- *Gelsemium sempervirens 5 C.* 2 granules every half an hour. The face is congested, and women become obsessed by the desire to be alone. The birth does not progress and the cervix remains closed.
- *Opium 5 C.* 2 granules every half an hour. The face is congested and women are tormented by shaking and convulsions, even though labour does not progress as it should.
- *Sepia 5 C.* 2 granules every half an hour. For slow labour, accompanied by shooting pains in the back and legs; yellow spots appear on the nose and other parts of the body. Sepia is also useful for countering the effects of post-natal depression.

Cystitis

Cystitis is an infection of the urinary system. It is characterized by sharp, acute pains in the urethra while urinating. In the inflammatory stage urinating becomes difficult, urine may be tainted with blood and accompanied by a viscous discharge. Consulting a doctor is an absolute necessity.

Women are more susceptible to the disease, which is usually triggered by the cold and is caused by an intestinal colibacillus (*E. Coli*). Women should take very hot (sitz) baths :37-38°C (98.6 - 100.4°F) for periods of half an hour.

Prevention

Since the disorder is often caused by a bacterium of intestinal origin, a simple preventive method is to clean the anus from front to back after defaecating. Not drinking enough creates conditions favourable for the proliferation of bacteria, since elimination occurs less frequently. It is a good idea to get used to drinking liquids at regular intervals. For chronic cystitis, consult a doctor.

3 granules once a day:

- *Cannabis Indica 5 C*. People have trouble urinating - discomfort occurs before, during and after - and may experience some dripping; they feel as if a hard ball were forming in the urethra or perineum, between the anus and the genitals.

  There is some degree of nervousness, as well as sexual arousal. Men experience painful erections.

- *Cannabis sativum 5 C*. Tension is painful, there is a burning sensation and a constant urge to urinate (every half an hour). Urinating is very painful.

  There is some yellow discharge and the urine contains pus. The urethra, and for men the penis, are very painful to the touch. Men may have trouble walking, experience painful erections and pain in their testicles.

- *Cantharis 5 C*. Symptoms closely resemble those of *Cannabis Indica,* but urine is less abundant, and searing and burning pains are more intense.

  Urine flows slowly, coming out in drops, the flow being interrupted by painful contractions. *Cantharis* cases are often sexually aroused, with painful erections in men and nymphomaniac tendencies in women.

- *Equisetum 5 C*. People experience discomfort in the bladder, which always feels full; the sensation is not soothed by urinating; the urge to urinate is intense, and accompanied by shooting pains in the urethra.

Urinating is difficult, and urine is full of mucus; pains are often worse when finishing urinating and the bladder is very sensitive to the touch. In some cases, urine contains pus.

- *Mercurius corrosivus 5 C*. Characterized by the presence of albumin in the urine, an intense, almost continual burning sensation and a constant urge to urinate. The disorder is aggravated by heat and gets worse during the night.

  Urinating is accompanied by a burning sensation in the urethra, which is so painful that patients sweat profusely; only a small amount of urine actually comes out.

- *Pareira brava 5 C*. There is a constant need to urinate. Urine is passed drop by drop, and patients often have to get down on all fours. Urine is mixed with blood and mucus, and is dark in colour.

- *Sarsaparilla 5 C*. Patients feel a constant need to urinate, but cannot always succeed in passing urine. If they do, urinating is accompanied by an intense burning sensation, especially when seated.

  They are able to urinate more easily when standing up. Passing urine, which may contain sediment, is difficult - children will often cry while urinating.

- *Terebinthina 5 C*. Once again there is a burning sensation while urinating; a small amount of urine is passed, it is very dark (sometimes as dark as coffee) with lots of blood; it smells something like violets; the tongue is red, dry, smooth and painful.

Dysmenorrhoea

Women who have painful periods - and there are many - find themselves severely handicapped for a few days every month, both at home and in the workplace. Painful periods place an added burden on these women. Fortunately, it is possible to do something about the problem.

In cases where cramps are frequent, try a preparation containing *Petasites* (butterbur). There are a number of homeopathic remedies which can ease the problem. Choose one that is appropriate to the individual's symptoms.

- *Actaea racemosa 5 C*. 2 granules every two hours unless otherwise indicated. Periods are irregular, exhausting, and blood flow contains black clots. Pains appear under the left breast. A characteristic of these cases is that the more abundant the flow of blood, the more painful the periods are, with intense shooting pains especially on the left side.

- *Belladonna 4 C.* 2 granules every quarter of an hour, for women who get their periods early; blood is bright red and abundant; pain seems to be dragging the organs downwards.
- *Borax 5 C.* For women who are agitated and hypersensitive, especially to noise; periods come early and are preceded by an acidic, warm and abundant discharge the colour of egg white.
- *Caulophyllum 5 C.* Intermittent spasmodic pains which resemble labour pains.
- *Chamomilla 6 C.* For women who are ordinarily high strung and irritable, and who become even more so before and during menstruation. Blood flow is abundant and accompanied by intense abdominal pains; blood is dark and coagulated; coffee seems to aggravate the symptoms.
- *Colocynthis 5 C.* Pain is so intense that women are doubled over and dig their fists into their abdomen; subjects are nervous and irritable.
- *Magnesia muriatica 4 C.* For nervous, irritable cases; blood is dark and contains clots, and flows more easily when patients rest; there is some pain in the kidney region.
- *Magnesia phosphorica 4 C.* 2 granules every quarter of an hour. When blood flow is dark and contains membranous tissue; women suffer from pains around the ovaries, especially on the right. The first day of periods is the most painful; pains are eased somewhat when women double up.
- *Platina 5 C.* Periods are accompanied by spasmodic nervous disorders; blood contains large dark clots; women tend to be melancholic.
- *Pulsatilla 5 C.* Periods arrive late, blood flow is scanty, intermittent and often accompanied by diarrhoea; women or girls shiver and tend to cry, and suffer from headaches and stomach-aches.

Enuresis (Bedwetting)

After about three years of age, bedwetting becomes abnormal and problematic for both parents and children. However, the problem should be treated discreetly, as it can have a profound effect on the process of growth and maturity. You may aggravate the problem by bringing it out into the open.

As you probably know, it's useless to blame or threaten children who suffer from enuresis. The problem, which is psychological, can be cured through homeopathic treatment combined with psychotherapy. But don't expect to see results overnight. It can take up to a year for a skilled homeopath to free a child, and parents, from this annoying disorder.

In the meantime, try and be patient and pay special attention to your child's behaviour because, through this abnormal behaviour, your child is trying to tell you something. Affected children are often nervous, highly emotional, and find it very difficult to express their emotions.

Before going to bed:

- *Belladonna 5 C.* 2 granules. Children's sleep is agitated; they talk and cry out in their sleep and are aware of urinating in their dreams.
- *Benzoicum acidum 5 C.* 2 granules. Urine has a strong characteristic odour.
- *Cina 4 C.* 2 granules. Sleep is agitated and children often have nightmares; they are bad-tempered, have rings under their eyes and dilated pupils; they often rub their nose or anus (make sure you're not dealing with a case of intestinal parasites).
- *Hyoscyamus niger 5 C.* 2 granules. For children who wet the bed and defaecate in their sleep. Administer with *Eupatorium purpureum 4 C,* 2 granules, every night before bed.
- *Kreosotum 5 C.* 2 granules. Children urinate in the first few hours after falling asleep; it's very hard to wake them up; they dream they are on the toilet when urinating in bed. In adult cases, people wake up too late and have no time to get to the toilet.
- *Pulsatilla 5 C.* 2 granules before going to bed. For rather shy children and also for children who constantly feel the need to urinate when in bed, but are so tired they fall asleep, at which point they wet the bed.

Genital Organs: Female

Congestion of the Uterus

The first thing you can do is take long sitz baths once or twice a week.

If pains occur outside of periods, use *Aesculus hippocastanum 5 C,* 3 granules per day. This remedy is also recommended if you feel a pulsing sensation behind the pubis or if you have any thick, sticky, irritating dark yellow discharge which gets worse after periods.

In cases of chronic congestion which leads to hardening of the uterus but without any haemorrhage, try *Aurum muriaticum natronatum 6 C,* 3 granules per day. Instead try *Aurum muriaticum 6 C,* 3 granules per day if the condition is accompanied by yellow, burning discharge. If the condition is accompanied by haemorrhage, use *Aurum muriaticum kalinatum 6 C,* 3 granules twice a day.

Pains During Menstruation
See Dysmenorrhea.

Pain in the Ovaries
3 granules twice a day:
- *Naja 6 C.* Pains are on the left side and get worse during menstruation; they seem to radiate right up to the heart; wearing tight clothes aggravates the condition.
- *Colocynthis 9 C.* Also for pains in the left ovary; these pains, however, are spasmodic and are triggered by annoyance or anger.
- *Platina 9 C.* For pains in either of the ovaries; subjects suffer from cramps, which get worse during periods; the genital organs are painful when touched.
- *Lycopodium 7 C.* For cases of pain in the right ovary.

Hypersensitivity of the Genital Organs
For cases of hypersensitivity of the female genital organs in general (whether during sexual intercourse or simply from the contact of clothing) use *Platina 6 C,* 3 granules twice a day. Also if you feel as if your period is about to start, or if it starts again after you think it's over, or if you suffer from insomnia accompanied by sexual arousal. Use *Staphysagria 6C* in cases of intense sexual obsession and where women are irritable in mood.

Genital Organs: Male

Congestion of the Prostate
- *Sabal serrulata compound,* ten drops three times per day. For inflammation of the prostate, accompanied by painful erections and discharge of semen at night, as well as some degree of sexual impotence. *Sabal* helps eliminate these problems without diminishing the volume of the prostate.

Zinc

Note: zinc is an essential nutrient for the proper functioning of the male sexual organs. It also helps prevent prostate disorders.

Hypersensitivity of the Genital Organs

3 granules twice a day:

- *Staphysagria 6 C*. For hypersensitivity of the genitals, sometimes accompanied by obsessive sexual arousal; masturbation or excessive sexual activity does not seem to ease the symptoms.

Inflammation of the Urethra

The urethra is the channel that carries urine from the bladder to the tip of the penis. When the problem, which is accompanied by discharge, is caused by a venereal infection, subjects must use antibiotics. But if the cause is not venereal, homeopathic treatment can cure the condition.

3 granules three times per day:

- *Petroselinium 5 C*. Discharge is accompanied by itching or an intense need to urinate.
- *Pulsatilla 5 C*. Discharge has a yellow colour.
- *Mercurius solubilis 5 C*. Discharge has a greenish colour.
- *Kali bichromicum 5 C*. When urine contains filaments of mucus.

Gonorrhoea

This infectious disease of the genito-urinary organs is caused by a microbe and is sexually transmitted. The condition produces inflammation of the urethra - the channel through which urine is carried from the bladder to the genitals.

Gonorrhoea is characterized by a burning sensation while urinating, which appears a few days after becoming infected. Other symptoms include a rather purulent discharge in men, and abdominal pains and discharge of pus through the vagina in women.

The best thing to do is to consult an allopathic doctor, who will prescribe penicillin. Once the symptoms have cleared up, begin a programme of homeopathic treatment, which can rid the body of toxins produced by the disease. Homeopathy is also helpful in fighting persistent cases which do not respond to repeated allopathic treatments.

Abstain from sexual intercourse while infected, unless you use a condom.

Wash your hands carefully after urinating. Take long warm baths and avoid excessive physical exertion.

3 granules three times per day:

- *Cantharis 9 C.* Patients experience intense searing pain before, during and after urinating. Urine, which comes in trickles, may be dark red in colour and may contain some sediment.

  In some cases, patients are agitated and even sexually aroused - men have painful erections.

- *Capsicum 5 C.* People often feel the need to urinate, which causes a burning sensation (as if they had eaten a lot of raw pepper) in the bladder and meatus (urinary orifice).

  Subjects also suffer from a creamy white discharge. Other frequent symptoms are a swollen foreskin and cold shivers immediately after drinking.

- *Gonotoxinum 9 C.* This is the basic remedy, which you can combine with one of the other remedies, depending on the individual symptoms.

- *Mercurius corrosivus 6 C.* Burning pain is intense, and gets worse at night and in heat. Men find their penis is inflamed, but not sensitive to touch.

Leucorrhoea

This term is used to describe the various kinds of vaginal discharge and blood flow, apart from menstruation, experienced by women and girls. These may also occur in prepubescent girls, in which case a foreign body may be lodged in the vagina. A specialist can carry out an ultrasound examination to locate the problem.

Girls normally have discharges, starting about two years before their periods start as the ovaries begin secreting. And in the first few periods after puberty, some discharge is inevitable and quite normal. However, this does not mean that proper hygiene around the vagina should be neglected.

White Discharge

This signals pathological and infectious cases of leucorrhoea. They affect the mucous membranes and may occur after exposure to cold or because of overwork or stress. As harmful bacteria take hold, the body reacts by producing mucus which is called "whites" - a thick, yellowish, foul-smelling, burning discharge.

How To React

To combat this problem, drink infusions of camomile to which you add 3 or 4 teaspoons of *Molkosan,* a natural lactic acid. This serves to replace the acid medium in the mucous membranes which is destroyed by the discharge.

Also take herbal (sitz) baths (thyme or juniper) at 98.6°F (37°C), for half an hour each time, 2 or 3 times a week. Stimulating blood circulation in the abdominal area helps the body react more effectively.

As for diet, consult the section on Gastritis in the chapter on digestive disorders. Make sure you get enough vitamins A, B_2, B_3 and C.

Also get a doctor to perform a cytological examination to test for bacteria.

Antibiotics - Anti-Life

The problem with antibiotics, which are considered a modern and easy solution to all kinds of infectious disorders, is that they destroy beneficial as well as harmful bacteria. This makes it hard for the body to re-establish a balance of bacterial flora, which is necessary for good health. Also, bear in mind that harmful bacteria reproduce much more quickly than beneficial bacteria. So before you resort to antibiotics, try to resolve the problem with a homeopathic remedy.

3 granules once a day:

- *Alumina 5 C.* Discharge is very abundant, transparent, acidic and corrosive. It starts suddenly in the middle of the day, and is soothed by washing with cold water.

  The genital area is inflamed, with burning and itching sensations; the skin and mucous membranes are dry; blood flow during menstruation is very limited; women tend to be weak, thin and somewhat depressed.
- *Borax 5 C.* The discharge resembles egg white (albumin) and runs like a hot liquid down the thighs, accompanied by a sensation of heat in the vagina. Subjects are very nervous; periods are abundant and painful.
- *Cubeba 5 C.* Discharge is creamy, thick and irritating; the condition occurs most often in young girls; discharge is often accompanied by a burning sensation in the vulva or vagina when urinating.
- *Kreosotum 5 C.* Discharge is yellowish in colour and irritating; it stains underwear, has an unpleasant odour and produces pricking and burning pains between the thighs and around the vaginal lips. Periods are intermittent or come on early; patients lack strength in their legs.
- *Mercurius 5 C.* Discharge is greenish and burning, and is more pronounced at night and while urinating. Patients suffer from intense

itching, which gets worse after urinating but is soothed by washing with cold water.

Periods are abundant and painful with blood which is black and contains clots; subjects have bad breath and perspire a lot at night.

- *Nitricum acidum 5 C*. Discharge is abundant, brownish in colour, viscous and contains filaments of matter and blood. Women tend to haemorrhage; periods often start early, blood flow is abundant and has the consistency of reddish coloured water.
- *Pulsatilla 5 C*. For discharge in girls, especially if gentle and passive by nature. The condition is not painful or irritating; it may be aggravated by cold weather, or when subjects are lying down; periods are late, blood flow is scanty and periods pass quickly.
- *Sepia 5 C*. Discharge is yellow and acidic, with the consistency of milk; it is more marked before periods, which are often late. Women are often melancholic and seek solitude.

Menopause

Menopause is a difficult period of transition which women must pass through before reaching what has been called one of the most serene of all the stages of life.

Various problems may accompany the menopause: hot flushes, headaches, ringing in the ears, floating spots before the eyes, respiratory tightness, personality problems like melancholy, irritability and even depression.

However, these symptoms are not inevitable: some women hardly notice that they're going through the menopause at all.

When problems do arise, it's a good idea to consult a doctor in order to avoid possible complications. But in certain mild cases, where the problems are tolerable, you can start by taking matters into your own hands.

A Healthy Reaction

Start with the body: exercise and fresh air, brisk walks and deep breathing can help to a great extent. Take sitz baths, adding hay flowers or *Alchemilla* (lady's mantle) to the water. Rub yourself down every day.

Avoid getting overtired and over-extending yourself. Also stop drinking coffee, tea and alcohol during this period. Replace them with infusions of thyme, marjoram and rosemary.

The better you sleep the more your body regains its strength every night, and this will help you remain in good humour and avoid getting nervous.

3 granules three times per day:

- *Aconitum 7 C*. For hot flushes.
- *Actaea racemosa 5 C*. For women who are melancholic, and who are afraid of going insane because of the incoherence they observe in their thinking. They tend to be very talkative. If periods resume, the psychological symptoms disappear.
- *Glonoinum 5 C*. Subjects feel their pulse beating in the veins all over their body and cannot tolerate light; pulse is rapid, sometimes strong and sometimes weak, and irregular.
- *Ignatia 5 C*. Women are very sensitive, very emotional, unstable, often sad and melancholic. They feel intense pulsations, especially around the temples. They suffer from headaches, and get dizzy when they stand up suddenly. Heat, especially around the head, seems to aggravate the problem. They also have trouble tolerating various odours, especially that of tobacco.
- *Lachesis 7 C*. Once a month only. For cases where women suffer from dizziness, headaches, nightmares, insomnia and hot flushes; they seem to alternate between states of euphoria and despair; sometimes accompanied by haemorrhoids and nosebleeds. *Lachesis* may re-start menstruation, as well as stabilizing the subject's personality.
- *Sepia 5 C*. For hot flushes, fatigue and slight faintness; subjects tend to be melancholic, lack motivation, and may become depressed.
- *Sulphur 5 C*. For women who are troubled by periodic depression and suffer from headaches and hot flushes; they feel too hot when in bed and need to get out in the fresh air; they are tired, especially towards mid-day, to the point where they can hardly stand up; lips and ears are very red, and they tend to itch in various parts of the body. This is a general remedy, along with *Lachesis*.
- *Thuja 5 C*. For women who feel they are getting old and who find themselves becoming more and more obsessed about various things.
- *Ustilago maydis 5 C*. Sudden hot flushes give these women the feeling that water is flowing down their back; they cannot tolerate hot stuffy rooms, and may even faint if they don't get enough fresh air; they tend to be depressive and irritable. Their condition improves when they start to move around, for example when they take a walk. They have a low pain threshold.

Metrorrhagia

Here blood flows from the uterus even when women are not having their periods. The condition may indicate cancer of the uterus (especially if bleeding is not abundant, and the blood contains impurities). But most often, it is simply indicative of a hormonal imbalance, or of a benign ulcer. Only a doctor can provide a clear diagnosis.

Menorrhagia, on the other hand, is characterized by too much blood flow during periods, and is generally caused by a tumour in the uterus (fibroma). In these cases, consulting a competent doctor is absolutely necessary.

While Waiting To See a Doctor

Stay in bed with your feet raised, and without a pillow under your head. Place an ice pack wrapped in a towel or pillow-case on your stomach.

3 granules every hour:

- *Bovista 4 C*. For accidents - blood flow is dark and contains clots; it is often accompanied by diarrhoea, or preceded and accompanied by discharge (leucorrhoea) which resembles albumin (egg white); subjects bleed when blowing their nose.
- *Erigeron 3 C*. Blood flow is bright red and does not contain clots; it comes out in spurts, and the condition is aggravated by movement.
- *Sabina 5 C*. 2 granules every two hours. Blood is bright red, contains no clots and comes out in spurts. Also for haemorrhaging in pregnant women, when a miscarriage seems imminent.
- *Thlaspi 4 C*. Women haemorrhage black, coagulated blood; uterine cramps are eased when subjects lean forward; if there is discharge before or after periods, it contains brownish coloured blood that has an unpleasant odour.
- *Trillium 4 C*. For haemorrhage of bright red blood.
- *Ustilago 4 C*. The blood is dark, containing blackish clots, and may smell bad; this type of haemorrhage is not painful, and oozes or flows very slowly; women are depressed and irritable, their periods usually come early, and are abundant and prolonged.

Miscarriage

This distressing event is usually the result of some kind of shock, accident or trauma. Women are in a state of shock, and ache all over their body. In all cases, women should take a vitamin E supplement, in the form of wheat germ or the medication *Ephynal*.

- *Arnica 5 C*. 5 granules. Administer immediately after miscarriage.
- *Caulophyllum 4 C*. 3 granules every half an hour. For miscarriage due to weakness of the uterus, with false labour pains and haemorrhage. This type of miscarriage usually occurs towards the end of the pregnancy.
- *China 4 C*. 5 granules. Administer immediately after a miscarriage.
- *Kali carbonicum 5 C*. 3 granules every three hours. After a miscarriage, for women who lack strength and suffer from back pains.
- *Millefolium 4 C*. 3 granules every half an hour. For cases of abundant haemorrhage after strenuous exercise or physical exertion. Pains may or may not be present.
- *Sabina 4 C*. 3 granules per hour. The most general remedy for miscarriage. The first signs are slight blood spots, which turn into profuse bleeding of bright red blood that contains clots. Pains occur in the lower back and increase in intensity, spreading into the pubic area. Bleeding increases with any movement.
- *Secale cornutum 4 C*. 3 granules every half an hour. For thin, fragile women who have suffered from trauma or had an accident in the first or last months of pregnancy.
  The problem starts with false labour pains, followed by haemorrhage. Blood is black, and any movement makes the condition worse. Women are fatigued, and may experience a sensation of pins and needles in their extremities.
- *Viburnum 4 C*. Sudden abdominal cramps signal the onset of *Viburnum* cases; the cramps ease painful spasms and uterine pains.

Pregnancy
(See Also Childbirth, Miscarriage, Vaccinations, Varicose Veins)

Since homeopathy is a science based on the concept that health is more than the simple absence of illness, this section on pregnancy is longer than might be expected. Our aim, after all, is to ensure that people gain the maximum possible benefits that life has to offer.

The advice and recommendations that follow are in no way meant to replace the work of a competent physician, who will monitor a woman's pregnancy closely throughout the nine months of pregnancy. This is something no book can hope to do. However, the advice we have to offer can make you better informed. Use it at your discretion.

Preventive Remedies for the Foetus

These remedies are designed to help infants get a head start in health by giving them all the benefits homeopathy has to offer during their in-utero period (their life before life, so to speak).

- *Hyperisan* is an extract *of Millepertius, Millefolium* (yarrow) and *Arnica montana,* to which a homeopathic concentration of *Pulsatilla pratens* (meadow anemone) is added. This preparation helps combat congestion of veins, varicosity and haemorrhoids, and regularizes circulation.

3 granules once a day:

- *Calcarea phosphorica 9 C.* One dosage per week helps restore minerals in future mothers and babies.
- *Sepia 5 C* and *Nux Vomica 5 C.* 3 granules after waking, in cases where prospective mothers' skin is sallow with yellow blotches, especially around the nostrils.
- *Sulphur 5 C.* Especially recommended in cases where one of the parents suffers from asthma, haemorrhoids, eczema or digestive problems.

Nervous Problems

These remedies are meant to help women deal with various mood changes associated with pregnancy which, although normal, are not necessarily desirable.

3 granules once a day:

- *Actaea racemosa 5 C.* For women who are afraid their pregnancy will go badly, who worry about all kinds of minor symptoms, exaggerating them out of all proportion - in other words, women who are hypochondriac.
- *Ignatia 5 C.* For women whose mood is rather capricious - they exhibit radical mood shifts which can be contradictory. For example, one day they say they can't eat a thing and the next day they stuff themselves to bursting point.
- *Sepia 5 C.* For women who are rather indifferent but sometimes

downright stunned by the idea of being pregnant.

Nausea and Vomiting

3 granules once a day:

- *Cocculus 4 C*. For nausea which occurs because of movement: travelling in trains, cars, planes, etc. Women have wind, and their feet get numb easily when they remain seated.
- *Ignatia 5 C*. For cases where nausea disappears while eating. But after meals, these subjects vomit. They are nervous to begin with, get upset or angry easily, and this produces their nausea and vomiting. As a basic treatment for vomiting during pregnancy, use *Ignatia 9 C,* once a week (since the effect of the remedy lasts for about a week).
- *Ipecac. 4 C*. This is the remedy most often recommended. Nausea is accompanied by excessive salivation, and vomiting provides no relief. The tongue remains clean and uncoated, but the stomach is upset.
- *Nux vomica 4 C*. 2 granules. This should stop the vomiting almost immediately. However, if it doesn't work, try *Ipecacuanha 3 C* or *Apomorphinum 4 C*.

Blood Loss

- *Sabina 4 C*. 2 granules every two hours. For cases of haemorrhage during pregnancy (metrorrhagia) indicating the possibility of an imminent miscarriage (consult the section on Miscarriage while waiting to see a doctor).

Future Mother's Diet

It's easy to understand why the diet you choose during pregnancy will have an important effect on the development of the foetus. Whatever you choose to eat, make sure you chew well, mixing a lot of saliva with your food. This will enable your body to absorb more of the nutrients, instead of just letting the food pass through your system undigested. It isn't really necessary to "eat for two" as was previously thought - eat better and not more. However, from the fifth month on, the amount of food should be increased to some extent.

Drink as little coffee as possible and make it decaffeinated if you can. Make sure to replace the minerals in your system by eating foods like cabbage, spinach, carrots and parsley (raw and chopped into a salad) and lots of fresh fruit; if you eat meat, roast or grill it instead of frying it. Cut down on fatty sauces, fish (unless it's very fresh), bread and cakes, pastries and starchy foods like noodles.

The complete list of foods to avoid is the same as for Gastritis, a digestive disorder (see section).

Milk and cheese provide calcium and protein. They help prevent cramps and dental cavities.

To provide the best possible growing conditions for your child, you should stop drinking alcohol completely during pregnancy. Also nicotine absorbed by mothers makes its way into the breast milk a few hours later. Smoking during pregnancy can only have a negative effect on the health of foetus and child.

Physical Activity

Get as much pure oxygen into your system as possible. Do breathing exercises and concentrate on filling your lungs with pure air. Taking walks in the countryside is ideal and is beneficial on both a mental and physical level.

You can continue with your normal level of physical activity for the first three months. But apart from prenatal exercises, don't start any new programme of physical training, except for very mild exercises designed to keep you in shape. As for walking, do it with friends or in company as often as possible throughout the course of your pregnancy.

Chemicals and Other Substances: as Little as Possible

Use natural medications as much as possible, in order to avoid the risk of possible complications for the foetus. Don't take drugs such as tranquillizers, certain antibiotics, anticoagulants and even aspirin (especially if you're close to the due date, since it can make labour longer and more difficult).

X-rays can be dangerous in the last three months. Some authors even recommend not watching too much TV. Vaccinations are also to be avoided during this period.

Homeopathic Vaccinations

On the other hand, there is a series of homeopathic vaccines (Nosodes) designed to arm the infant against various hereditary disorders. Consult the section on Vaccination for more information.

The Ninth Month

Five or six weeks before the due date, as a kind of preparation for giving birth:

Actaea racemosa 5 C, 3 granules on waking up, and *Caulophyllum 5 C,* 3 granules before going to bed.

Also consult the section on Childbirth.

Note: none of these methods will be of much use if the mother is anxious and feverish, and has to deal with negative influences in her immediate environment. Homeopathy is just one more reason to rely on nature. And in the final analysis, what nourishes babies the most is the affection and care of the parents.

Sexual Arousal

Sexual arousal in itself is not a problem. However, it is not always welcome, for example when no suitable partner is available, or when people remain aroused after masturbating or after normally satisfying sexual relations.

Being mentally obsessed with sex can cause psychological imbalances and lead to all kinds of aberrant behaviour which people are likely to regret later on. It is sometimes better to take the necessary steps to curb sexual arousal because any kind of excess is likely to cause us harm.

Work Is Healthy

Working until you're exhausted, or doing hard physical exercise in the open air, can bring your sexual appetite back to normal. Diet should be as vegetarian as possible (see the diet outlined in the section on Gastritis).

3 granules three times per day:

- *Calcarea phosphorica 6 C.* When sexual arousal occurs during periods or breast-feeding.
- *Cantharis 9 C.* For cases of excessive sexual arousal and erotic fantasy, both psychological and physical, usually occurring in excitable, agitated and hypersensitive people. In men this causes prolonged and painful erections (priapism). Women experience uterine spasms, which get worse during menstruation; people may have a lot of erotic dreams and make obscene comments and propositions.
- *Cannabis Indica 6 C.* Symptoms are the same as for *Cantharis,* but with more cerebral activity, aggravated by coffee and liqueurs.
- *Kali carbonicum 5 C.* People are in a constant state of sexual arousal, but find the actual act of sex exhausting.
- *Platina 5 C* with *Murex purpurea 5 C.* 2 granules on alternate days, for excessive sexual arousal in women.

- *Staphysagria 7 C* with *Bufo 7 C*. 2 granules of each on alternate mornings, for excessive sexual arousal in men.
- *Stramonium 9 C*. Subjects are mostly women; the condition is aggravated before and during periods; blood flow is heavy; women tend to get over-excited and talk a lot.
- *Veratrum album 6 C*. For pronounced sexual arousal during periods or pregnancy.

Sexuality

You can seek professional help (psychologist, psychotherapist, sex therapist) to resolve sexual problems. But this should not stop you doing your own work in the form of honest self-examination, reading, informal exchange of ideas or participating in organized workshops.

The progress you make through your own efforts can only help the eventual work of a therapist, if and when you decide to consult one.

On the other hand, in the context of a couple, healthy communication between partners is an essential element for achieving sexual and sensual fulfilment. And finally, in many cases, homeopathic remedies can be of great help.

Food as Stimulants

Seaweed (Kelp) is an excellent natural stimulant of sexual activity. Add it to your salads in the form of granules, or take it in the form of tablets (sold in health food shops).

Also *vitamin E,* the basic anti-stress vitamin, is recognized for its regenerative and stimulating effect on sexual and reproductive functions, in both men and women. It is also reputed to have cured many cases of impotence in men and frigidity in women.

Finally, certain foods are considered to be aphrodisiacs: lemons, asparagus, oats, caviar, celery, oysters, onions and truffles, for example.

Female Sexual Problems
Self-restraint

For cases of prolonged sexual self-restraint, 3 granules twice a day:
- *Conium 7 C*. When the condition is accompanied by melancholy and depressive tendencies.

- *Thuja 7 C*. If subjects tend to perspire around the genital area (or if there are greenish yellow, irritating secretions).

Pains
When intercourse is painful and followed by bleeding, use *Argentum nitricum 5 C*.

Frigidity
Frigidity refers to the difficulty some women have in experiencing pleasure during sex, and in having orgasms. We shouldn't forget that the quality of a sexual relationship is not measured by the frequency of orgasms - even though sexual satisfaction is a prerequisite for a satisfactory relationship.

Instead of waiting for a problem to resolve itself - which often leads to the breakdown of the relationship - it is sometimes a good idea to take concrete steps to resolve the problem, to compromise in some way, in order to improve matters. Personal development, however, requires a lot of motivation. (Also refer to the section above on stimulating foods.)

Nothing To Fear Except Fear Itself
In some cases, it may be necessary to overcome one's fear of the opposite sex. To do this, you can take *Pulsatilla 5 C*, 2 granules twice a day. Other remedies include:

- *Natrum muriaticum 5 C* or *Causticum 5 C*, both useful when the vagina remains dry during intercourse, which makes sexual activity painful.
- *Onosmodium 9 C*. Sexual desire is greatly diminished or non-existent; usually accompanied by depression.
- *Platina 5 C*. Recommended for women with a superiority complex, who think they're better than their partners.
- *Sepia 5 C*. Intercourse is painful, and women's general health is not very good; periods are irregular, they experience a feeling of heaviness in the uterus and lower back pains, often accompanied by anxiety and obsessive thoughts.
- *Turnera 5 C*. For women who are prostrate.

Nymphomania (See Also Sexual Arousal)
The problem of constantly seeking sexual pleasure without ever being really satisfied can be due to physical disorders: cystitis, herpes, leucorrhoea, vaginitis, poor hygiene, etc. When the cause is psychological, a therapist should be consulted.

- *Murex purpurea 6 C.* 3 granules three times per day. An active remedy for women. This substance has a calming effect on all mammals, including human beings (it can also be administered to pets to calm them down when on heat - 2 granules three times per day).
- *Ovarinum 9 C.* 5 granules once a week.
- *Platina 5 C.* 2 granules every two days, to calm excessive sexual desire.
- *Rana bufo 5 C.* 3 granules three times per day. When sexual arousal is accompanied by a tendency to epileptic fits and a strong desire for solitude.

Obsession

- *Staphysagria 5 C.* The genitals are hypersensitive; subjects are often in a bad mood and irritable; they are more prone to take their pleasure alone (masturbation) which they do very frequently, rather than engage in a sexual relationship; subjects often seek solitude.

Male Sexual Problems
Self-restraint

- In cases of prolonged abstinence from sexual activity take *Conium 5 C* and *Ovarinum 5 C,* 2 granules of each once a day.

Premature Ejaculation

- *Agaricus muscarius 9 C.* 3 granules every three days. For premature ejaculation without orgasm; after intercourse, men feel weak, experience pains in their thighs, and have no appetite.
- *Caladium 5 C.* 3 granules twice a day. For men who do get sexually aroused, but who feel weak - erections are weak, despite intense desire; ejaculation sometimes occurs without an erection.
- *Caladium* is also recommended after sexual excesses.
- *Conium maculatum 5 C.* 2 granules twice a day. Erections are weak and do not last long; men suffer from a kind of moral or mental depression; these cases often occur after prolonged sexual abstinence.
- *Gelsemium 5 C.* 2 granules twice a day. For men who are nervous, anxious and afraid of not being able to perform; they are emotional and are unable to retain their sexual arousal when they become emotional, or think about failure.
- *Lycopodium 5 C.* 2 granules twice a day. For men who lose interest in sex

and are generally inactive; they don't want to work, become depressed, taciturn, intolerant and authoritarian; erections are weak.

- *Selenium 9 C*. 3 granules every three days. For men who are in a generally weak condition, who still have sexual desires but who ejaculate too easily, and tend to be impotent.

Sexual Exhaustion

If the case is one of general exhaustion, then the person's general condition must be treated before concentrating on the sexual aspect. Take a look at the person's diet, lifestyle and level of physical activity. Is the person sufficiently active? Is he comfortable with his body? Consult the section on Overwork.

Pollen has a strong influence on the function of the sexual glands - a teaspoon of pollen can get rid of sexual (as well as other kinds of) fatigue. Also, wheat germ cures and Kuhne baths can have a beneficial effect on sex drive. Also refer to the section on stimulating foods above.

3 granules once a day:

- *Calcarea carbonica 6 C*. For sexual coolness in men with balanced personalities, who are calm, methodical, responsible; desire is low, and they feel weak after sexual intercourse.
- *Graphites 9 C*. For men who have a tendency to obesity, dry skin and hard nails; their character is rather apathetic, and they lack direction.

Impotence

A prolonged wheat germ cure, accompanied by *Kuhne baths,* can go a long way towards curing impotence. In fact, wheat germ contains a high level of *vitamin E,* which is essential for the proper functioning of the reproductive organs.

3 granules every two days:

- *Agaricus 9 C*. For cases where impotence is due to general nervous exhaustion, and mental and physical weakness.
- *Agnus castus 7 C*. Men are depressed and sad, and feel that they're at the end of their tether; intestines are pulled downwards and ankle joints are weak.
- *Gelsemium 9 C*. For impotence caused by psychological problems like nerves, anxiety, etc.
- *Onosmodium 9 C*. For men who experience a decrease or complete disappearance of sexual desire; erections are very weak and ejaculation occurs too rapidly; at the same time, these men are mentally depressed,

they have trouble concentrating and comprehension is slow.

Sterility

Hormonal problems can lead to sterility. Women may make use of natural methods instead of resorting to hormones, which can involve some risk. In any case, why not start by trying the natural physical methods at your disposal, before turning to more radical treatments?

Physical Methods

Start by taking sitz baths, hot and cold showers, and Kuhne baths (see section). Also, remedies like *Hyperisan* stimulate circulation and improve blood flow to the abdominal area, which can lead to increased production of hormones.

Supplements like wheat germ and wheat germ oil are excellent complements to a balanced diet. They contain high levels of vitamin E_1, called the reproductive vitamin, which plays an essential role in the development and function of our reproductive organs, both male and female. 100 grams of wheat germ contain close to 30 grams of pure vitamin E. Soya beans and watercress also contain high levels of vitamin E.

- *Natrum muriaticum 7 C, Medorrhinum 7 C* and *Luesinum 7 C*. 5 granules every day on alternate days, one after the other.

Problems in conceiving are just as likely to be caused by the male as by the female partner. Men can become sterile for various reasons: diabetes, hyperlipidaemia, chronic pancreatitis, varicocele (varicose condition of the spermatic cord), orchitis, etc. Wearing underwear that is too tight heats up the testicles and can produce temporary sterility. So men should wear underwear and trousers that are not too tight - the testicles must remain a few degrees below normal body temperature. If they get too warm, the sperm are destroyed.

Another helpful measure is to cut down on your intake of tobacco and alcohol.

Also see remedies for Impotence.

Testicles

Hydrocele

The skin of the testicles in infants is swollen because of a secretion of liquid.

3 granules three times per day (see Directions for Use - Infants):

- *Aurum 5 C*. For infants who are taciturn, rather fat and sometimes violent.
- *Calcarea 5 C*. For fat babies who are quiet, soft and easily frightened.
- *Pulsatilla 5 C*. For sensitive children who are easily upset by heat, and who hate milk and drink very little.
- *Silicea 5 C*. For thin, nervous, fragile children who feel the cold and who perspire a lot through their feet.

Swollen Testicles

Testicles are swollen, red and painful. The condition may be caused by an accident, or by twisting a testicle. A doctor must be consulted immediately.

General Disorders

3 granules three times per day:
- *Mercurius solubilis 5 C*. For cases of herpes of the scrotum or penis.
- *Rhododendron 5 C*. A liquid, which is visible and transparent, spreads in the scrotum around the testicles. This condition is called hydrocele.
- *Spongia 5 C*. Testicles are swollen and painful, and very sensitive to the touch.

Urine

Urine, and especially its appearance, can be a valuable indication of our state of health. If the urine resembles the descriptions below and if there are no other symptoms, try the appropriate remedy for a while. If the anomaly persists, consult a doctor.

3 granules once a day:
- *Berberis 5 C*. Urine is sandy red and sticky.
- *Chelidonium 5 C*. The urine is dark yellow.
- *Cina 5 C*. For cases where urine is abundant and milky white.
- *Lycopodium 5 C*. Urine leaves a non sticky, sandy red deposit.
- *Pareira brava 5 C*. Urine contains a white sediment.
- *Solidago 4 C*. For cases where urine is passed in small quantities, leaves deposits, contains sediment, or is a darker colour than usual.

Chapter 7

Respiratory System

Aphonia (Loss of Voice)

Aphonia is a common disorder. It starts with a tickling sensation at the back of the throat, which becomes more and more sensitive to the passage of air. A cough usually follows, after which people lose control of their voices - it goes high or low on its own - or they may lose their voice completely.

Precautions

It's better to prevent aphonia, which often develops along with, or after, a severe sore throat. Those who use their voices professionally (singers, actors, politicians, salespeople, etc.) are more likely to develop the condition and should therefore take more precautions to prevent it.

2 granules three times per day:

- *Aconitum 5 C.* When aphonia develops after exposure to dry cold. This remedy should be taken as soon as the first signs appear.
- *Argentum nitricum 5 C.* For chronic cases, especially singers, actors, etc.
- *Arum 5 C.* This type of aphonia develops after exposure to dry cold. It is accompanied by itching sensations around the lips, nose and larynx.
- *Arum triphyllum 5 C.* For cases where people cough up a lot of mucus, or when aphonia develops after catching a cold.
- *Causticum 5 C.* After catching cold in dry weather, especially if the throat is sensitive and burning, and accompanied by chest pains. A good remedy for singers, speakers and others who use their voice professionally.
- *Gelsemium 5 C.* For aphonia which develops after menstruation.

Asthma

This disorder, which is characterized by difficult breathing, has a variety of possible causes: nervousness, bronchial asthma (which depends to a great extent on weather conditions) and cardiac asthma. In all cases, people feel as if they are suffocating; attacks often occur in the middle of the night; subjects make a bronchial rattling sound but do not have fever.

The room where the asthma sufferer sleeps should be clean and kept free of dust. Keep the temperature fairly low. Avoid contact with pets - even their presence may set off an attack. Try not to be over-protective of children suffering from asthma - they should be allowed to lead normal lives as much as possible.

Except when caused by allergies, asthma is difficult to treat in a radical way. Treatment is tricky and long-term, especially in cases of bronchial asthma which develops after a pulmonary illness that has healed badly. If treatment continues during winter, try to get patients to a sunny environment, preferably at a high altitude.

3 granules twice an hour:

- *Aconitum 4 C.* For children who are the victims of sudden attacks, accompanied by crying and anxiety.
- *Arsenicum album 4 C.* Patients show signs of exhaustion and agitation. Attacks occur between midnight and three in the morning. Patients feel a burning sensation in the chest; they suffer from anxiety, are agitated and nervous, and constantly need to move around
- *Antimonium tartaricum 4 C.* Attacks occur in the middle of the night, with a large accumulation of mucus in the chest, which causes people to snore loudly when asleep; they cannot, however, expel this mucus. This type of asthma typically appears after a bout of bronchitis.
- *Bryonia 5 C.* Pain is aggravated by the slightest respiratory movement.
- *Chamomilla 5 C.* These asthma attacks characteristically occur during or after subjects become angry.
- *Cuprum 5 C.* 2 granules. To be administered as soon as the first signs of an imminent attack appear.
- *Drosera 5 C.* For asthma in people who have had tuberculosis. Alternate with *Moschus* and *Sambucus*.
- *Ipecac. 5 C.* When attacks are accompanied by coughing, nausea and wheezing in the chest. This is a tuberculous type of asthma, which often occurs after a bout of bronchitis. *Ipecac.* is recommended when the condition is aggravated by humidity. Subjects also produce an abundance of saliva.
- *Kali carbonicum 5 C.* Attacks usually occur between one and three o'clock in the morning, and are accompanied by wheezing and shooting pains in the chest. Patients have to sit up in bed or lean forward. Attacks may follow a bout of bronchitis.
- *Lachesis 5 C.* Attacks are aggravated by sleep.
- *Moschus 5 C.* Especially for cases of asthma caused by nervousness or when people are very upset.
- *Natrum sulphuricum 5 C.* Attacks occur between four and five o'clock in the morning, and coincide with damp weather. *Natrum sulphuricum* can

be used as a basic remedy.

- *Nux vomica 5 C*. People are irritable, and attacks usually occur at the end of meals.
- *Sambucus 4 C*. For attacks that occur around midnight, accompanied by a feeling of suffocation and hoarse coughing, especially in young children.
- *Phosphorus 4 C*. People feel heat in the chest area. Phosphorus is a basic remedy, but should be used with discretion, after consultation with a specialist.
- *Psorinum 5 C*. A skin rash accompanies the asthma attacks.

Bronchitis

The alveoli in one or sometimes both lungs become filled with blood plasma or serous fluid. Infection then causes congestive inflammation. Remedies aim to free the pulmonary passages of congestion.

It should be noted that complications arising from bronchitis can be serious. On the other hand, the spread of the disease depends, to a great extent, on the patient - on his or her attitudes and general state of health. Typical attacks last for about ten days, as if the body were finally able to rid itself of the problem after that time.

People should stay in bed as long as fever persists, except to take very hot foot baths. Also get the patient out of the sick room every day so that it can be properly aired. Call a doctor if symptoms become acute.

3 granules every three hours:

- *Aconitum 5 C*. After exposure to dry cold. Fever rises rapidly; patients shiver, are agitated, but do not perspire; they have to deal with a high level of anxiety; they are agitated and suffer from dry coughing. *Aconitum* is a good remedy to prescribe at the outset of a bronchial attack and generally helps avoid complications.
- *Antimonium tartaricum 5 C*. Most often prescribed for chronic cases. Mucus accumulates, but cannot be expectorated; patients are drowsy, sometimes prostrate; wheezing and rattling sounds originate in the chest. Coughing is less dry than in other cases, but patients often suffer from painful nausea and vomiting. Children feel oppressed. Also for cases where coughing is thick and heavy, and breathing is noisy with wheezing. Patients feel better when seated; the tongue often has a white coating. *Antimonium tartaricum* is also a remedy that can be prescribed

for chronic cases of capillary bronchitis and bronchopneumonia, where mucus accumulates in the lungs.

- *Belladonna 5 C.* An initial remedy to be used after the first phase, following *Aconitum*. Patients perspire, tend to remain prostrate and seem almost numb; the skin is hot and flushed, especially around the face, with slight perspiration.

  Headaches may develop, accompanied by some degree of mental confusion, especially in children. The throat is itchy, talking is painful and the eyes are bloodshot. Children often suffer from insomnia or sleep badly, groaning, tossing and turning all night long.

- *Bryonia 4 C.* Dry coughing tickles the throat, but this occurs only during the day. On the other hand, patients feel acute pains (similar to stitch) in the chest area; patients remain immobile, and simply breathing is uncomfortable.

  Patients also develop high fever, headaches, hot sweats and intense thirst. *Bryonia* is usually prescribed following or in conjunction with *Aconitum* treatment.

- *Ferrum phosphoricum 5 C.* Patients are exhausted, feel a heaviness in the chest area, are congested, suffer from a dry cough and have waves of fever accompanied by flushing. Administer *Ferrum phosphoricum* for the duration of the illness, as well as in cases of chronic bronchitis.

- *Carbo vegetabilis 5 C.* For bronchitis in older people. Persistent coughing occurs, usually at night. Patients have trouble breathing, feel a heaviness and burning sensation in the chest area, sometimes accompanied by bluish discolouration of the mucous membranes and skin on the face, lips and fingers.

  Subjects are exhausted and their voice is weak, sometimes disappearing completely.

- *Hepar sulphuris 4 C.* People catch cold after exposure to dry wind; coughing makes breathing extremely difficult, to the point of suffocation; these people cannot tolerate draughts; there is, however, no expectoration.

- *Ipecac. 5 C.* For cases of acute bronchitis and capillary bronchitis. Symptoms resemble those of *Antimonium tartaricum,* except that the tongue remains uncoated. Mucus is not expectorated by coughing; patients suffer from nausea and vomiting, are often short of breath and feel as if they are suffocating; they also avoid moving around and cannot tolerate cold air; nosebleeds (blood is bright red) sometimes accompany the cough. This remedy may be alternated with *Antimonium tartaricum* and *Ferrum phosphoricum,* but this should be under the supervision of a specialist.

- *Kali carbonicum 4 C.* For cases of bronchial paralysis, capillary bronchitis and bronchitis in older people. A dry cough occurs, usually at night about two o'clock in the morning; subjects are weak, eyelids are swollen, and they feel acute pains, especially on the right side.

  Subjects are not able to expel mucus; they perspire a lot and tend to suffer from asthma; sitting up in bed and leaning forwards provides some relief. *Kali carbonicum* is often prescribed during convalescence, along with *Pulsatilla.*

- *Mercurius 4 C.* After inflammation and congestion occur, patients start coughing up large amounts of yellow phlegm; they perspire at night, have some fever, accompanied by successive hot and cold flushes. The condition seems to become permanent. *Mercurius* should be administered with caution.

- *Phosphorus 5 C.* For cases of acute or capillary bronchitis, and hepatization (lung becomes solidified like the liver). Fever does not affect the patients' appetite or thirst, and they sometimes experience heat or a burning sensation in the chest.

  The cough is aggravated by speaking and patients have difficulty breathing, especially when lying on the left side. If rasping sounds and the feeling of oppression persist, administer *Phosphorus* with *Bryonia, Ferrum phosphoricum* and *Antimonium tartaricum.*

- *Pulsatilla 5 C.* For persistent or chronic bronchitis. The cough is dry at night, but phlegmy in the morning, accompanied by expectoration. Subjects are feverish but not thirsty, and feel the need to urinate when coughing.

  Patients may also lose their sense of taste and smell, alternating with shivering and pain. In fact, *Pulsatilla* cases are characterized by extreme instability and variation of symptoms: fever goes down, and the next day subjects start shivering and coughing; this is followed by hot flushes and rising temperature . . . and so it goes on. Use *Pulsatilla* towards the end of a bout of bronchitis, if the condition is not accompanied by otitis.

- *Sanguinaria 5 C.* When pulmonary congestion, in its initial phase, is accompanied by prolonged shivering. Expectorations are sticky;

sensations of oppression and burning in the chest are eased when patients lie on their back.

- *Sulphur 5 C.* During a bout of bronchitis and also during the convalescent phase. Expectorations are greenish and purulent; patients feel as if there were a weight on their chest, and need to breathe fresh air; they may also experience a burning sensation in the chest area.

  Sulphur may be administered as a follow-up to *Aconitum* or *Phosphorus,* when skin rashes appear. Also for cases of acute bronchitis: the face is congested, patients have high fever, and suffer from diarrhoea.

  Patients' appetite seems to disappear at meal-times; they suffer from chronic fatigue, sleep lightly and perspire a lot at night.

Common Cold

Everyone has caught a cold at some time or other, so there's no need to describe the collection of annoying symptoms that characterize the common cold, symptoms that tend to persist for days or even weeks.

One way to get rid of the disorder, which has proved so resistant to modern medicine, is to cut a thin slice of fresh onion and soak it for a few seconds in a glass of hot water. Then sip small amounts of the water throughout the course of the day.

You can also place an onion that has been cut in half on your bed-head overnight, and apply onion compresses to the throat and chest, which will reduce the flow of mucus in the nasal passages.

3 granules twice a day:

- *Aconitum 5 C.* Take this remedy at the slightest exposure to cold, especially dry cold. *Aconitum* is characterized by a sudden onset of symptoms, sometimes accompanied by headaches. Coughing is dry and painful; the face is red, skin is dry; fever is accompanied by shivering; patients are anxious.
- *Belladonna 5 C.* Patients suffer from headaches in addition to a runny nose; they sweat profusely, are anxious and fatigued.
- *Hepar sulphuris 5 C.* Patients have a dry cough and hoarse voice, and wheeze when they breathe. *Hepar sulphuris* cases are aggravated by cold air, or when patients are uncovered; the cough gets worse when they speak; heat and hot compresses generally provide some relief.
- *Pulsatilla 5 C.* The nose is very runny; coughing comes in fits, especially

in the morning, and is dry at night; the condition is aggravated in overheated rooms; the nose is blocked and dry during the day. A characteristic *of Pulsatilla* cases is the loss of the sense of taste and smell, and an absence of thirst.

- *Nux vomica 5 C*. The nose is blocked at night and runny during the day, with non-irritating yellow mucus.

Coryza (Head Cold)

In its acute form, coryza - a head cold - starts with an itching, prickling sensation in the nose, which may be accompanied by a dripping nose; people start wiping and blowing their nose incessantly. The disorder is harmless, but it's better to nip it in the bud instead of letting it develop, so as to avoid possible complications like sinusitis, laryngitis, sore throat (tonsillitis) and bronchitis.

Keep the patient's head raised on pillows while sleeping. Lying down promotes congestion and blocks the nasal passages, especially in babies. A cold should not be taken lightly in new-born infants and very young children. If the cold persists, or the nasal discharge is streaked with blood, it's better to call a doctor.

Use soft tissues to wipe the nose (instead of a handkerchief) to avoid spreading the infection.

3 granules three times per day:

- *Aconitum 5 C*. An initial remedy, to be administered at the first signs of an impending head cold, or after exposure to dry cold. The nose remains dry, but violent sneezing produces a burning sensation in the throat. Patients feel general discomfort, develop fever and become agitated, but there is no sweating as yet.

- *Allium cepa 4 C*. For excoriating colds which appear after people have stayed in the cold with wet feet. Runny nose, eyes full of tears and difficult breathing are characteristic symptoms. Sneezing is frequent, and both nose and mouth are irritated. *Allium cepa* cases get worse at night, and in hot, stuffy rooms; they are soothed by fresh air; the left side of the body seems to be more affected.

- *Ammonium carbonicum 4 C*. For babies and young children (see Directions for Use - Infants). Typically, babies have trouble feeding; they sleep with their mouth open because the nose is blocked, and turn over suddenly so as not to suffocate. If children wake up during the night, use

Sambucus nigra 5 C.

- *Arsenicum album 5 C.* For colds caused by hay fever, or spasmodic head colds. Patients sneeze a lot, the nose drips and becomes irritated, as does the upper lip. The condition seems to get worse after midnight, and is soothed in a warm room, or by taking a hot bath.

- *Camphora 4 C.* For colds which develop after sudden changes in temperature. The nose is blocked and dry, and the air patients breathe feels cold; they shiver and can't get warm, and complain of headaches in the upper part of the forehead.

- *Chamomilla 5 C.* Children who are teething may develop a cold; they become agitated and nervous, and demand to be carried and rocked; nostrils are inflamed and irritated, and lips are chapped.

- *Euphrasia 5 C.* Because of incessant, corrosive crying, eyelids become puffy, and irritating conjunctivitis sets in. The right side of the body is more affected.

- *Gelsemium sempervirens 5 C.* For the kind of head cold that creeps up on you slowly, after exposure to cold weather. People seek solitude, suffer from headaches and a very watery discharge from the nose.

- *Kali bichromicum 5 C.* To be administered when the cold is at its worst. Long filaments of greenish yellow mucus flow from the nose; these tend to solidify, forming crusts which block the nasal passages almost completely.
  The nose is difficult to unblock, especially in the morning, and breathing though it causes a burning sensation; the root of the nose is painful, and the formation of crusts may precede the development of frontal sinusitis.

- *Kali iodatum 5 C.* A basic remedy for cases of abundant, burning, yellowish-green mucus which tends to harden in places.

- *Kali sulphuricum 5 C.* For those who lose their sense of taste and smell. An abundance of mucus accumulates in the chest; breathing is rasping and resembles bronchitis; expectoration is watery and yellowish and very abundant; the condition gets worse at night and in overheated rooms, and is improved by fresh air.

- *Lycopodium 5 C.* For cases of hepatic congestion, sometimes accompanied by moroseness. *Lycopodium* is a basic remedy for people who catch cold at the drop of a hat, and who tend to develop tenacious head colds; to get rid of the condition permanently, a general cleaning out of the body is required.

- *Mercurius 5 C. Mercurius* patients shiver incessantly and sweat profusely, especially towards the end of the day and during the night. Breath is fetid, and the characteristic sore throat is irritated by a constant need to clear the throat and expel or swallow excess saliva.
- *Mercurius solubilis 5 C.* Incessant and irritating nasal drip of a yellowish colour characterizes this type of head cold. Patients have some fever, and tend to sneeze a lot, especially out in the sun.
- *Natrum muriaticum 5 C.* A basic remedy for cases of repeated colds due to allergies; symptoms include a runny watery nose, cold sores on the lips, and/or eczema. The cold lasts for two or three days and is punctuated by excessive sneezing and a stuffy nose.
  Patients lose their sense of smell and taste; they feel weak and exhausted, especially in the morning, and are often thirsty. Administer at the onset of the cold, once only, when the nose starts to run.
- *Nux vomica 5 C.* This type of cold is characterized by incessant sneezing, especially in the morning. *Nux vomica* cases can be recognized by the fact that they always get worse in dry weather. Patients shiver when they have to move, or when covers are removed. They suffer from headaches, especially around the forehead; the throat is painful, and the nose, which is blocked up at night, tends to become runny during the day.
- *Sulphur 5 C.* The nose is dry with reddish irritation around the inside of the nostrils; the sense of smell is affected; patients are tired in the morning, have trouble standing up and suffer from hot flushes.
- *Pulsatilla 5 C.* Symptoms include inflammation of the mucous membranes, clear or yellowish nasal secretions which are sometimes thick and abundant during the day but are not irritating; the condition is soothed by fresh air and aggravated in overheated, dry rooms; patients lose their sense of smell and taste, and are not thirsty. This is a basic remedy for persistent colds which do not appear to clear up.
- *Thuja 5 C.* For cases of chronic coryza (head colds) accompanied by infection. The flow of mucus is thick and brownish-green in colour; it may contain pus or blood, and is aggravated by cold air; when patients blow their nose, they feel pain in their teeth.

Croup
(See Also False Croup)

Some forms of croup are cases of diphtheria (see section) which has spread to the larynx. For cases of acute laryngitis, homoeopathic treatment may be used as a temporary measure, but a doctor should be consulted. Breathing is severely restricted by both croup and false croup; patients sit up in bed and feel as if they're suffocating; the face is pale, patients are usually agitated and anxious.

In cases of true croup, the larynx and vocal cords are coated with a membrane-like substance; the voice is hoarse, the cough is rasping and subsides gradually; a characteristic of true croup is a wheezing, whistling sound in the throat and a persistent feeling of suffocation.

During Attacks

For children, apply hot compresses around the neck and get them to take mustard footbaths. Keep the sick room humid (use a humidifier, or boil eucalyptus leaves to produce a vapour). When convalescence begins, disinfect the room completely.

2 granules three times per day:

- *Aconitum 5 C.* Patients cough and clutch at their throat; the ribs are painful, fever is high, they are agitated, anxious and afraid. The face is flushed when they lie down, but goes pale when they stand up.
- *Hepar sulphuris 5 C.* A follow-up to *Aconitum* at the outset of croup. Patients develop a burning dry cough, which gets worse in the middle of the night; they feel a tickling sensation at the back of the throat, and breathing is laboured and noisy; they perspire when coughing; the condition is aggravated when subjects are uncovered or exposed to cold air.
- *Hepar sulphuris* when combined with *Spongia 5 C, Aconitum 5 C* and *Nigra 5 C,* can cure croup within a few hours, in some cases.
  The alternative to these remedies is that offered by allopathic medicine, which involves inserting a tube down the patient's throat, or performing an emergency tracheotomy.
- *Kali bichromicum 5 C.* Patients keep clearing their throat, trying to dislodge the membranous phlegm coating; the cough becomes more and more irritating, as if something were stuck at the back of the throat.
- *Sambucus nigra 5 C.* Patients wake up suddenly in the middle of the night to avoid suffocating, their faces are blue and they are sweating profusely all over their body.

Cough

No lengthy description is necessary - we all know that coughs come in a variety of forms and are often indicators of other disorders.

3 granules three times per day:

- *Bryonia 5 C*. For a dry cough, aggravated by movement and deep breathing, and when people enter overheated rooms. Bryonia coughs typically originate in the stomach region

  There is no expectoration, although patients feel as if their chest cavity were full of mucus. Coughing is triggered by a feeling of irritation or dryness; if fever develops, *Bryonia* cases will become intensely thirsty; the condition is frequently aggravated by eating or drinking.

- *Belladonna 5 C*. For a sharp dry, cough which begins suddenly, accompanied by congestive fever which gets worse after midnight; cases suffer from respiratory spasms, the voice is hoarse and the throat is dry.

- *Aconitum napellus 5 C*. For cases which develop after exposure to dry cold; coughing is sharp and dry, and patients tend to be both physically and mentally agitated.

- *Kali bichromicum 5 C*. The cough is phlegmy and occurs when people undress or after meals; they have difficulty expelling mucus; crusts form in the nose; phlegm is greenish; this form of sinusitis often appears in older people.

  As in cases of chronic sinusitis, the cough stems from mucus from the respiratory passages; patients also experience pains in their chest.

- *Ipecac. 5 C*. For a violent, dry cough caused by irritation in the form of a tickling sensation at the back of the throat; accompanied by nosebleeds or vomiting; the face is congested and bluish; people are constantly and intensely nauseous; streaks of blood appear in vomit and phlegm; the tongue is clean; patients experience constriction in the chest.

- *Coccus cacti 5 C*. Coughing comes in fits and is phlegmy; *Coccus cacti* patients immediately go red in the face; they expel filaments of mucus, which are transparent and sticky; they often vomit; the condition is worse in the morning after waking, and is soothed in well-ventilated, cool rooms.

- *Drosera 5 C*. Coughing fits are spasmodic, congested and suffocating; the condition gets worse at night, especially after midnight, or when patients breathe cold air; it is also aggravated by using the voice (talking, laughing, singing, crying, etc.)

Coughing fits are accompanied by purplish flushing of the face, nosebleeds, as well as acute pains at the base of the chest; patients clutch their stomach while vomiting; they are agitated, and the condition is aggravated by hot air.

- *Spongia tosta 5 C.* A barking cough which is dry during the day and phlegmy at night; accompanied by a feeling of suffocation of cardiac origin; the condition is aggravated when eating or drinking; the feeling of burning dryness in the larynx tends to get worse after eleven o'clock at night.

  This type of cough is aggravated by sweets and nervous agitation but improves when eating; *Spongia tosta* patients feel as if they're suffocating and feel anxious in overheated rooms.

- *Antimonium tartaricum 5 C.* The cough is phlegmy, accompanied by a rattling sound; there is no expectoration, but patients vomit, and nostrils are constantly flaring as they try to breathe; they experience bouts of suffocation after which they feel exhausted; extremities are bluish, the tongue has a yellow coating; the condition is aggravated between one and five o'clock in the morning and after meals.

- *Arsenicum album 5 C.* The cough is phlegmy and attacks are set off by cold air; if the cough is worse at night, patients become asthmatic; the condition is improved by heat and movement, and aggravated when patients lower their head or when they are lying on the side that is painful; they are agitated and thirst for water, which they sip in small quantities.

- *Rhus tox 5 C.* Patients cough during the night; the cough is dry and slightly wheezy; attacks come on when patients are only slightly uncovered, for example when their hands are out of bed; the condition is soothed by movement.

- *Hepar sulphuris 5 C.* The cough is rough, and comes in sporadic bursts; as in *Rhus tox* cases, the condition is aggravated when patients are uncovered.

- *Ignatia 5 C.* For coughing triggered by cigarette smoke.

- *Pulsatilla 5 C.* The cough is phlegmy during the day and dry at night; fits are often set off by physical exertion; in women the condition is accompanied by an absence of menstruation.

  Coughing gets worse in overheated rooms and is soothed by fresh air;

patients weep and expectorate clear or yellowish phlegm.

- *Aralia racemosa 5 C.* Coughing starts as soon as people go to bed, and can continue until about 11 p.m.; accompanied by irritation and abundant nasal discharge, the condition is aggravated by cold air or draughts, and improved by expectoration of salty mucus; patients frequently feel is if they have a foreign body lodged in their throat.
- *Sanguinaria Canadensis 5 C.* Patients have red cheeks, and expectorate phlegm the colour of rust; this type of cough is identifiable by the fact that it is improved by belching and/or passing wind.
- *Rumex crispus 5 C.* For a dry cough, caused by a tickling sensation in the throat, aggravated by the slightest draught of cold air; the condition gets worse around eleven o'clock at night, then calms down and gets worse again between two and five in the morning.

  Patients feel as if their head were going to burst; they suffer from urinary incontinence, and expectorate small amounts of thick mucus which is difficult to dislodge from the mucous membranes.
- *Rumex 5 C.* For violent, dry coughing fits accompanied by sharp pains in the side; aggravated while eating and by draughts of cold air; people are generally nervous, and suffer from diarrhoea.
- *Aconitum 5 C.* Coughing sets in after people catch cold, have been exposed to wind or stayed outside in cold weather without moving; the cough is hoarse and appears around eleven o'clock at night; the face is flushed when lying down, but goes pale when patients sit up; accompanied by anxiety and fear of dying.
- *Phosphorus 5 C.* Dry, painful coughing, aggravated when people breathe cold air, or when they go from a warm room into cold; the condition is worse on getting up and after drinking; it is also aggravated when people are lying on their left side.

Diphtheria

Although diphtheria, which is rare nowadays, is usually contracted by children between the ages of two and eight years, it is by no means limited to children. It is caused by a microbe which reproduces in nasal secretions even after the disease is cured.

The incubation period lasts from two days to a week, after which subjects develop tonsillitis (sore throat). There is s a slight fever and a dirty grey membrane-like coating appears, first on the tonsils, and then the entire throat. A laboratory test can confirm whether or not the diphtheria bacillus is present by analysing a throat swab. However, do not wait for the results to come back to start the treatment. Once the diagnosis is confirmed, patients must be kept in isolation because of the contagious nature of the disease, and will undergo conventional treatment (antibiotics, antitoxin) because of the serious potential complications of diphtheria.

If the larynx is affected, then you're dealing with a case of croup (see section) and its attendant risk of asphyxiation. However, this complication is relatively rare.

- *Ammonium causticum 3 C.* 2 granules every three hours. Administer this remedy to try and dissolve the characteristic grey pseudomembrane and coating on the throat.
- *Apis 4 C.* 2 granules every two hours. When the disease appears suddenly; patients are exhausted and drowsy; the throat is so constricted that they cannot swallow; they are not thirsty; the uvula (the small protrusion up at the back of the throat) is swollen; if the throat has a white coating, use *Mercurius cyanatus* or *Kali bichromicum*.
- *Belladonna 5 C* and *Mercurius cyanatus 5 C.* 2 granules of each, alternating every hour. Swallowing is painful, the throat is red, with white patches on the grey coating.
- *Kali bichromicum 5 C.* 2 granules every three hours. The pseudomembrane appears to be developing ulcers and spreading towards the nose and the back of the throat.
- *Lachesis 5 C.* 2 granules every three hours. The disease first attacks the right tonsil; hot drinks aggravate the pain.
- *Lycopodium 5 C.* 2 granules every three hours. The disease first attacks the left tonsil; hot drinks soothe the pain, while cold drinks make it worse.

Dyspnoea (Shortness of Breath)

When not caused by intense exertion or emotion, shortness of breath accompanied by laboured breathing can have a variety of origins, for example croup, false croup or, if exhaling is difficult and causes coughing, asthma (see sections).

In cases of shortness of breath accompanied by accelerated breathing (either inhaling or exhaling) with coughing fits and abundant expectoration, you may be dealing with acute oedema of the lungs. If symptoms are accompanied by intense pain in the side, the condition may be due to a pulmonary embolism.

False Croup

This disorder usually affects children between the ages of two and seven who have been exposed to dry, cold wind. The first symptom is a hoarse voice which lasts for a few days. Then a cough develops, and patients suffer fits of coughing especially in the middle of the night.

Mucus descends into the throat, causing spasmodic contractions and a feeling of suffocation. Young patients lose their voice completely, and develop a high fever (104-105.8°F or 40-41°C). Respiration remains normal but difficult, coughing becomes intense, barking and hoarse, the voice remains clear.

Children may exhibit signs of anxiety and cry often. To calm the spasms, keep a night light on, and apply hot-water compresses to the throat area.

3 granules every three hours:

- *Belladonna 5 C*. Patients feel an intense itching or tickling in the throat, and spasms of the glottis; the throat is red and they have trouble swallowing even liquids.
- *Sambucus nigra*. Children wake up suddenly in the middle of the night and have to sit up in order not to suffocate; the face goes blue and they sweat profusely over their whole body.
- *Spongia 5 C*. As with *Aconitum*, the symptoms appear after exposure to cold, dry wind. The cough is hoarse and violent; children are afraid and agitated; spasms appear slowly, and breathing is difficult between spasms.

Hay Fever
(See Also Allergies)

Not to be confused with spasmodic coryza (head colds), which are caused by other types of allergies, hay fever patients are often hypersensitive to certain types of grasses and flowers, to dust and various odours. Hay fever is actually a passive way for the body to eliminate toxins.

3 granules twice a day:

- *Allium cepa 5 C*. For acute attacks; sneezing gets worse when people sleep in a warm room and gets better out in the fresh air; a constant flow of mucus irritates the nostrils and upper lip; eyes are sensitive to light.

- *Kali iodatum 5 C.* Another treatment for acute attacks of hay fever. The mucous membranes in the nose are inflamed and secrete abundantly; secretions have a fetid odour and create tiny, irritating ulcerations. Symptoms improve in warm rooms, but are worse early in the morning and for extreme heat; patients feel shooting pains in the lungs, and quickly become short of breath after any physical effort.

- *Naphthalinum 5 C.* Characterized by a flow of thick mucus; symptoms improve out in the fresh air.

- *Sanguinaria 5 C.* Eyes and nose are dry; mucus is burning, abundant and yellowish; cheeks are red; patients experience hot flushes, especially towards the end of the day, and suffer from diarrhoea; at night, coughing is incessant; they feel constriction and oppression in the chest area, as well as pain at the base of the nose.

- *Sabadilla 5 C.* Sneezing comes in spasms, accompanied by watering eyes and watery, runny nose; patients feel pain in the frontal sinus region, and eyes are bloodshot. The condition is aggravated by fresh air, cold and cold drinks, and soothed by heat and hot drinks. Patients are not thirsty when the hay fever is at its peak, which is generally indicated by an itching sensation on the palate.

Influenza (Flu)

The major difference between a simple cold and influenza is that the latter is accompanied by high fever, aches and pains throughout the body and headaches. In general, flu is spread by nasal secretions.

After an incubation period of between two and five days, the characteristic symptoms of influenza make their appearance: headaches, shivering, fatigue, aches and pains; it generally lasts four or five days and is accompanied by fever of between 100° and 102.2°F (38-39°C).

Bronchitis is the principal potential complication, and appears around the fourth day. For normal cases, the most difficult period seems to be the convalescent stage, which seems to drag on indefinitely - people wonder if they'll ever regain their health completely.

- *Oscillococcinum 200* is the homoeopathic remedy most often prescribed for influenza, and it's a good idea always to keep a supply in your medicine cabinet, instead of having to rely on aspirin or similar medication.

- *Sulphur 7 C. 5* granules. A useful precaution at the outset of the flu, to help clean out the body.

2 granules every three hours for specific cases:

- *Allium cepa 5 C.* The nose drips constantly, especially on the left side; the face is swollen, eyes are red. Patients may be hungrier than usual, develop stomach pains and wind which, when expelled, eases headaches.
- *Belladonna 5 C.* The flu starts with a headache; the face is characteristically flushed, the eyes are shining and red; patients cannot tolerate being moved; they sweat profusely when sleeping under covers, and may then become very excited and even aggressive.
- *Bryonia 5 C.* Patients crave quiet - any movement produces nausea - and sitting up in bed makes them dizzy; the mouth is dry, and they have acute pains which are aggravated by movement.
- Patients are very thirsty for large quantities of cold water; they have twinges in the side; the stomach is painful, and they suffer from diarrhoea; they also have a dry cough, which comes in fits, and shakes them from the head right down to the stomach.
- *Camphora 5 C.* Patients suddenly start shivering intensely; they feel frozen, but may throw off their covers; the tongue is cold, and they feel as if the air they're breathing is icy.
- *Eupatorium perfoliatum 5 C.* Patients are exhausted and feel completely racked with aches and pains; muscles are stiff, especially in the calves; they have pains around the eyes, the nose runs incessantly (coryza); they are always thirsty, but when they drink something they vomit.
- *Gelsemium 5 C.* For muscular influenza, characterized by general aches and pains; patients are very fatigued and weak, with moderate fever; they sometimes feel as if their head were being squeezed in a vice.

Laryngitis

The major symptoms of laryngitis are relatively easy to recognize, since they are so typical. After exposure to cold, people develop a rasping, noisy cough characterized by a constant tickling sensation at the back of the throat.

After a while, the voice gets progressively more hoarse, until it is reduced to a whisper. In some cases it may disappear completely.

Be Careful

You have to be especially careful if any respiratory problems arise with a characteristic wheezing sound. Small children may start suffocating, so be on the lookout for any difficulties inhaling or exhaling.

On the other hand, if the laryngitis is just starting, and is not accompanied by fever, a non-specialist can attempt to reduce it by homoeopathic treatment. But if the condition is advanced or if there is any fever, a professional should be consulted.

In cases of tubercular laryngitis, care from a professional is essential. In cases where people have forced their voice too much, get them to remain silent, and administer hot mustard footbaths (mustard powder mixed with water). Alcohol and tobacco should be avoided (also dusty places, as is the case for all forms of laryngitis). Also avoid exposure to cold.

Instead, try to build up your resistance to freezing weather through physical exercise or taking cold showers, for example. Try to react as quickly as possible when symptoms appear, since the best results are achieved if treatment is begun at the very outset.

Finally, avoid inhalation devices and never ignore a hoarse voice or persistent aphonia.

2 granules three times per day:

- *Aconitum 5 C.* For acute laryngitis, caused by sudden exposure to dry cold; may or may not be accompanied by fever. The throat is red and dry, the cough is rasping and tends to get worse shortly after patients fall asleep.
  Patients develop fever and feel hot, but do not perspire; the skin is dry, and the face, which is red when lying down, goes pale when patients sit or stand up; coughing is painful, and they tend to clutch at their throat, which is very sensitive to the air being inhaled.
- *Allium cepa 5 C.* In children, *Allium cepa* is characterized by insomnia; children cry for no apparent reason; the condition is aggravated in overheated, humid rooms, as well as by inhaling cold air, and soothed by fresh air. The voice is hoarse, and patients feel as if their throat were being torn apart when they cough. *Allium cepa* is also the remedy for acute laryngitis, complicated by head colds (coryza). In these cases coughing is also painful, and aggravated at night and by the passage of cold air through the throat; patients have a constantly runny nose which irritates the nostrils,

and breathing is laboured.

- *Argentum metallicum 5 C*. The voice is hoarse or completely lost, especially in the morning - this may be caused by straining the voice, and *Argentum metallicum* is recommended for those who use their voice professionally (singers, teachers, actors, etc.) Talking seems to aggravate the pain, which is felt most intensely below the sternum; pain is also aggravated when they lean forward; mucus is abundant and expectorated easily.
- *Argentum nitricum 5 C*. There appear to be ulcers on the vocal cords, as if splinters were sticking out of them. *Argentum nitricum* is prescribed for cases of chronic laryngitis or when the voice has been put under a severe strain. Trying to reach high notes sets off a coughing fit, and these people are constantly clearing their throat.
- *Arum triphyllum 5 C*. After exposure to cold wind or after straining the voice (singing very high notes, for example, or speaking at outdoor meetings); the voice is hoarse and irritated. The cough is dry, and the voice goes high and low without patients being able to control it; they may sometimes experience intense pain, as if the larynx were inflamed and burning; pain is aggravated by talking or singing. Take this remedy before a performance or conference where you know your voice will be put under a strain.
- *Belladonna 5 C*. After exposure to draughts; patients perspire, suffer from a dry, spasmodic cough and develop high fever. The voice becomes weak, and the larynx is painful; fever is not accompanied by agitation, but by exhaustion and drowsiness. The skin is damp, pupils are dilated.
  Belladonna is very helpful at the outset of the condition, as well as in damp weather, or when people's head or feet have stayed wet for a long period of time.
- *Bryonia 5 C*. Patients are anxious and seek solitude; the face is pale, and they sweat profusely; in children, hoarseness is painful; after an attack, they tend to sleep a lot and sweat profusely.
  Changes in temperature, as well as eating and drinking, tend to aggravate *Bryonia* cases; the voice becomes more hoarse in the fresh air; the dry cough gets worse at night, especially when patients have to sit up in bed in order to breathe.
- *Drosera 5 C*. For cases of chronic laryngitis. The cough, which is especially bad at night and after midnight, resembles whooping cough.

Patients clutch their stomachs and remain very agitated between coughing fits.

- *Hepar sulphuris 5 C.* For cases of laryngitis that appear after exposure to dry cold, with or without fever; when the body is partially or entirely exposed to cold air, a dry, violent cough begins; expectoration, when there is any, is fetid and yellowish.
- *Phosphorus 5 C.* Often the result of straining the voice, which becomes hoarse; the larynx is sensitive and painful to the touch.

  A burning sensation at the back of the throat forces patients to remain silent; pain caused by the hoarse voice is worse at night, and when there are sudden changes in temperature; the cough is dry and spasmodic, triggered by an acute tickling sensation at the back of the throat, and aggravated when lying down, especially on the left side. Patients have fever, perspire at night, and feel a kind of burning between their shoulders.
- *Populus candicans 5 C.* For cases of acute laryngitis with total loss of voice (aphonia). The remedy can also be used as a preventive measure.

  A hoarse voice is accompanied by a burning sensation in the throat and nostrils; patients tend to lean forward during coughing fits, and the chest area is sensitive.
- *Rhus toxicodendron 5 C.* Caused by straining the voice, and aggravated by humidity and improved by talking; *Rhus toxicodendron* cases are characterized by a prickling sensation.
- *Sambucus 5 C.* The voice goes hoarse, and is accompanied by spasms and abundant mucus, which is difficult to expectorate; the condition gets worse around midnight with a suffocating cough. Children wake up suddenly, usually around midnight; they sit up in bed, their face blue, their mouth gaping, and sweat profusely; they are constantly sniffing.
- *Spongia 5 C.* For cases of stridulous (shrill and harsh), acute laryngitis; accompanied by a rasping and wheezing cough; mucous membranes are dry; the larynx is also dry and burning; coughing is aggravated by breathing movements. *Spongia* is also prescribed for cases of stridulous laryngitis associated with thyroid problems. Patients are agitated and anxious, suffer from a dry wheezing cough, and cannot keep their head down. As in *Sambucus* cases, children wake up in the middle of the night with the feeling that they're suffocating; they have a wheezing dry cough and are very anxious; in general, the respiratory passages are dried out; immobility and rest tend to soothe the condition.

Pleurisy

Although pleurisy constitutes a group of disorders which can be effectively treated with homoeopathic remedies, proper diagnosis should be carried out by a competent homoeopathic doctor.

Pleurisy refers to inflammation of the pleura - a double wall which envelops each lung. One wall, the parietal pleura, sticks to the lung itself, while the other is in contact with the chest. After inflammation - which can be very painful - sets in, the two walls, which under normal conditions slide easily over each other during breathing, become irritated and produce a liquid effusion.

Note that there are different types of pleurisy: dry pleurisy, serofibrinous pleurisy, empycma, and finally haemorrhagic pleurisy.

The practice of puncturing a lung to drain fluid is not recommended, unless it is done for purposes of analysis. Draining is considered useless from a homoeopathic point of view, since getting rid of the effusion - which after all is only a sign being sent by the body - does not cure the disorder, and in fact stimulates the production of more fluid and tires patients out even more.

2 granules every three hours:

- *Aconitum 5 C*. Administer at the outset of the disorder, before effusion begins, or in cases of dry pleurisy, where there is no production of liquid; patients have difficulty localizing the pain in their side; the condition often occurs after exposure to cold. The temperature is high, patients are intensely hot and the skin is dry. *Aconitum* patients are typically agitated and fearful.

- *Apis mellifica 5 C*. For the second phase of the disorder, termed serofibrinous; patients are short of breath and have difficulty breathing; they are generally not thirsty, suffer from a dry, sharp cough; the face is pale, the tongue is red and swollen; urine is expelled with difficulty, and in small amounts; hot air aggravates the condition, while cold air and cold compresses ease symptoms to some extent.

- *Arsenicum album 5 C*. For cases where an additional pulmonary cavity forms during the course of the illness, filled with abundant pleural effusion, which is produced very rapidly. Patients have a dry cough and a sense of oppression that causes panting and a feeling of suffocation.

  Although the condition is not especially painful, patients' heartbeat accelerates rapidly with the slightest movement; lower eyelids are frequently puffy (oedema); they are agitated and anxious, and usually have very low morale, bordering on desperation.

- *Asclepias tuberosa 5 C*. Administer when the illness is at its worst, i.e. when the pleura is being rubbed and irritated, in cases where the pleurisy was caused by prolonged exposure to damp cold.

   A dry cough is accompanied by sensitivity all along the sternum, and intense pain on the left side, which is aggravated by movement; pains are eased when patients lean forward; the throat is constricted; patients are very short of breath with a tiring cough, but do not expectorate.

- *Bryonia 5 C*. For dry pleurisy, or pleurisy during the rubbing stage; a dry cough produces headaches; respiration is accelerated and painful.

   Patients have twinges in the side, which are soothed by pressure or by lying on the side. Pain is acute, and patients try to avoid all movement; they thirst for cold water, and the tongue and lips are dry.

- *Cantharis 5 C*. The illness has reached its peak (with profuse effusion - the acute phase of serofibrinous pleurisy). *Cantharis* may be administered in conjunction with *Bryonia*.

   Patients have palpitations and perspire. Effusions increase in quantity, urinating becomes difficult, urine is sometimes red and is expelled in small quantities; pain is felt in the chest, in the larynx and in the urinary tracts (in men this causes spontaneous erections).

- *Hepar sulphuris 5 C*. For serofibrinous pleurisy or empyema characterized during the second phase of the illness by profuse effusion.

- *Ranunculus 5 C*. Administered during the stage where the pleura is rubbing, this remedy soothes pains in the ribs, and acts on the skin, muscles and intercostal spaces in the thoracic wall; patients feel a prickling sensation between the shoulder blades; pains felt in the chest are aggravated by cold, damp weather, by movement and by variations in temperature.

- *Sulphur iodatum 5 C*. Administer after a bout of pleurisy. *Sulphur* works on the adhesions (areas where the pleura has rubbed together) and prevents them from reforming. *Sulphur iodatum* lessens the tendency to chronic inflammation.

   Use *Sulphur iodatum* along with *Pulsatilla* when breathing remains difficult even after effusion ceases, and as long as pain is still felt in the affected side of the body.

Pneumonia

Pneumonia (from the Greek "pneuma" - lung) is inflammation of the lungs, accompanied by chest pains and expectoration of blood. The initial phase can be recognized by a characteristic shivering, which may last as long as half an hour. This is followed by breathing difficulties.

Lips become blue, and patients sweat profusely; they feel sharp twinges in the side; a dry cough sets in, punctuated by expectoration of a reddish colour, which becomes yellowish after about a week; fever is steady at about 102.2 to 104°F (39-40°C).

Pneumonia seems to last for a set length of time - fever starts coming down around the tenth day, so it can be assumed that it takes that long for the body to mount its own defence.

2 granules twice a day:

- *Antimonium tartaricum 5 C*. Breathing produces a rasping sound in the chest; patients gasp for breath and expectorate with difficulty; lips and fingers turn blue, and the tongue is coated white.

  Coughing fits are sometimes followed by nausea and vomiting. *Antimonium tartaricum* is especially recommended for older people, in whom the illness is harder to detect.

- *Arsenicum album 5 C*. Burning pain is aggravated by cold, especially after midnight; the condition is improved by dry warm compresses, hot drinks and food, and when patients are in a sitting position with the head up.

- *Belladonna 5 C*. For sensitive or hypersensitive patients of a delicate constitution. Draughts and movement aggravate the condition, while resting in bed in subdued light soothes the discomfort.

  Patients are not agitated but sweat profusely; they are drowsy and, in some cases, exhausted (characteristic of *Belladonna* cases). This is an appropriate remedy to administer at the outset of bronchopneumonia and may also be given to small children.

- *Bryonia 5 C*. This is one of the important remedies for curing pneumonia and is often used as a follow-up to *Belladonna*. Patients are thirsty, they have a dry cough, and any movement -breathing and especially coughing - causes extreme discomfort.

  Pain is soothed by lying on the affected side and remaining immobile. Patients frequently suffer from headaches and hot oily sweating. They thirst for cold water, the tongue is coated yellow, and they expectorate rust-coloured phlegm.

- *Carbo vegetabilis 4 C*. This remedy is recommended for older people whose bodies have been weakened by one or a number of illnesses - subjects have lost their strength and vital heat.

  Lips are purple, the extremities are cold and the pulse is weak. Patients are generally cold and suffer from violent coughing fits.

- *Lycopodium 4 C*. Digestive problems appear, especially in the liver. Nostrils quiver, the skin is dry and patients are generally weak; they suffer from a distended stomach, intestinal wind and constipation. The right lung (close to the liver) is affected.

- *Phosphorus 4 C*. The entire body is hot; patients sweat profusely and are agitated and anxious; they feel a burning heat in the chest cavity; they are short of breath, racked by a dry, painful cough, and thirst for cold water.

  Pain is often localized on the left side; hot flushes are accompanied by a feeling of heaviness and pressure on the chest; in some cases the pulse is weak and rapid.

  Phlegm contains blood and patients become delirious; they develop digestive problems, especially diarrhoea.

Rhinopharyngitis (Nasopharyngitis)

Rhinopharyngitis is inflammation of the respiratory mucous membranes, which become very irritated and therefore subject to spasms. They secrete an abundance of filament-like mucus which is difficult to expel.

The walls of the respiratory passages (mucous membranes) are very sensitive to touch - the nose and back of the throat are inflamed. Fever is what distinguishes rhinopharyngitis from a common head cold (coryza). If there is fever, you must act quickly, either by consulting a doctor or by administering a homoeopathic treatment, in which case you should be on the lookout for rapid results (if they do not appear, consult a doctor).

3 granules twice a day:

- *Coccus cacti 5 C*. For acute cases of rhinopharyngitis. A characteristic remedy for those who are sensitive to cold and catch cold easily. Respiratory passages are sensitive to the touch; mucus is colourless and the nostrils are dry.

  Patients feel as if their throat is being torn apart every time they try to cough up mucus; nostrils are dried out, coughing is spasmodic and comes in fits; the condition is aggravated in overheated rooms and soothed by drinking cold liquids.

- *Hydrastis 5 C.* In addition to general physical weakness, people tend to become depressed. Mucous membranes (mucosa) produce a tenacious, thick, viscous, yellowish discharge which gives the impression of burning without parching the throat (large balls of phlegm form, especially at the base of the throat). *Hydrastis* is also recommended for cases which seem to take a turn for the worse, or where a patient's general condition seems to be deteriorating.

- *Kali bichromicum 5 C.* Subjects experience a sensation of weakness and slight burning in the mouth and pharynx; saliva is stringy and viscous, the tongue is red and dry, or covered with a yellowish coating.
Patients feel thirsty and need to clear their throat every morning, trying to expel globs of phlegm. Ulcerations are surrounded by a coppery-red halo.

- *Pulsatilla 5 C.* When patients are in an overheated room, their nose gets blocked and the condition worsens; fresh air seems to improve the symptoms; nasal suppuration is intense, especially at night; expectoration decreases in the morning; slight fever is accompanied by shivering.

- *Sambucus 5 C.* The nose is blocked and dry, and patients can only breathe with their mouth open. Infants who are affected cannot feed and come close to suffocating. *Sambucus* cases are characterized by constant sniffling, a feeling of suffocation especially around midnight, fever, sweating and hoarseness; the condition is aggravated by exposure to dry cold air.

Sinusitis

Inflammation of the sinuses in the face starts in the nose after a cold, throat infection or influenza. Initial symptoms are congestion and an accumulation of excreted liquid.

This causes the sinuses to start suppurating rather quickly, which becomes apparent as a purulent liquid starts to flow from the nose, usually from one nostril at a time.

Painful pulsing is felt in the forehead or around the jawbone. In its chronic form, sinusitis does not cause extreme suffering, but merely signals its presence by colds or hoarseness for no apparent reason. The type of cough is an indicator of which specific remedy to administer.

Onion poultices, although unpleasant, are effective. Cut an onion into small pieces, and wrap them up in some gauze; secure this to the nape of the neck and leave it there overnight. Compresses and hot foot baths can also alleviate pain. But don't forget that each case of sinusitis has its own unique "personality."

3 granules twice a day:

- *Belladonna 5 C.* For cases of acute sinusitis, without a runny nose; symptoms appear suddenly, accompanied by shooting pains; the nose is blocked, the face is flushed, pupils are dilated and patients develop nosebleeds; the condition is aggravated by light, noise and jolts; patients tend to suffer from fatigue, and have some fever.

- *Hepar sulphuris 5 C.* A recognized remedy for sinusitis; especially suited for cases where people experience prickling pains; the condition is aggravated by extremes of temperature, by touch and by cold draughts. Symptoms are improved by local application of heat (a warm scarf or compresses, for example). Do not use *Hepar sulphuris* if there is no suppuration.

- *Hydrastis 5 C.* In these particular cases, secretions are watery and cause irritation of the nostrils and lips; patients sweat profusely; the condition is aggravated by overheated rooms and soothed by fresh air but this will increase the flow of mucus.

- *Kali bichromicum 5 C.* Similar to *Hydrastis* cases, except that symptoms are soothed by heat and aggravated by cold; secretions are viscous yellow (thicker than *Hydrastis* cases) and tend to form crusts; patients feel painful pressure at the base of the nose, which is usually blocked.

- *Kali iodatum 5 C.* The tip of the nose is red and inflamed; the discharge is clearer than in *Kali bichromicum* cases, but is more irritating; patients suffer from headaches, centred around the base of the nose; the condition is aggravated by fresh air.

- *Mercurius solubilis 5 C.* For sinusitis which occurs after a head cold (coryza). Symptoms include a persistent runny nose producing a greenish discharge which irritates the nostrils; sinus pains get worse at night; the condition is aggravated by cold damp weather and soothed by rest.

- *Cinnabaris 5 C.* Patients have very bad breath, and a purulent running nose; they are very sensitive to touch and to darkness; they experience painful pressure at the base of the nose, especially at night; the condition is aggravated by extremes of temperature and soothed by fresh air and sunshine.

Tonsillitis (Throat Infection)

Although not very serious in itself, inflammation of the throat requires careful treatment, since it can lead to serious complications, from inflammation of the kidneys (nephritis) to cardiac problems and otitis.

The condition generally produces small, isolated white spots on the throat. If, instead of the white spots, you observe a grey pseudomembrane which covers the throat area, then you may be dealing with a case of diphtheria (see section).

As for all throat disorders, washing and gargling with *Molkosan* (a whey concentrate) is essential and may cure the problem completely, as it is a powerful disinfectant.

Make sure you maintain proper oral hygiene by brushing your teeth regularly, and gargling with salt water. Also, infusions of *Solidago* help fight toxins in the throat. You can take syrup made from *Santasapina pine buds*.

Poultices made from cabbage leaves and diluted clay make a good external treatment, accompanied by horsetail infusions and sweat baths which help eliminate toxins produced by the inflammation.

Finally, diet should be low in salt and protein, and rich in calcium. Make sure you include two or three teaspoons of honey per day.

2 granules every two hours:

- *Belladonna 4 C*. This is the most common remedy. The inflammation is severe; the throat is dry and bright red, and lymph nodes are swollen; patients suffer from thirst, and swallowing is painful.
- *Dulcamara 4 C*. For repeated sore throats that appear suddenly; lymph nodes in the neck increase in volume; people salivate a lot.
- *Kali muriaticum 4 C*. Although the throat is red, the tonsils are white; there may also be black spots on them.
- *Mercurius cyanatus 4 C*. These people have slight fever, the throat is dark red; white spots are visible on the tonsils, and lymph nodes are very sensitive; patients clear their throat continually, trying to expel an object that isn't there; as in *Belladonna* cases, subjects are very thirsty.

Whooping Cough (Pertussis)

Perceived as a benign disorder, whooping cough is in fact much less dangerous now than it used to be. However, it should be treated as soon as the first symptoms appear, to avoid complications. Homoeopathy can usually cure the illness in about a fortnight, if the right treatment is chosen at the outset. If this is the case, a progressive decrease in the severity of characteristic symptoms will be observed.

Whooping cough usually affects children under ten years of age. After an incubation period of between one and two weeks, the first symptoms, which resemble those of an ordinary cold, appear. However, subjects also tend to lose their appetite and become generally apathetic.

Sneezing is replaced by a dry cough. After a fortnight, coughing fits become violent, and this phase can last more than a month. The frequency and intensity of the coughing fits are indicative of the seriousness of the situation. If patients have more than one coughing fit per hour, or more than thirty in a 24-hour period, a doctor should be consulted.

Keep children warm, but ventilate the sickroom regularly (put the child in another room while airing it out). To avoid complications, make sure the patient's diet is supplemented with appropriate nutrients to help the body resist complications.

Complications develop if the patient's body is weak. It must be stated that homoeopathic treatment does not suppress the whooping cough, but does help reduce the duration and intensity of the disorder, as well as avoid complications.

3 granules three times per day:

- *Antimonium tartaricum 5 C.* Breathing is noisy, with rasping in the lungs; the voice is hoarse, but there is little expectoration. Children tend to be drowsy between coughing fits. This remedy should be administered at the height of the disorder, and as it declines.
- *Arnica 5 C.* Children feel the cough coming on and start crying beforehand. Afterwards, they are exhausted, and can't get comfortable in bed, which feels too hard; they suffer from fatigue and irritation of the larynx.
- *Belladonna 5 C.* The cough is more phlegmy and occurs especially at night; brought on by a tickling sensation in the throat, it is accompanied by congestion and agitation; mucus is thick and colourless; coughing fits are accompanied by sneezing; children shiver, and may lose their voice for a while. The face is red, eyes are bloodshot, skin is clammy. In some cases the cough is dry, and the throat is red and painful.
- *Carbo vegetabilis 5 C.* A remedy to be administered when the illness is at its peak, or in case of an epidemic as a preventive measure, when children start coughing; they are soon exhausted and suffer from hot

299

flushes; the cough is dry. In some cases, coughing fits are accompanied by sneezing and cold sweats, as well as vomiting after meals. Personality changes may also become apparent. Patients tend to become more hoarse at night and may experience a burning sensation in the chest.

- *Coccus cacti 5 C.* Coughing fits are punctuated by expectoration of dribble and thick viscous mucus. Patients sometimes suffer from headaches and tend to haemorrhage - nosebleeds, or blood mixed with mucus. Abundant urine is a characteristic symptom of *Coccus cacti.*

- *Coral rubrum 5 C.* A basic remedy. Coughing fits are preceded by gasping for breath or bouts of suffocation, and the face goes almost purple; coughing is violent and suffocating, and leaves patients exhausted; they seem to go on and on without any intervals; they may also vomit mucus which contains blood.

- *Cuprum 4 C.* Coughing is convulsive, fits are prolonged and repeated; the face is red and patients feel as if they are suffocating; they have a tendency to faint and are overcome with anxiety between attacks. Drinking cold water between coughing fits provides some relief. Extremities (especially lips and fingers) are bluish.

- *Drosera 5 C.* Attacks often occur after midnight. A characteristic sign of *Drosera* is that patients hold their stomach while coughing - dry coughing produces spasms which are so intense that patients have to press on the stomach for some relief. Coughing may be accompanied by nausea and vomiting, and mucus may be mixed with blood; patients often have fever at the beginning or end of the day, and suffer from hot sweats at night; they are sad, lose their appetite, and their voice becomes hoarse.

- *Ipecac. 5 C.* Patients are in good moral and physical shape. Coughing fits are violent, causing them to shake with spasms; they tense up, go pale and are covered in cold sweat. After a coughing fit, they may sneeze continually or vomit, both of which leaves them feeling exhausted. The tongue is not coated; expectorated mucus is slimy; patients tend to be anxious.

- *Mephitis 5 C.* The cough is violent and is preceded by spasms. Fits usually occur during the night, or when patients are eating, in which case they are accompanied by vomiting. *Mephitis* types want to bathe in cold water, have difficulty breathing, are feverish and have bloodshot eyes.

- *Pertussinum 4 C.* This remedy can be used in cases of persistent coughing, as an aid to *Pulsatilla* or as a preventive measure in times of epidemic. When prescribed early on, it reduces the risk of complications.

- *Pulsatilla 5 C.* The basic remedy for whooping-cough, *Pulsatilla* can also be used as a preventive measure during epidemics. During convalescence with *Pulsatilla,* patients characteristically expel a lot of mucus. It is during convalescence that bronchitis may develop - there will be no more vomiting or coughing fits, but frequent expectoration of yellow mucus.

  During the illness, the cough is dry at night and phlegmy during the day; patients are not thirsty, and lose their sense of smell and taste.

- *Sulphur iodatum 5 C.* An initial remedy, to be administered at the outset of the illness after *Pertussinum* (unless the throat is delicate and tends to suppurate). Also administer at the end of the illness, to prevent it from becoming chronic.

Chapter 8

Skin Disorders

Abscess
(See Also Boils)

An abscess is an accumulation of pus in tissues, or sometimes in natural cavities such as the lungs or even the liver, which then becomes harmful to surrounding tissue.

To help an abscess come to a head more quickly, suck 5 granules of *Hepar sulphuris 7 C* (especially if the abscess suppurates, is sensitive to touch and causes the person to sweat profusely from even minor effort), or *Lachesis mutus 7 C*. You can also apply compresses made with *Calendula* solution (one teaspoon of *Calendula T.M.* dissolved in a glass of water that has been boiled and cooled) or *Calendula* ointment. You can also make a poultice using onion slices.

3 granules once a day:

- *Belladonna 4 C.* An initial remedy, when inflammation progresses rapidly, causing intense pain, which tends to irradiate with heat.
- *Ferrum phosphoricum 6 C.* Alternate every hour if *Belladonna* does not produce results, or if patients are of a frail constitution.
- *Hepar sulphuris 4 C.* The most effective homeopathic remedy for cases of suppuration; the slightest touch is painful; pain gets worse at night and when exposed to cold; when the abscess is open, pus is often mixed with blood and has an odour of old cheese.
- *Lachesis 7 C.* Administer every two hours, to help the abscess come to a head more quickly.
- *Tarentula Cubensis 9 C.* Used successfully for abscesses of the nails, especially in cases where affected areas take on a bluish colour.
- *Pyrogenium 5 C.* A general remedy. Patients are prostrate, have a slight fever, and their pulse is very rapid; they suffer from bad breath, and perspiration (as well as urine) also has an unpleasant odour.

Dental Abscess

- *Hepar sulphuris 7 C.* Once the affected tooth has been pulled.

Acne

In this day and age, a lot of emphasis is placed on appearance. An unhealthy looking skin can create many problems, not the least of which is a loss of self-confidence. This is even more true during adolescence, an age where acne commonly appears on the face, shoulders, back and chest.

It is well known that diet plays an important role in maintaining healthy skin. To get rid of impurities that affect the skin, start by eating less greasy food (especially animal fat) to the point where you cut out fried foods completely. Also, sweets, pastries, eggs (including egg-based recipes) and spicy foods should be avoided whenever possible.

On the other hand, certain foods are recommended because they are rich in vital nutrients: white cheese, soft ripe cheese, fresh vegetables, natural whole grain rice, potatoes (not to be eaten with rice).

An essential point is to eat slowly and chew your food well in order to avoid facial congestion after meals and prevent the build-up of fatty substances that are eliminated through the skin and increase secretion by the sebaceous glands (the glands which provide the skin with its natural oils).

3 granules once a day:

- *Antimonium crudum 4 C*. For overweight people.
- *Antimonium tartaricum 5 C*. Pimples leave a bluish scar.
- *Eugenia jambosum 5 C*. For acne that gets worse during menstruation.
- *Graphites 5 C*. Pimples suppurate and produce viscous, sticky, thick yellowish pus which forms crusts; pimples are often situated behind the ears, between fingers and toes, and even on or around the genitals.

  Two further symptoms characterize *Graphites*: constipation and dry unhealthy skin which suppurates easily.
- *Kali bromatum 5 C*. For acne on the face, back of the neck and shoulders; children who develop this type of acne suffer from night terrors and may walk in their sleep; adults may suffer from memory loss and constant agitation of the hands.
- *Natrum muriaticum 5 C*. A basic remedy, often prescribed during adolescence; spots concentrate around the hairline, and small dry crusts form soon after the rash.
- *Pulsatilla 5 C*. A basic remedy, especially prescribed during puberty, and for those with delicate constitutions, who tend to blush easily.
- *Sulphur 5 C*. For rather thin people with dry, rough, unclean skin; acne develops on the forehead and back, and suppurates easily; these people also suffer from gastric problems after meals; the tongue has a thick white coating; the corners of the mouth are chapped, and subjects are constantly thirsty.

Acne Rosacea (Blotchiness)

This inflammation of the cutaneous glands of the face produces characteristic red blotches.

The condition is caused by improper functioning of the digestive system, certain chronic heart or lung disorders, problems of the tonsils or the menopause.

While waiting to see a doctor, care for your liver, eat slowly, drink little between meals and avoid alcoholic beverages and hot drinks, especially tea. Adopt a sober diet (see the diet prescribed for eczema) and drink fresh fruit juices. Avoid extreme temperatures, the sun, sea air and clothes that are too tight. Replace your normal soap with an antibacterial skin-cleansing lotion.

- *Radium bromatum 5 C* and *Sulphur iodatum 5 C,* 5 granules every seven days, alternating.
- *Nux vomica 5 C and Ledum palustre 4 C*, 2 granules of each on alternate days, for alcoholic cases.

Aphthae (Mouth Ulcers)

Aphthae are small ulcers which develop on the mucous membranes of the mouth or throat.

Drink infusions of thyme or mother-of-thyme, rinse the mouth with *Calendula T.M.* (10 drops dissolved in a glass of water that has been boiled and cooled). After meals, brush your teeth with M.C. toothpaste (30 percent hydroxydase). Children should take 1 to 3 teaspoons of *Scientia vitamin C* every day. Adults should take a capsule of 500 mg ascorbic acid per day.

3 granules once every two days (Also see Directions for Use - Infants):

- *Borax 7 C. Borax* babies start crying as soon as they are made to lean forward, and when defaecating (they suffer from clear yellowish diarrhoea) or urinating; ulcers appear as very painful, burning blisters, which bleed easily; the mouth is hot and sensitive.
- *Mercurius cyanatus 5 C.* People have bad breath, their face is pale and their body is cold.
- *Mercurius solubilis 4 C.* The mouth is very wet from abundant saliva, yet people are always thirsty; they have a slight metallic, coppery and sweetish taste in their mouth.
- *Natrum muriaticum 5 C.* A basic treatment for people who develop these mouth ulcers repeatedly.
- *Sulphuric acid 4 C.* For aphthae which appear in people who are

generally weak or suffer from fatigue, and who use stimulants like alcohol.

Blepharitis (Palpebritis)

Although a minor disorder, blepharitis, which causes inflammation of the edge of the eyelids, is unpleasant and tenacious. In cases of ciliary blepharitis, the eyelashes stick together and sometimes fall out.

Blepharitis often accompanies a head cold, conjunctivitis or eczema. Women sometimes develop the disorder after using certain brands of eye pencil or mascara.

- *Graphites 9 C.* 5 granules once a week, in the morning after waking up, with *Staphysagria 7 C* and *Pulsatilla 7 C,* 2 granules around six o'clock in the evening, alternating one with the other.

Boils

Boils are the body's reaction to microbes which become lodged at the base of a hair follicle. They are like volcanoes, filled with pus. In more serious cases, when a cluster of boils forms, the condition is called a carbuncle.

Take supplements of vitamins A, B_1 and C. Avoid wearing clothes that rub. Do not touch or press on the boil, especially if it's on the face, not only for aesthetic reasons, but because you risk spreading the microbe through the blood and causing a generalized infection (septicaemia). Don't take baths, for the same reason.

Don't apply hot or wet compresses, unless prescribed by a doctor. Finally, abstain from sugar and starchy foods for the time being (see the diet outlined for Gastritis, in the chapter on digestion). Instead, boil ground fenugreek or ground linseed, and apply the solution to the boils.

This will bring the boil to a head and open it up more quickly (boiled, mashed potatoes will have the same effect). Once the boil is empty, wash the wound well, and spread a little biological lime powder (or fine sugar) on it. Then apply mashed cabbage leaves. Take brewer's yeast extract to accelerate the healing process (in small quantities). Also take brewer's yeast to prevent boils from reappearing.

2 granules twice a day:

- *Anthracinum 5 C.* For cases of large boils or carbuncles; skin around the boil(s) is hard; the centre of the boil may be black.

- *Apis mellifica 4 C,* every twelve hours, after *Hepar sulphuris* if the inflammation gets worse and swells up, forming a burning, red blister.
- *Arnica 5 C.* For boils that are very painful and seem to contain dark-coloured blood instead of pus.
- *Arsenicum album 4 C.* 2 granules every six hours, accompanied by *Hepar sulphuris* if the boil is bluish-black and causes burning pain, especially at night; subjects are agitated.
- *Hepar sulphuris 4 C.* As soon as the first signs of a boil or carbuncle appear; follow up with *Apis mellifica, Arsenicum album* or *Lachesis.*
- *Lachesis 5 C* with *Hepar sulphuris 4 C.* The boil is a dark purple colour, and seems to get worse during the night.
- *Tarentula Cubensis 7 C.* An effective remedy for boils and abscess. When injected, healing occurs even more rapidly.
- *Pyrogenium 5 C.* When the pulse is rapid, and patients feel physically agitated.

Corns (On the Feet)

Corns usually develop because of constant rubbing of shoes on a toe or between the toes. So in most cases, improperly fitting shoes are to blame.

Actually, we are at fault and not our shoes! Many people tend to place fashion above comfort, and many parents do not replace their children's shoes to keep pace with quickly growing feet.

Wear shoes with thick, firm, flexible soles, which give the feet enough room to spread lengthwise and sideways. Avoid high heels. If you do have corns, you may be forced to buy shoes that are a size larger than usual, to fit the new shape of your feet.

3 granules every two days:

- *Antimonium crudum 5 C.* The corn is painful, very sensitive to touch, and the heat of being indoors aggravates the pain, as does walking. Footbaths soothe the pain.
- *Radium bromatum 6 C.* For verrucas, corns or calluses that are not inflamed, but which grow larger and are painful to the touch. They are soothed by hot and moist compresses.
- *Thuja 5 C.* For inflammation that is less painful and less sensitive to touch.

Cosmetics
(See Also Skin Hygiene)

Certain types of lipstick can cause eczema. Eye-shadow can cause dermatitis of the eyelids and even corneal ulcers. Hair-removing creams, medicated soaps and creams used without medical advice can also cause skin problems.

In other words, you should be careful in your choice of cosmetics. Use natural products as much as possible, in which the perfumes are made from natural essential oils instead of synthetic products. The skin usually does not react well to chemical-based beauty products.

Powders, some oil-based foundation creams and concealers block the pores and prevent the skin from breathing. Skin that is covered with cosmetics too much of the time begins to fade and age prematurely.

In fact, strictly speaking (and leaving fashion aside for a moment) a healthy skin does not need to be cosmetically enhanced at all, except to protect it from severe weather: sun, wind, cold and water. *Bioforce* cream is an excellent protection for all kinds of inclement weather.

Testing Lipstick

To avoid problems, you can test a new brand of lipstick by applying a small amount onto your arm (which has been cleaned of grease). Wait for 24 hours, then clean the skin. If there is any redness, try a different brand.

Dermatitis (In Infants)

Starting on the buttocks, redness spreads to the stomach, the back, the chest, up to the folds of the neck and armpits until it finally reaches the face and scalp.

The skin becomes wrinkled and covered with scales. Choose one of the following homeopathic remedies while waiting to consult a doctor. This seemingly harmless disorder can result in serious complications, especially if accompanied by fever (see Directions for Use - Infants).

3 granules every two days:

- *Euphorbium 5 C.* When redness is intense and complicated by inflammation; the skin seems thick and peels off in scales (desquamation).
- *Graphites 5 C.* Lesions appear in the folds of the skin, with oozing that forms crusts.

- *Rhus tox 5 C.* For agitated infants who can't stop scratching themselves. Especially for dermatitis that produces pimples.

Eczema
(See Also Allergies and Rashes)

Eczema is not an illness in itself, but rather a surface indication that something is wrong inside the body. It might be an intestinal or liver disorder, an allergy, nervousness, etc.

But don't be fooled. Eczema, like many skin problems, is very difficult to cure, and you may have to consult a dermatologist if the descriptions that follow do not address your specific case (it would be impossible to predict all the potential causes of eczema, which is why the knowledge and experience a professional practitioner can offer is always preferable to the information you can find in books).

Allergies: Fighting Fire With Fire

When inflammation is due to an allergy, start by identifying the substance or product that causes the reaction. You can then undergo a form of treatment called "Isotherapy": you provide a laboratory with a sample of the substance in question, where it is then "triturated" and "dynamized" scientifically. A single dose of this isotherapeutic medication may be enough to cure a person of a very unpleasant allergy.

If you cannot identify the substance in question, administer *Histaminum 9 C.*

Baths and Compresses

Bathing affected areas with *Molkosan* is an effective way to cure eczema, if the condition is not caused by an allergy, or an intestinal, liver or kidney disorder. *Molkosan,* a whey concentrate, contains a natural lactic acid that destroys harmful bacteria, irrigates the epidermis and regenerates the skin through the action of its mineral salts and enzymes.

Complete the local treatment with compresses of *Urticalcin* powder (a calcium complex) and *Bioforce* cream.

Diet

Lactic albumin in the form of white cheese, buttermilk, butter or almond milk (especially in cases where cow's milk itself causes problems) are all foods that can help the condition. Base your diet on natural whole grain rice and add foods that are rich in calcium (white cabbage, raw natural sauerkraut, rape leaves, etc.).

Avoid pastries since white sugar, and to some extent white flour, have a harmful affect on people with skin rashes.

Urticalcin, a tested biological, calcium-based preparation, can compensate for any calcium deficiency, while *Nephrosolid* will ensure proper functioning of the kidneys. Also drink myrtle, blackberry or grapefruit juice. It is essential that the liver and kidneys function properly, and that kidneys are always protected against cold and damp.

Spinach and Lemons

Food poisoning or a vitamin deficiency can also cause eczema rashes. Prepare salads with lemon, spinach and young nettle leaves (using organically grown ingredients, if possible). The vitamins contained in these foods should clear up the eczema rash rapidly. To this you can add infusions of dandelion leaves and yarrow.

External Care

Apply *Molkosan* and *Usneasan* directly to affected areas. Since skin suffering from eczema tends to dry out, use St. John's wort oil and *Bioforce* cream as moisturizers.

2 granules once a day:

- *Apis 5 C.* For eczema that appears suddenly; patients are hot, not thirsty, and urinate in small amounts.
- *Anagallis 4 C.* For eczema on the palms of the hands.
- *Arsenicum album 4 C.* The skin is scaly (desquamation); the condition improves with heat and gets worse when exposed to cold; patients scratch themselves (which always causes them to bleed).
- *Belladonna 5 C.* Inflammation appears suddenly; the skin is hot, swollen and shiny.
- *Bovista 5 C.* For eczema that is aggravated during the summer months.
- *Carbolicum acidum 5 C.* For eczema around the eyelids.
- *Cistus 5 C.* For eczema that is aggravated during the winter months.
- *Croton tiglium 5 C.* For eczema of the genital organs.
- *Dulcamara 5 C.* When eczema is aggravated by humidity.
- *Graphites 5 C.* A thick, sticky, irritating liquid oozes from crusts. Combine with *Calcarea carbonica 5 C* if the eczema affects the face, the

scalp or the area behind the ears.

- *Hepar sulphuris 4 C.* For purulent, fetid and painful eczema.
- *Mezereum 5 C.* For eczema that forms crusts or when the rash appears on the scalp. Also for cradle cap in infants.
- *Mercurius 5 C.* For eczema that produces a foul-smelling pus, often accompanied by fever.
- *Natrum carbonicum 4 C.* For eczema that affects the back of the fingers.
- *Natrum muriaticum 5 C.* For dry and crusty eczema of the tubercular type.
- *Petroleum 4 C.* For eczema where the skin is cracked, dry and thick, and rashes are often found in the folds of the skin; chapping and fissures may become established between the fingers; the condition is accompanied by neck pains, diarrhoea and dizziness, and is aggravated in winter.
- *Pix liquida 4 C.* For eczema on the back of the hands.
- *Sulphur 5 C.* The skin is dry and unhealthy looking; eczema is aggravated by washing.
- *Rhus toxicodendron 5 C.* For painful eczema (more painful when exposed to cold air) accompanied by blisters or pustules oozing a clear liquid; the condition tends to get worse at night.
- *Sepia 5 C.* For eczema in the folds around the elbows.
- *Viola tricolor 4 C.* One of the most effective remedies for eczema and crusting. Also for cases where the eczema affects the face, and crusts are the colour of honey.

Erysipelas (Facial)

Eruptions in the form of blisters (vesicles) form against a reddish background and are accompanied by itching. Scratching only aggravates the condition.

2 granules once a day:

- *Mezereum 3 C.* For cases which conform to the above description.
- *Carbolicum acidum 5 C.* If vesicles produce a burning sensation.

Erythema (Buttocks)

Redness on the buttocks appears during an acute but temporary illness or during a bout of diarrhoea, especially in infants. If the redness spreads rapidly or if pimples or blisters form on the stomach, back or thighs, consult a doctor.

The following remedies are designed to treat the most common types of erythema (see Directions for Use - Infants for correct preparation of dosages).

A thick paste, applied locally, will isolate the affected area from faeces and urine, and prevent further irritation.

2 granules twice a day:

- *Borax 5 C.* Where redness appears, the skin is thick, inflamed and painful. If *Borax* alone is not enough to cure the disorder, add *Mercurius 5 C,* especially in cases where stool smells very strongly.
- *Cantharis 5 C.* Buttocks are red and burning; babies cry as soon as they are wet; urine aggravates the condition.
- *Kreosotum 5 C.* When streaks of blood appear in the nappies, and stool has an especially unpleasant smell.

Erythema Nodosum

This disorder, which in the past was considered a form of tuberculosis and then of rheumatism, still has not been classified satisfactorily. It is characterized by the appearance of about a dozen hard nodules on the skin; these are rounded and clearly defined, and measure between one and five centimetres in diameter.

These nodules resemble those of ecchymosis; they disappear after about ten days and are usually accompanied by fever. Erythema nodosum usually appears in springtime and winter, and affects women more than men, especially between the ages of twenty and thirty.

It's best to consult a doctor and get a general check-up, to make sure the erythema nodosum is not a forerunner of a more serious disorder, like tuberculous meningitis or pulmonary tuberculosis.

A local treatment consists of massaging the affected area with *Arnica* oil.

2 granules twice a day:

- *Apis 5 C.* Administer for a few days, when redness is still not very apparent; pains are burning and prickly, are soothed by cold and aggravated by heat.
- *Carbolicum acidum 5 C.* For cases of burning erythema nodosum, accompanied by itching.
- *Euphorbia lathyris 5 C.* Erythema starts, or predominates in exposed parts of the body (especially the face) with redness, swelling, and burning sensations; nodules are painful to the touch and are aggravated by exposure to cold air.

- *Rhus tox 4 C*. 2 granules every three hours, alternating with *Sulphothiazole 4 C*, also every three hours. The erythema has a dark red colour.
- *Pulsatilla 5 C*. Alternated with *Sulphur iodatum 5 C*, will accelerate convalescence.

Face
(See Also Skin and Wrinkles)

Certain skin problems of the face like redness, oedema and burns can be treated in their initial phase with *Apis 5 C* and *Iodatum 5 C*.

Hair

Beautiful hair is a sure indication of good general health and depends on diet, exercise, fresh air and sunshine.

General Care

A simple way to remedy scalp problems consists of rubbing it with half a raw onion before shampooing. You can then apply a lanolin-based cream (oil extracted from lamb's wool). You can also buy onion lotion if you don't want to use raw onions! Wash your hair with camomile or onion water.

Good hair care, however, is not just a matter of external treatment. A preparation of silicic acid and biological calcium can do wonders for the scalp, which often falls into bad condition due to a lack of calcium and silicic acid in the body.

For rashes affecting the scalp, try a decoction of nettles or fresh nettle extract.

Split Ends

- *Fluoricum acidum 5 C*. 2 granules every two days. Hair is dry, the ends are split and the hair lacks shine and body.

Greasy Hair

Girls and women with hormonal problems who have greasy hair can remedy the problem by taking hot sitz baths every night, and wearing warm underwear.

- *Phosphoricum acidum 5 C*. 2 granules every two days.

Dry Hair

- *Thuja 5 C.* 2 granules every two days.

Hair Loss (Alopecia)

- *Arnica 20 C.* 3 granules once a week. For hair loss due to shock, or psychological trauma.
- *Fluoricum acidum 5 C.* 2 granules once a day. For localized hair loss.
- *Graphites 5 C.* Once a day. Hair falls out by the handful.
- *Natrum muriaticum 20 C.* 3 granules once a week. When hair loss occurs following grief or worries.
- *Phosphoricum acidum 5 C.* 2 granules every two days. When hair loss occurs after a period of depression or a debilitating illness. Also for general hair loss in nervous people and people with greasy hair.
- *Sepia 5 C.* 3 granules every two days. For hair loss after giving birth.
- *Thuja 5 C.* 3 granules every two days. People suffer from seborrhoea (excessive secretion by the sebaceous glands); their hair has split ends, and eyelashes also fall out. Also for cases of dry hair.

Dandruff

- *Phosphoricum acidum 5 C.* 3 granules every two days.

Seborrhoea

- *Oleander 5 C.* 3 granules every two days. When sebaceous glands excrete too much, follicles get blocked up and the hair falls out. Also for those who have itchy or painful scalps.

Herpes

We often develop herpes symptoms after catching a cold or getting flu (hence the common name of "cold sores") and they sometimes appear during menstruation or when we are under a lot of stress. Developing herpes seems to have a lot to do with our psychological state.

This disorder is caused by a virus, and is situated on the lips and genitals in particular, but may also appear on any other parts of the body. Approximately 30 per cent of people do not have anti-herpes antibodies, which creates an ideal environment for recurrent herpes, recognizable by a red area on the skin where a number of transparent blisters (vesicles) form, which ooze a murky, non-purulent liquid. Itching is frequently present.

In pregnant women, herpes can cause a miscarriage - consult a homeopathic doctor as soon as possible. The same goes for herpes contracted by infants and young children.

Treat herpes locally (as a complement to internal treatment) by applying *Calendula tincture* mixed with *Calendula talc* to the vesicles. When the case concerns painful genital herpes, add *Vaccinotoxinum 7 C,* one dose every two weeks. Clay compresses are also effective. *Capsicum T.M.,* one drop on the vesicle every night before going to sleep, combats herpes of the lips.

3 granules once a day:

- *Anagallis 6 C.* Vesicles are grouped together and people experience intense itching.
- *Croton tiglium 5 C.* Herpes sores are very itchy, but scratching only aggravates them. Also for genital herpes in males, with *Graphites 5 C.*
- *Lachesis 5 C.* For women who are approaching their period.
- *Psorinum 5 C.* When the herpes sore oozes liquid.
- *Rhus tox 7 C.* For herpes that causes intense itching which is soothed by heat; the area around the vesicle(s) is red. Recommended for genital herpes.
- *Sepia officinalis 5 C.* For female genital herpes.

Ichthyosis

Ichthyosis is a congenital disorder characterized by dry skin which forms scales.

In some cases you can treat the condition by applying *Homeodora* cream locally to the affected area. This will help soften the skin. A daily bath with starch additive also helps.

Diet is a crucial factor (consult the section on Eczema). Drinking diuretic infusions and *Solidago tea* is recommended, as are supplements of vitamins A, C, D, F and H.

- Kali arsenicum 9 C, Plumbum metallicum 9 C. 5 granules per day on alternate days.
- Petroleum 5 C, Arsenicum album 5 C, Hydrocotyle 5 C.
- Platanus occidentalis 5 C. 2 granules once a day.

Impetigo

Impetigo is a purulent skin disorder that most often affects children. The skin develops blisters, which eventually burst open. Then crusts form on the wounds. Children scratch the crusts, which open and then crust again, and blisters spread over the body.

Impetigo is contagious and is transmitted easily in schools. Intertrigo is the same disorder, except that blisters appear in the folds of the skin behind the ears, knees and in the folds of the neck. The remedies for the two disorders are the same.

Clean open blisters with a medicated, antibacterial liquid soap and then apply an antiseptic ointment (e.g. Neomycin cream). Instead of soap, you can also use a 45 per cent alcohol solution, to which you add a few drops of *Arnica*. Then dab the affected areas with *Molkosan* to kill bacteria, and with *Echinaforce* to reduce inflammation. Take a tablet of *Kelpasan* to accelerate the function of the glands within the dermis. Eat at least 150 grams of fresh carrot pulp per day.

3 granules once a day:

- *Antimonium crudum 5 C*. Wounds ooze an irritating liquid, which forms thick, yellowish crusts; often for cases of over-eating; itching is aggravated in bed and by heat.
- *Antimonium tartaricum 4 C*. Honey-coloured scabs form around the mouth and nostrils, causing an intense burning sensation.
- *Dulcamara 4 C*. When itching is intense, and inflammation of the lymph glands can be easily observed; crusts are brownish yellow, and pustules bleed easily when scratched.
- *Hepar sulphuris 10 C*. Wounds ooze a purulent liquid; eruptions are sensitive to the touch and to cold air. *Hepar sulphuris* cases are generally passive and lethargic.
- *Graphites 6 C*. Eruptions are aggravated in summer; wounds suppurate a honey-coloured liquid. Irritation and itching are less intense.
- *Mercurius 5 C*. When itching is aggravated by heat or cold, and scabs are wet and soft. *Mercurius* patients are rather lethargic, and often have clammy skin.
- *Mezereum 6 C*. Eruptions are severe, and itching is aggravated by touching the wounds, as does the heat in bed and washing.
- *Viola tricolor 5 C*. For impetigo of the face and scalp, accompanied by itching; wounds ooze an abundance of thick, irritating liquid; crusts are thick and yellowish, and bleed easily.

Itching
(see Pruritus)

Itching sometimes indicates improper functioning of the liver or kidneys. If neither of these is the cause, an effective external treatment consists of massaging affected areas with sliced or grated raw potato.

Lips

You can find specific remedies for certain disorders of the lips and their surrounding area.

Chapped Lips

- *Petroleum 5 C, Antimonium crudum 5 C* and *Oleander 5 C*, 2 granules per day on alternate days. For fissures or chapping along the lateral edges.

Impetigo

- *Antimonium tartaricum 5 C* with *Aurum tartaricum 5 C,* 3 granules once a day on alternate days. Add to these the medications recommended in the section on Impetigo.

Hypersensitive Lips

- *Arum triphyllum 5 C* and *Sanicula 5 C,* 2 granules once a day on alternate days.

Dry Lips

- *Arsenicum album 5 C, Kreosotum 5 C, Lac caninum 5 C and Kali sulphuricum 5 C*, 2 granules once a day on alternate days. For the lower lip.
- *Natrum muriaticum 5 C, Sepia 5 C and Nitricum acidum 5 C*, 2 granules per day on alternate days. When skin on the lips peels off in scales. Especially for people who are dehydrated and underweight.
- *Arum triphyllum 5 C and Sanicula 5 C,* 2 granules each day on alternate days. When lips are dry and split, or develop fissures.

Pustules and Thick Scabs
- *Graphites 5 C* for people who habitually over-eat; *Antimonium crudum 5 C, Condurango 5 C* and *Nitricum acidum 5 C,* 2 granules of each per day on alternate days.

Mycosis (Fungal Infection)

Mycosis refers to any fungal disorder. The condition produces eruptions which are well-defined, do not cause itching, and are not painful. However, it isn't easy to get rid of the problem once it has taken hold.

Bathe affected areas with a little *Calendula tincture.* Also use *Molkosan,* which sometimes cures mycosis of the feet and nails that has resisted other forms of treatment.
- Arsenicum album 5 C, Baryta carbonica 5 C, Psorinum 5 C and Sepia 5 C, 2 granules once a day on alternate days.

Athlete's Foot

For mycosis of the feet, disinfect shoes every night with a 10 per cent *Formalin* solution. Wear socks made from cotton instead of synthetics like nylon or acrylic (which do not absorb perspiration and therefore favour the spread of mycosis). Wash your socks separately every day, and dry them with *Formalin*.

Mycosis of the Nails: See Nails.

Nails

Like hair, the condition of our nails is a good indication of our general state of health. Sick nails that break, crack, split or become ingrown indicate a lack of calcium in the system (also when white spots appear on the nails) or a disorder that is accompanied by fever, or a nutritional deficiency. If you are suffering from one of these symptoms, then you should review your diet to make sure it isn't lacking any essential nutrients.

Care

If the cuticle at the edge of the nails is torn or lifted, cut it off with a pair of clean scissors, and apply *Calendula ointment* locally. Take *Calendula officinalis 5 C,* 2 granules twice a day.

Nail polish, and especially acetone-based nail polish remover, can damage or deform the nails by attacking the roots. To remove nail polish, use the following solution: 80 cc. of *ethyl acetate* mixed with 20 cc. of *methyl glycol*.

Mycosis (Fungal Infection) of the Nails

The disorder can be contracted from populated beaches or swimming pools, or by coming in contact with affected people. Cut the nails very short, coat them with *Bioforce* during the day, and soak them in *Molkosan* at night.

Brittle or Fluted Nails

Every 2 days:

- Thuja 5 C, Calcarea fluorica 6 C, Silicea 5 C or Graphites 5 C (the latter for brittle nails only).

Ingrown Toenails

Ingrown nails are usually caused by the rubbing of shoes that are too tight. Start by wearing comfortable shoes that suit the shape of your feet. When you cut your nails, cut them square instead of pointed. If the nail starts to penetrate the skin and flesh, insert a piece of cotton wool soaked in *Calendula tincture* between the nail and the skin.

- *Eugenia jambosa 5 C* and *Ledum palustre 5 C,* 3 granules once a day on alternate days. To put a stop to ingrown nails that recur.

Biting the Nails

Homeopathy can provide that little extra push to help people who can't get rid of this unseemly habit, which usually starts during childhood.

- *Cuprum oxydatum 5 C* and *Baryta carbonica 5 C,* alternating 2 granules of each every two days

Perspiration

Perspiration in itself is healthy. It is one of the ways the body gets rid of waste products from the functioning of all the organs, i.e. metabolism. In fact, 30 per cent of all waste is eliminated through the skin (representing about 1 to 1.5 litres of water per day) without perspiring excessively.

Chemical analysis of perspiration has shown that it is composed of elements which are very close to those which constitute urine. It's no surprise that the skin is called the third kidney!

Saunas or strenuous exercise increase the skin's cleaning action by stimulating sweat glands and therefore perspiration. And certain homeopathic remedies can also stimulate these functions, when the body does not perspire enough.

Saunas, taken at least once a week, can be very beneficial, especially for people who have sedentary jobs where they hardly perspire.

On the other hand, perspiring too much, or producing unpleasant smelling sweat, is a problem, especially in this day and age where body odours have been deemed unacceptable, to the point where many women feel it is necessary to use artificial products to change the natural odour of their private parts.

External Treatment
Drink infusions of sage or bathe in water scented with sage and rosemary.

3 granules once a day:
- *Baryta 5 C*. For problems caused by suppression of sweating (like palpitations). Also for unpleasant smelling perspiration, cold sweats and excessive perspiration of the feet.
- *Belladonna 5 C*. For perspiration caused by fever.
- *Bryonia 5 C*. For excessive or sour perspiration, or both.
- *Calcarea carbonica 5 C*. For perspiration from the head; some children perspire from their head while sleeping.
- *Kali carbonicum 5 C*. For people who perspire too easily, from the slightest physical exertion. Also for cold sweats, or for those whose perspiration is localized in the armpits.
- *Magnesia carbonica 5 C*. For acidic, sour perspiration.
- *Psorinum 5 C*. For sweating that soothes all kinds of symptoms.
- *Nux moschata 5 C*. For people who never perspire.
- *Sanguinaria 5 C*. For sweats during the menopause, with *Lachesis 5 C* and *Thuja 5 C*.
- *Sanicula 5 C*. For excessive sweating through the feet.
- *Sepia 5 C*. For excessive hot sweats and under the armpits.

Perspiration Through the Feet
Various techniques to stop the feet from perspiring can cause other problems like dry patches on the skin or palpitations. However, in cases of excessive

perspiration, measures should be taken - the smell of the perspiration is usually very unpleasant and can be uncomfortable for other people.

Ideally, opt for the surest and most long-term method - internal treatment designed to stimulate skin and kidney functions - using medications like *Solidago* or *Nephrosolid,* for example.

Take frequent foot baths, using herbs whenever possible. Also, rub the feet with aromatic essential oil in order to stimulate circulation. Change your socks frequently.

- *Silicea 5 C.* For excessive perspiration from both feet and hands.

Pruritus

Pruritus is the medical term for itching, which is usually a sign of some more significant disorder, often indicating a problem with the liver or kidneys. A corresponding remedy or solution must be found. Also, when itching occurs, the possibility of parasites should be taken into consideration.

An original and effective external treatment consists of massaging affected areas with a raw potato, cut into slices or grated.

In some cases, a homeopathic remedy may actually aggravate the itching. After all, itching is a way for the body to get rid of toxins. Of course, a homeopathic doctor will be able to evaluate a given situation but, while waiting to see a doctor, or for temporary conditions, you can administer one of the following remedies.

3 granules once a day:

- *Agaricus 5 C.* For pruritus of the fingers and toes; itching is burning, and aggravated by cold weather.
- *Arsenicum album 6 C.* For itching of scaly skin (desquamation) which is soothed by heat, and irritated by scratching.
- *Caladium 5 C.* For genital pruritus.
- *Cina 6 C.* For itching that mainly affects children, and is caused by intestinal parasites; children often rub their nose, face and anus (see Parasites).
- *Dolichos 5 C.* For itching suffered by constipated people. Also for cases of intense itching with no skin eruptions, particularly affecting the armpits, knees, elbows and scalp; the condition usually gets worse at night.

Dolichos is especially recommended for itching that is caused by nervous or digestive disorders (constipation, haemorrhoids), and for pruritus in older people.

- *Granatum 6 C*. For pruritus on the palms of the hands, caused by intestinal parasites.
- *Graphites 5 C*. For pruritus that accompanies anal fissures. Also for pruritus of the vulva which precedes menstruation.
- *Hepar sulphuris 5 C*. For itching aggravated by wool.
- *Ignatia 6 C*. For nervous people who are very sensitive and emotional. Itching may be accompanied by erratic skin eruptions on various parts of the body.
- *Mezereum 5 C*. Itching is burning, or aggravated by heat; also for senile pruritus, which gets worse at night.
- *Rumex 5 C*. For itching that is aggravated by eating meat.
- *Scrophularia 5 C*. For pruritus accompanied by swelling of the lymph nodes.
- *Selenium 6 C*. For pruritus between the fingers.
- *Sulphur 6 C*. For itching that accompanies skin eruptions, aggravated by scratching or washing, by heat or by lying in bed. Also for cases of anal pruritus accompanied by a burning sensation.

Psoriasis

Like eczema, psoriasis is a complex disorder which is difficult to cure and which,for that reason, usually requires the competence of a doctor, preferably a homeopathic one.

Psoriasis may be caused by emotional problems, metabolic problems (diabetes, gout), genetic immune deficiencies, or even personality problems (especially in nervous, irascible types).

Clearly defined patches of varying size appear in areas where the skin has dried out and formed dry, shiny, silvery scales which fall off easily. Beneath that, the surface is shiny, red and bleeds easily. Psoriasis patches usually develop around the elbows, knees, scalp and coccyx (more precisely, the sacrum). Psoriasis is not contagious.

Itching is intense, and makes patients extremely nervous - some scratch until they bleed. Homeopathic treatments may take up to three months to effect a cure. However, allopathic treatment presents certain problems. In fact, some experts claim that treating the disorder with ointments of sulphur, tar or mercury becomes practically impossible after a patient has been treated with X-rays (see Pollution).

Preventive measures for children consist of maintaining proper skin hygiene, and making sure their diet is rich in vitamins and calcium.

As a local treatment, apply *Molkosan* and *Urticalcin* in powder form and *Bioforce* cream. Powdered *Graphites* also provides excellent results, as does *Nerisone* (diflucortolone valerate) cream.

Note: combine basic remedies, administered once four or five days beforehand, with symptomatic remedies, which should be given in dosages of 2 granules twice a day. Of course, there are other remedies that can be used which are not mentioned here. Your homeopathic doctor will be able to establish a precise diagnosis, in cases where symptoms do not correspond to the following descriptions.

Basic remedies: 3 granules twice a day:
- *Sulphur 7 C*. The initial remedy (draining cutaneous tissue) to which you add a specific remedy.
- *Arsenicum album 6 C*. When skin comes off as fine white powder, or when itching is soothed by heat.
- *Calcarea carbonicum 7 C*. For people with blond hair and blue eyes, who tend to perspire from the slightest physical exertion; they develop scaly areas on the legs, and itching causes an intense burning sensation.
- *Graphites 4 C*. For overweight people, or for women whose periods tend to be late.
- *Phosphorus 7 C*. For psoriasis of the hands, arms, knees and elbows, with abundant desquamation (scales).
- *Sepis 7 C,* every ten or fifteen days. For psoriasis that affects the face and scalp, and causes hair loss; patients are often melancholic, and have red, rough skin.

Symptomatic remedies: 3 granules twice a day:
- *Arsenicum album 4 C*. For psoriasis of the lower back (sacrum).
- *Fluoricum acidum 6 C*. For psoriasis on the forehead, above the eyebrows.
- *Graphites 7 C*. For psoriasis that produces fissures, on the palms of the hands, the feet and in the folds behind the knees and in the elbow joints.
- *Hydrastis 5 C*. Psoriasis of the head, around the hairline.
- *Manganum 6 C*. For persistent psoriasis.
- *Mercurius solubilis 6 C*. For acute cases. The condition covers the hands, with patches on various other parts of the body; the scalp is painful when touched. *Mercurius solubilis 30 C* can be administered for cases which have lasted a long time.

- *Natrum arsenicosum 6 C*. The scaly layer is very thin and skin is slightly pinkish underneath.
- *Pulsatilla 4 C*. For diffuse psoriasis, forming large plaques (especially on the palms of the hands); the condition is aggravated by heat.
- *Sepia 4 C*. For psoriasis of the nails, tongue, face, bend of the elbow and knee folds; also for psoriasis in the form of round patches.

Quincke's Oedema

The onset of Quincke's oedema is signalled by a sudden swelling of the face, caused by an allergic reaction.

Warning

If the oedema extends to the mouth, tongue and pharynx in children, the condition can become very dangerous. Administer *Apismellifica 5 C* every five minutes while waiting for a doctor to attend as a matter of urgency.

- *Apis mellifica 5 C*. 3 granules. Administer at the first sign of oedema, every hour until the condition is cured.
- *Sulphur 30 C*. 3 granules only once, for cases where *Apis mellifica* does not produce the desired effect.

Rashes (Eruptions)
(Also see Allergies, Eczema, Erysipelas of the Face)

Infant Rashes

If pimples filled with liquid appear and tend to get larger day by day, a doctor must be consulted. While waiting, squeeze the blisters and rub the affected area with a 2 per cent *Eosin* solution. Also administer *Ranunculus bulbosa 5 C* if pain does not seem to be too bad, *Cantharis 5 C if* pain is intense, and *Arsenicum album 5 C* if the child seems to be in general ill health (See Directions for Use - Infants).

Scars

For scars that don't heal, use a topical application *of Homeodora* cream. Make sure your diet is varied and nutritious, and take supplements of vitamins A, C, D,

E, K and P.

2 granules once a day:

- *Arnica 5 C*. When the scar is painful. *Arnica* helps speed up healing, as does *Calendula 5 C* and *Causticum 5 C*.
- *Calendula 5 C*. When healing is slow and the wound does not close up. You can add *Radium bromatum 5 C* and *Nitricum acidum 5 C* (2 granules per day, on alternate days).
- *Causticum 5 C*. For an old scar that continues to cause discomfort, or for wounds that refuse to close.
- *Graphites 5 C*. To heal an old inflamed scar. Also use as a preventive measure against infection after a wound or surgical operation.

Shingles (also Herpes Zoster)

The burning sensation that precedes the rash is misleading: people think they've been bitten by an insect. This infectious disease is a form of herpes, and is characterized by the appearance of small blisters (vesicles) along a nerve pathway and always on one side of the body only.

Shingles is a painful and highly unpleasant disorder, especially in older people. Among all the possible varieties, herpes zoster ophthalmicus is the most dangerous, since it often results in lesions on the eyes.

Allopathic medicine responds to herpes zoster with antibiotics, which can cure the condition in a few days. Homeopathy can also be effective for people with allergies or people who are resistant to antibiotics or suffer from serious side-effects (nausea, stomach-aches, dizziness).

One homeopathic remedy consists of administering injections of *Formisoton 6 C* and *Rhus tox 12 C*. In these cases, of course, a doctor should take charge of the treatment.

Shingles can be contagious: infected people can pass on herpes zoster as well as chicken-pox, so they should be kept out of contact with children who have not had chicken-pox.

External treatment consists of bathing affected areas with fresh extract of *Melissacitri* and *Calendula*. As for diet, it should be low in salt and protein, and rich in vegetables and whole grains like rice, wheat, barley and buckwheat. Infusions *of Solidago* and *Cynorrodon* are also useful, since they stimulate kidney function and help eliminate toxins.

3 granules three times per day:

- *Arsenicum album 5 C.* For cases where pain is intolerable, and soothed by applications of hot water; attacks are most intense between one and three o'clock in the morning; crusts itch intensely and patients scratch their skin off to try and find some relief, they are usually very agitated.
- *Mezereum 3 C.* For cases where vesicular eruptions occur against a background of red splotches, accompanied by itching which is aggravated by scratching; also when burning pains are severe, and eruptions form thick, purulent crusts.
- *Ranunculus bulbosus 5 C.* For shingles of the eyes or around and on the chest area; eruptions are burning and intensely itchy.
- *Ranunculus scleratus 5 C.* Symptoms are the same as for *Ranunculus bulbosus,* but pains are extremely violent.
- *Rhus tox 4 C.* The typical remedy for herpes diseases and this type of eruption.
- *Sulphur 5 C.* Used to clean out the system after an acute attack.

Skin (Appearance of)

Certain homeopathic remedies can influence the appearance of the skin:

3 granules every two days:

- *Alumina 5 C, Nux moschus 5 C and Petroleum 5 C.* For dry skin.
- *Calcarea carbonica 5 C.* For skin that appears chalky and dull.
- *Chelidonium 5 C or Lycopodium 5 C.* For sallow skin.
- *Iodum 5 C.* For brownish, dry skin.
- *Natrum muriaticum 5 C or Psorinum 5 C.* For greasy, oily skin that has a lot of blackheads.
- *Thuja 5 C.* For skin that is too oily.

Skin (Hygiene)
(See Also Cosmetics)

If skin is to stay healthy, it must be well irrigated with blood. Anything that is likely to block pores (like cosmetics) prevents the skin from breathing.

A Young Skin

Plants that contain carbohydrates (mucilages), like borage, keep the skin looking young and prevent wrinkles. This allows the skin to regain or maintain its firm tone. After washing, dab the skin with cotton wool soaked in *Symphosan*. St. John's wort *(Hypericum),* available from health food shops, stimulates circulation and irrigates capillary vessels.

Toiletries

For dry skin or sores, wash daily with infusions of wild pansy. Avoid over-use of creams, oils and other perfumed products. Instead, use *St. John's wort oil,* or prepare your own pure and economical toilet water by mixing olive oil and a little lemon oil.

Finally, don't forget that fresh air and sunshine are the two natural ingredients our skin needs most.

Baby Skin Care

There's nothing more delicate than a baby's skin. Use specially formulated baby soaps. However, you don't have to wash babies with these soaps every day - doing so could interfere with the proper functioning of the sebaceous glands which moisturize the skin naturally.

Like adults, babies benefit greatly from a twice weekly massage with pure, natural oil (like *Bioforce* oil).

Bath Herbs

You can add certain herbs to a baby's bath (just be careful to avoid any irritating herbs):

- *Horsetail (Equisetum)* is rich in silica and has a beneficial effect on the skin.
- *Lemon balm (Melissa)* helps infants who are nervous and need to be calmed.
- *Marigold (Calendula)* is suitable for infants with a delicate skin, or who develop eczema.

Dry Skin

Use a cream made from vegetable essences, and which contains lanolin. Make sure you're getting enough vitamin F. *Bioforce* cream is also useful.

Strophulus (Tooth-rash, White Gum)

Strophulus refers to prurigo in children, and both conditions require the same treatment. Small lesions the size of pinheads appear and become slightly inflamed. Itching is intense, and when scratched some cases develop into impetigo.

In breast-feeding infants, the mother's diet is the decisive factor. Older children should not be fed eggs, chocolate or strawberries. The condition may also be due to an allergic reaction. Adults should stick to the diet outlined for Gastritis.

- *Sulphur 7 C,* once only. Then *Antimonium crudum 4 C,* 2 granules twice a day.

Stye (Hordeolum)

This is a common inflammation of the eyelid.

3 granules three times per day, unless otherwise indicated:

- *Aconitum 5 C.* For a stye that appears suddenly, causing burning pain accompanied by weeping.
- *Apis 4 C.* 3 granules every hour. An initial remedy, when the skin is swollen, and pain is aggravated by heat.
- *Mercurius solubilis 5 C.* 3 granules per hour. When the stye is on the point of bursting; the eyelid is red, while the stye itself is yellowish white.
- *Pulsatilla 4 C.* 2 granules four times a day. When administered at the outset, *Pulsatilla* can help prevent a stye from developing.
- *Staphysagria 5 C.* For a stye that is accompanied by conjunctivitis; patients are often shy and withdrawn, and have dilated veins. Also for a persistent stye that becomes a hard swelling on an inflamed eyelid.
- *Staphysagria 30 C* and *Silicea 30 C.* 5 granules only once. Administer when the stye is healing, to prevent it from recurring.

Sunstroke

Sunshine is good for your health. But if you spend long hours in the hot sun with your head uncovered, you run the risk of getting sunstroke. In fact, hundreds of people die every year from cerebral apoplexy, after working or exercising in the hot sun.

When you go out in the sun at the beginning of summer, do it gradually, whether you're ill or in good health. Our skin has become accustomed, over the centuries, to clothing that protects us from extreme climatic conditions.

Think about women in the Middle Ages, who spent most of their lives indoors, and for whom a milky white skin was the aesthetic ideal. Times have changed, of course. But they will change again. The generations of sun worshippers are already seeing the effects of over-exposure on their skin, which becomes wrinkled and ages prematurely.

This is true for all people who, because of their work or pastimes, spend a lot of time exposed to the elements. But these people do it out of necessity or pleasure, and not because they are trying to imitate some aesthetic ideal.

For severe sunstroke, consult the section on Apoplexy (Stroke).

Simple Sunburn

Apply *Calendula-Hypericum* ointment, which is antiseptic and speeds up the healing process (1 granule of *Calendula T.M.*, 1 granule of *Hypericum T.M.*, mixed with 28 g of vaseline.)

- *Glonoinum 4 C.* 2 granules every two hours. The face is red and congested; the pulse is visible in the neck and temples; people are unsteady on their feet and seem to have trouble concentrat-ing.
- *Opium 4 C.* 2 granules per hour while waiting to see a doctor. This is for serious cases, where they are almost in a coma; they are in a deep sleep, with snoring breathing; the face is red and bathed in hot sweat.

Tanning
(See Also Sunstroke)

There's nothing like a good tan to make your skin look healthy. And up to a point, it is true that exposure to fresh air and sunlight, which provides the body with vitamin D, is beneficial. The natural light of the sun increases elasticity of the skin and improves muscle tone, both of which are important for well-being and a healthy appearance.

Needless to say, over-exposure to ultraviolet light cancels out these advantages, especially when the light is artificial (as with sunbeds). It causes unnatural pigmentation (often unsightly), not to mention premature ageing of the skin, which is exactly the opposite of the desired effect.

Before doing any intensive tanning (especially with artificial ultraviolet light) consult a doctor or dermatologist to see if tanning will be good for your skin or not, especially if you have dry or sensitive skin.

Urticaria (Hives)

This common allergic reaction is very unpleasant. Red patches dotted with small white blisters or isolated pimples appear on the skin, accompanied by intense itching or burning sensations.

Sometimes caused by contact with nettles (hence the name "nettle rash"), urticaria is often an allergic reaction to some food (especially seafood, strawberries, pork, eggs or cheese).

Urticaria is usually not accompanied by fever, but if it is you should consult a doctor. It may be complicated by burning inflammation, as is the case with Quincke's oedema.

One way to combat the effects of certain substances that cause attacks is to ingest lime. Lotions or bathing with *Viola tricolor* also help reduce sensitivity. Isotherapy should also be considered as a possible treatment (see Eczema).

When attacks occur, stay in bed and drink nothing but water for 24 hours. Then drink vegetable broth for a few days, as you slowly get back to solid food.

Basic treatment: 3 granules three times per day:

- *Apis 5 C*. Pains are aggravated by heat and soothed by cold; eruptions are more swollen (oedema) and less red than *Urtica urens* cases; also for attacks that occur before menstruation.
- *Calendula T.M.* and *Arsenicum album 5 C*. If eruptions are obviously caused by a specific food (signalled by an incubation period of 6 to 48 hours, followed by diarrhoea, fever and vomiting). Stick to a rigid and simple diet for the next few days.
- *Gardenal 7 C*. Red eruptions are itchy and sometimes burning or prickly. These cases frequently occur when people are exhausted and/or drowsy.
- *Lycopodium 5 C*. For urticaria related to rheumatic problems.
- *Natrum muriaticum 5 C*. For urticaria caused by nervousness or by a non-food allergy; these cases are of a more "psychological" nature.
- *Rhus toxicodendron 5 C*. If small white blisters (vesicles) appear on the red patches, which are more painful and are accompanied by a burning sensation.
- *Sulphur 5 C*. Irritation is itchy and produces a burning sensation; scratching soothes the itching, but aggravates the burning; eruptions are aggravated by washing in cold water; heat in bed and contact with bedclothes (especially wool) makes the itching worse.
- *Urtica urens 5 C* or *mother tincture*. This is the treatment most often

prescribed. Red or pink inflammation is accompanied by intense itching, burning and prickling sensations; the condition is aggravated by application of cold; also recommended for urticaria caused by allergies, by eating seafood or fish, or coming in contact with stinging nettles.

Symptomatic Treatments:

- *Aconitum 5 C*. For urticaria caused by the cold.
- *Antimonium crudum 5 C*. When urticaria is accompanied by indigestion.
- *Apis 5 C*. For urticaria accompanied by oedema, or caused by over-exposure to the sun (in the latter case, keep patients out of the sun completely).
- *Astacus 5 C*. For generalized urticaria that appears very suddenly. Fresh air aggravates the itching.
- *Bombyx 4 C*. For allergic urticaria with intense itching around the joints; patients feel as if they had insects crawling under their skin.
- *Homarus 5 C* with *Vespa crabo 5 C*. When small pimples appear that become very itchy.
- *Pulsatilla 5 C*. For urticaria accompanied by diarrhoea.

Children and Fruit

Children who eat too much fruit may develop urticaria. Cure the problem by treating the kidneys: administer *Solidago*.

Warts

Warts are protuberances of flesh, usually yellow, dark brown or grey. They can appear on any part of the body, but the hands and face are the areas most often affected.

Although the exact cause of warts is still unknown, homeopathy considers them to be an important indication of a person's temperament. The nervous system is certainly involved, except for contagious warts (flat warts), some of which may be caused by microbes or parasites.

Apart from these cases, getting rid of a wart only gets rid of the symptom and not the cause. If you do decide to get rid of a wart, don't do it yourself by cutting or scratching the wart off - it will only grow back again, worse than before, and may even become malignant.

External Treatment

Get your homeopathic pharmacist to prepare a collodion solution for you (cotton powder dissolved in ether and alcohol) made with *Thuja tincture* or *Chelidonium tincture*. Apply a little of this solution to your wart(s) every evening, after first cleaning the skin around the affected area with a little ether.

For cases of simple warts on the hands, the following procedure may be effective: use a magnifying glass to focus the sun's rays on the wart for a few seconds each day - after a few days, the wart should fall off.

Basic Remedy:

- *Sulphur 7 C, 5* granules once only, followed a week later by 5 granules of *Dulcamara 7 C*.

Symptomatic remedies: 3 granules once a day unless otherwise indicated:

- *Antimonium crudum 6 C*. For hardened warts and for all crusty growths on the skin (warts, corns, calluses, etc.) which are very hard and sensitive, especially to humidity and contact with water. *Antimonium crudum* is appropriate for heavy eaters who often suffer from digestive problems.
- *Berberis vulgaris 1 C*, 1 granule twice a day, for flat, smooth warts.
- *Causticum 5 C*, 3 granules morning and night. For fissured, bleeding warts that are painful, as well as for warts that are large and tend to spread. *Causticum* warts become more painful in cold damp weather.
- *Thuja 6 C*. For warts that grow on the feet (verrucas); they are fissured, fluted on the surface, and sensitive to humidity or cold weather. Also for red warts.

Local remedies:

- *Antimonium crudum 6 C*. For warts on the fingers.
- *Calcarea carbonica 5 C*. For warts on the arms.
- *Causticum 5 C*. For warts on the face, eyelids, nose, eyebrows and tips of the fingers.
- *Dulcamara 7 C*. Warts on the hands, palms and under the nails.
- *Lycopodium 4 C*. For warts on the penis.
- *Natrum sulphuricum 5 C*. For warts that spread all over the body.
- *Sabina 5 C*. Warts on the genitals or around the anus.
- *Sepia 5 C*. For warts situated around the nails.
- *Spigelia 5 C*. Warts on the toes.
- *Thuja 5 C*. Warts on the feet.

Whitlow

The term refers to all purulent infections of the fingers.

Soak fingers in hot water (98.6 to 104°F or 37-38°C) for at least one hour two or three times a day. Protect affected fingers from cold.

3 granules three times per day:

- *Eugenia jambosa 5 C.* For recurring whitlow that develops under the nails. People are sometimes psychologically over-excited, and suffer from mood swings including depression.
- *Formalin 5 C.* When nails get soft and turn dark brown; skin around the nails is swollen and begins to suppurate.
- *Rana bufo 5 C.* Burning pain spreads to the forearm.
- *Tarentula Cubensis 8 C.* An extremely effective remedy for whitlows and boils.

Wrinkles

There are various ways to prevent the appearance of premature wrinkles: first, make sure you get enough rest, eight hours per night being the norm, from which you should deviate only occasionally. Try to avoid frowning, or maintaining a worried expression: it's not an accident that people who are serene appear to age more slowly.

Don't always sleep on the same side, or lose weight too rapidly, or abuse alcohol or tobacco.

Symphosan helps fight wrinkles and crow's feet, and revives skin that has been covered with cosmetic products too often or for too long. You can also use *Symphytum* cream.

As for diet, make sure you eat foods rich in the following vitamins:

- *Vitamin A:* prevents the skin from drying out and getting rough.
- *Vitamin B$_1$:* improves circulation.
- *Vitamin B$_2$:* prevents the skin from collapsing.
- *Vitamin C:* keeps the skin elastic.

Foods rich in these vitamins include fresh fruit and vegetables, wheat germ, brewer's yeast, milk, eggs and cheese (see the diet outlined for Gastritis).

Chapter 9

Accidents
Emergencies
General Disorders

> *This section is an emergency handbook, designed to help you react quickly to crisis situations and to deal with unexpected events as effectively as possible. It's always helpful to have quick access to homeopathic remedies when faced with health problems ranging from simple discomfort to acute depression to pleurisy.*
>
> *The commentary in this chapter has been kept to a strict minimum - in an emergency, speed is a factor; and there is no time to sit down and start studying.*
>
> *In some cases, the recommended remedy is only meant to help calm the patient until a doctor can be reached. In other more common cases, you can probably avoid consulting a doctor altogether; since you'll be able to deal with the problem yourself. To make full use of this section, obtain the remedies mentioned in the Emergency First Aid Kit section in the Appendix, and keep them at home in your homeopathic medicine cabinet.*
>
> ### Warning
>
> *If you don't get rapid results by administering a homeopathic remedy, or if the patient's condition gets worse, then you should consult a doctor as quickly as possible. As soon as symptoms start to improve, you can space out the doses.*

Accidents

(See Also Wounds, Cuts, Haemorrhage and Other corresponding sections)

Arnica is a remedy that it is always useful to have for a variety of accidents - blows, falls, open wounds, contusions, etc. Administering 20 granules of *Arnica 30 C* as soon as possible can provide precious relief.

Once you've seen the effects for yourself, you'll automatically turn to *Arnica* for any unpleasant occurrences - and rightly so. After the accident, administer *Arnica* once a week for a month or two. Also apply cold (ice pack, damp cloth, etc.) to the affected area in the case of contusions, sprains, etc. Treat open wounds with *Calendula tincture* or cream ointment.

Add one of the following remedies, depending on which part of the body is affected:

3 granules every hour:

- *Arnica 9 C*. When the injury affects muscles or the skin.
- *China 4 C*. If there is any haemorrhage.
- *Hypericum 9 C*. For injuries to the spine.
- *Ledum 9 C*. An eye is affected.
- *Natrum sulphuricum 9 C*. For injuries to the head.
- *Opium 9 C*. For people who suffered from shock or fear during an accident, or if people lost consciousness - slide 2 granules under the tongue.
- *Ruta 9 C*. For damaged bones but without any fracture.
- *Symphytum 9 C*. A bone is affected, it is fractured.

Aches

Aches can have all sorts of causes, including excessive exertion, fever, flu, etc.
- *Arnica I5C*. 5 granules once only.
- *Rhus tox 9 C*. 5 granules once only.
- *Bellis perennis 15 C*. Very similar to *Arnica,* this remedy can help if *Arnica* alone does not do the trick. More specifically for aches of the abdominal wall, or in the thighs.

Note: A sure way of getting aches and pains is not to warm up before doing physical exercise. The more strenuous the activity, the more complete the warm-up should be. Warming up stretches the muscles and makes them pliable.

Altitude Sickness

Discomfort due to altitude is characterized by a fainting feeling; breathing accelerates and the pulse becomes weak. The face is congested, and people may bleed from their nose or ears.
- *Ignatia 7 C,* 2 granules only once, followed by 5 granules of *Coca 4 C* and *Arnica 5 C,* alternating every hour.

Anger

Even the most peaceful people become angry at some point in their lives. It's better to accept anger than try and suppress it. If it becomes physical, direct it at some inanimate object (smash a tennis ball or batter a punch-bag - but be careful not to strain your muscles!). People who know how to meditate can use this is a long-term method for curbing anger.

- *Colocynthis 7 C*. 10 granules only once. After anger has been let out instead of suppressed (preferably directed at an inanimate object).
- *Staphysagria 7 C*. 10 granules only once. For people who have contained or suppressed their anger, but the contained emotions eat away at them.

Animal Bites

Dog Bites

Clean the wound carefully while waiting to see a doctor, and apply a compress using 30 drops of *Calendula tincture*. (If this is not available, use diluted bleach.) Avoid using iodine, which prevents elimination of toxins.

- *Arnica 15 C*. 10 granules as soon as possible.
- *China 5 C (15 C* for children and infants). 5 granules immediately and then twice a day. For bleeding wounds.
- *Pyrogenium 9 C*. 2 granules per day. To prevent infection.

Whenever possible, make sure the dog is examined by a vet (e.g. from the RSPCA) to test for rabies (although this is very rare).

Snake Bites

Slow down blood circulation (do not cut it off completely) by applying a tourniquet between the bite and the heart. Do not give patients any alcohol. Get them to rest, and keep them warm.

If no serum is available, you can use Dr. Chavanon's formula for snakebite: 10 grams of *Cedron tincture,* 20 grams of *Calendula tincture* and 3 grams of *Guaco tincture,* in addition to an injection of high-dose cortisone (given by a medical professional).

Anxiety

Anxiety is a psychological manifestation of a problem with an identifiable cause: fear of losing a job or a loved one, for example. These things happen, and people fall prey to all kinds of doubt, apprehension, fear - and feel a general sense of misgiving. Many people turn to tranquillizers to solve the problem. These may diminish their unease for a while, but will also make them dull and insensitive. So tranquillizers are not a real solution. They just make the symptoms disappear for a short time. People may think they feel better, but in the long run it will be harder to get rid of the real cause of the anxiety if it is suppressed at the outset.

Administer 3 granules of the appropriate remedy per hour to calm people down. As soon as there is an improvement, extend the period of time between doses.

- *Aconitum 15 C*. For those who are usually lively and active.
- *Argentum nitricum 15 C*. For hurried individuals who act without thinking.
- *Arsenicum album 15 C*. For those who are generally agitated.
- *Gelsemium 7 C*. For people who are paralysed by anxiety.
- *Ignatia 7 C*. For anxious people (they feel like they have a lump in their throat) who suffer from sudden mood changes.

Appendicitis

Acute pains are felt on the right of the lower abdomen and are accompanied by general discomfort, then vomiting; the tongue is coated, and temperature varies between 99° and 101°F (37.5-38°C); pulse is rapid, often rising above 100 beats per minute.

To be sure you're dealing with a case of appendicitis: the appendix is located below and to the left of the navel. Press firmly on the area. If, when you release the pressure, pain spreads to the right, you can assume it is appendicitis. The following treatment is meant to prepare patients for surgery, which should be carried out as quickly as possible.

Administer 5 granules of each, at half-hour intervals:

- *Colocynthis 7 C, then Pyrogenium 7 C*, followed by *Belladonna 4 C, Arsenicum album 7 C* then *Bryonia 9 C*.

If surgery has still not taken place, administer *Colocynthis 7 C* every three or four hours, *Belladonna 4 C* every 11 hours and *Pyrogenium 7 C* every 24 hours.

Asphyxiation

Call the emergency services as quickly as possible - they should have the proper equipment to resuscitate asphyxiated people.

Asphyxiation by Gas

For asphyxiation by carbon monoxide in unventilated rooms (for example, a malfunctioning heating system). People have trouble breathing, suffer from dizzy spells and nausea; a period of exaltation is followed by a phase of severe depression.

Get the patient out into the fresh air, and raise the head and chest. For serious cases, carry out artificial respiration. When patients revive, get them to suck 20 drops of *Soludor* placed on a cube of sugar.

- *Lauroverasus 4 C*. 2 granules three times in a 24-hour period.
- *Carbo vegetabilis 9 C*. 2 granules immediately.

Asphyxiation From Drowning

Place victims with their head down to clear the mouth of weeds, sand and other foreign bodies. Then carry out mouth-to-mouth artificial respiration if breathing apparatus is not available.

- *Carbo vegetabilis 4 C,* 2 granules every half an hour. Place the granules under the victim's tongue. If the case is less serious, administer 2 granules of *Carbo vegetabilis 7* C once.

Asphyxiation by Strangulation

Give mouth-to-mouth artificial respiration as quickly as possible.

- *Arnica 7 C*. Place a few granules on the person's tongue.

Infant Asphyxiation

This can happen if milk goes down the wrong way or if infants vomit up food. Keep the head down, pull on the tongue and clear the mouth and throat of obstructions with your finger. Call a doctor if there is no immediate improvement.

Prevention: after feeds, place infants on their side and not on their back.

Asthma Attacks

Asthma can be cured by homeopathy. Doing so requires the help of a doctor (see the section on Asthma under Respiratory Disorders). For an acute attack:

Children and Adults:

- *Sambucus nigra 9 C* and *Ipecac. 4 C,* alternating 2 granules every hour. Continue the treatment for a few days.

Infants

- *Belladonna 4 C, Ipecac. 4 C* and *Sambucus nigra 4 C,* one after the other twice a day (see Directions for Use - Infants).

Black Eye
(See Also Contusions)

- *Ledum palustre 7 C.* 2 granules immediately, with *Arnica montana,* 2 granules. Repeat once a day.

Blisters

When a blister develops from rubbing, for example, try *Cantharis 5 C.* If the blister is caused by a burn, use *Rhus toxicodendron 5 C.*

Blows
(See Also Contusions, Wounds)

A moist, cold compress soaked in five to ten drops of *Bellis tincture* will help reduce swelling and soothe pain caused by a blow.

- *Arnica 15 C.* 10 granules. For all cases.
- *Ruta 5 C.* 10 granules. In addition to *Arnica* if bones are affected by the blow.

Broken Teeth
(See Also Teeth)

It happens a lot to children - they fall, or get hit by a ball, and come running home with a broken tooth, sometimes in floods of tears.

If it's a milk tooth, don't do anything, even if the root is still in place. Let a dentist remove the root if necessary.

If it's a permanent tooth, leave the stump in place, even if it is jagged and painful. It may stay in place, although it might go rather yellow.

Dab the painful area with a little *Calendula tincture*. Then administer the appropriate remedy.

- *Arnica 15 C.* 2 granules per day for a few days, in all cases.
- *Hypericum 7 C.* 5 granules. When pain is very intense.

Burns

Start by cleaning the burn and surrounding area with *Calendula tincture* (20 drops in a glass of boiled water which is then cooled). If this is not available, use a 90° alcohol solution. Then apply a dressing with *Calendula* ointment.

- *Cantharis 4 C*. 2 granules twice a day.
- *Pyrogenium 7 C*. 5 granules per day.

For very localized burns, when you don't have any medication available, immerse the affected area in cold water or apply an ice pack.

If blisters appear add:

- Rhus toxicodendron 5 C, Echinacea 4 C. 2 granules of each once a day.

Then proceed by applying *Cantharis 1 C* (dissolve 10 drops in a glass of water that has been boiled and cooled) and a sterile dressing with *Calendula* ointment.

Chilblains

Certain individuals are predisposed to chilblains. They require a more basic treatment, specially designed to arrest congestion of capillaries and veins in the skin.

An effective preventive measure consists of taking hot and cold footbaths, alternating three minutes of hot water with three seconds of cold (repeat the process 7 or 8 times); also administer rubs with thyme and *Symphosan*.

- *Aesculus hippocastanum 5 C,* 2 granules every two days, alternated with *Hyperisan 5 C,* 2 granules every two days. To treat circulatory problems.

External Treatment

Apply *Arnica* ointment (1 gram of *Arnica 1 C*, mixed with 20 grams of pure sterilized vaseline) if there is redness of the skin accompanied by a burning sensation.

If itching is intense, especially at night, with a prickling sensation like pins and needles, use the following ointment: 1 gram of *Rhus tox T.M.* mixed with 20 grams of pure sterilized vaseline.

For cases of chapping, cracks and ulcerated chilblains, prepare a dressing with *Calendula T.M.* ointment.

Internal Treatment

2 granules every hour:

- *Agaricus 7 C.* A prickling, burning sensation predominates; chilblains are very sensitive to cold air and pressure.
- *Arsenicum album 7 C.* Chilblains are swollen, burning and itching; the skin is cold and dry; blisters appear and turn brownish-black.
- *Arnica 7 C.* Chilblains are bluish or purple and very sensitive, like severe bruises.
- *Nitricum acidum 7 C.* For extremely cold weather; chilblains cause a sensation of pins and needles; affected areas are ulcerated and bleed easily.
- *Pulsatilla 6 C.* For those who often develop symptoms of congestion of the veins; in these cases, heat and rest will aggravate the chilblains.

Coma

The condition pertains to people who have lost consciousness, feel nothing, cannot move, but continue to breathe normally and maintain a regular heartbeat. A doctor must be called as soon as possible.

First, let's look at cases of diabetic coma.

Hypoglycaemic Coma

Preceded by spasms, muscular contractions, convulsions and profuse sweating, coma sets in suddenly.

- *Opium 5 C,* 2 granules, and *Insulinum 5 C,* 2 granules. While waiting for a doctor, follow-up with *Cuprum arsenicum 4 C,* 2 granules a quarter of an hour later, and then once every hour.

Hyperglycaemic Coma

Breathing troubles are characteristic; patients are dehydrated, their skin is dry; their breath smells of acetone; coma sets in gradually.

- *Opium 5 C.* 2 granules while waiting for a doctor. Then *Senna 4 C,* 2 granules a quarter of an hour later, followed by *Acetonum 4 C,* 2 granules a quarter of an hour after that.

Apoplectic Coma

The face is puffy, breathing is noisy and laboured, the sphincter muscle may open. While waiting for a doctor:

- *China 4 C*. 2 granules placed under the tongue (and then three times per day); then *Opium 5 C*, 2 granules a quarter of an hour later, followed by *Glonoinum 4 C* a quarter of an hour after that; then alternate *Arnica montana 5 C* and *Ethyllicum 5 C*, 2 granules twice a day.

Concussion

Before seeing a doctor:

- Arnica montana 5 C, Gelsemium 5 C and Opium 5 C. 2 granules of each once a day.

Contusions (Bruises)

Apply compresses soaked in *Calendula T.M.* (one teaspoon dissolved in a cup of boiled and cooled water). If the skin is not grazed or wounded, apply *Homeodora* cream. While waiting for a doctor:

- *Arnica 5 C* and *Bellis perennis 4 C*. Alternating 2 granules every hour.
- *China 4 C*. In addition to the above, if there is any haemorrhage.

Convulsions (In Infants)

Lay the child flat and ventilate the room. While waiting for a doctor, administer 2 granules of the following remedies every 5 minutes:

- *Cicuta virosa 4 C*, followed by *Cuprum metallicum 5 C* and *Oenanthe crocata 5 C*.

Then, depending on the case:

- *Chamomilla 5 C*, five minutes later, for children who have just thrown a tantrum.
- *Cina 5 C, 5 minutes after Oenanthe crocata*, for children suffering from worms.

Long-term remedy:

Infusions of chickweed *(Stellaria media)* can cure these febrile convulsions in infants.

Cramps

Cramps can be very painful, especially if they occur after some strenuous physical exertion. It's very helpful to have a handy remedy, especially if you do a lot of sports.

- *Cuprum 5 C.* 3 granules as quickly as possible. Repeat every five minutes, if necessary.

Cuts

To clean cuts, use a mixture of 10 drops of *Calendula T.M.* in a little pure water.

- *Staphysagria 7 C.* 3 granules. When the cut is clean, caused by some sharp object. Alternate with *Arnica 15 C* (10 granules for the first dosage, and then 3 granules).

Complications: See Tetanus.

Delirium

People may become delirious during the course of an ordinary illness, or after giving birth. Depending on the case, administer:

- *Belladonna 4 C.* 2 granules. When people develop fever and facial congestion, are agitated and have dilated pupils. Also for delirium caused by rage, where they are very talkative and become violent.
- *Hyoscyamus 4 C.* People giggle a lot, laugh and behave in an exhibitionist way.
- *Stramonium 4 C.* For violent delirium; people are overcome by insane agitation, scream and shout, and cannot stop talking.

Dislocations

The first thing to do is put the dislocated thigh or shoulder bone back into its socket. This is not possible unless patients are anesthetized, or completely relaxed despite the pain. If not, contracted muscles will prevent the bone from returning to its normal position.

Try to find a position where the patient does not feel any pain. Experience is required to replace the limb - you have to know exactly how hard and in which direction to exert pressure.

- *Aconitum 15 C.* 10 granules immediately.

Ecchymosis
(See Also Contusions)

After a blow, swelling appears and the skin around the affected area turns dark blue and brown. If you think there might be some internal injury, especially in the areas of the head, abdomen or lungs, consult a doctor.

Soothe the pain locally with a damp compress made with 10 drops of *Arnica T.M.*, dissolved in a glass of boiled and cooled water.

However, do not apply a compress if the skin is grazed or cut open.

- *Arnica 30 C. 3* granules every half an hour. For the majority of cases.
- *Conium 7 C.* 2 granules per day, if the skin around the affected area is showing a tendency to become hard.
- *Hypericum 7 C.* 5 granules. For fingers that get crushed in a car door, or smashed by a hammer.
- *Ledum palustre 7 C. 5* granules. For black eyes, if the eye itself is not affected.
- *Ruta 7 C. 5* granules twice a day. For contusions on the front part of the tibia, which are very painful.
- *Symphytum 7 C. 5* granules twice a day while waiting to be seen by a specialist.
- *Sulphuric acidum 7 C. 5* granules. Add this remedy if people go into a state of shock, or suffer from extreme fatigue.

Electrocution

The skin is cold and bluish, breathing is shallow, the heartbeat is weak. Call the emergency services and give mouth-to-mouth resuscitation if the person loses consciousness.

- *Carbo vegetabilis 4 C.* Slip 4 granules under the tongue of the electrocuted person, and repeat every half an hour.

Embolism

People spit up black phlegm, full of blood; they start suffocating and feel intense pain in the chest area.

Keep the patient completely immobile.

- *Arnica 5 C*. 2 granules every half an hour while waiting to see a doctor.

Epilepsy

There are few disorders which are as dramatic as an epileptic fit. Fortunately, we no longer believe that epileptics are possessed by the devil.

Patients begin convulsing and fall to the ground; they may foam at the mouth; while unconscious they may bite their tongue, clutch their stomach and shout.

If possible, get the person to lie down on a mattress or carpet, put something soft under his/her head, loosen any tight clothing and clear away any obstacles which might cause injury to the person having convulsions.

Administer medication by placing granules under the tongue:

- *Cicuta virosa 5 C*. 3 granules as soon as possible.

Faintness

A strongly felt emotion, very hot temperatures and a host of other factors can cause people to experience general discomfort. Symptoms include dizziness, nausea, and may cause actual fainting for a few minutes; pulse is often accelerated and people sigh deeply as they come round after fainting.

General discomfort can also indicate a more serious disorder, which only a doctor is in a position to determine.

Get people to lie down with their head down, in a calm, well ventilated place. Tap them vigorously on the face to stimulate the superficial circulation, and loosen any tight clothing.

Fatigue
(See Also Weakness, Overwork)

That feeling of utter exhaustion that leaves us feeling weak and powerless is all the more disconcerting in that it often occurs when we are at our busiest (which may not be a coincidence).

Don't forget that stimulants like coffee, Coca-Cola, tea or alcohol may provide a temporary lift (if the body has not already become immune to their effects) but then leave us feeling even more tired than before, so that they must be taken in ever increasing doses.

3 granules once a day:

- *Argentum nitricum 6 C*. For those who are melancholic, impulsive and always in a hurry.
- *Coca 30 C*. For people suffering from palpitations, shortness of breath after the slightest exertion, anxiety and insomnia (and sometimes headaches). Also administer 5 drops of *Coca tincture* every half an hour for two hours before an important meeting or a performance for singers and actors (make sure they don't take too much).
- *Gelsemium sempervirens 6 C*. For fatigue suffered by students during examination periods, and by others who have a heavy intellectual workload (teachers, conference speakers, actors, etc.) These people are weak and tend to feel dizzy.
- *Ignatia 30 C*. 2 granules every two or three hours. For cases of nervous fatigue, especially in women. Also for men who suffer from "paradoxical fatigue", i.e. they get tired quickly when engaged in work they do not like.
- *Kali phosphoricum 6 C*. 3 granules immediately, and repeated as required; fatigue is accompanied by memory loss and a feeling of repugnance towards even minor tasks; also for mental exhaustion from overwork.
- *Nux vomica 15 C*. 2 granules immediately. For cases of nervous fatigue, especially in men; a sudden feeling of exhaustion occurs after lunch; short naps help somewhat (for these cases, give 2 granules before lunch).
- *Phosphoricum acidum 6 C*. For nervous exhaustion characterized by apathy, discouragement, confusion, occasional memory loss and dizziness.

Fear

For people suffering from fear after an accident or shock, administer 3 granules of *Opium 7 C*.

Fever (Sudden)

If the fever is not accompanied by any other symptoms, administer *Sulphur iodatum 5 C*, 5 granules immediately. Then consult the section on Fever in the chapter on General Disorders.

Fractures

Of course, a doctor should be consulted. To soothe pain, administer *Ruta 4 C*. 2 granules four times a day.

Closed Fracture
- *Arnica 7 C*. 2 granules once every two days, *Calcarea carbonica 7 C*. 2 granules once a day, and *Symphytum 5 C*, 2 granules per day.

Open Fracture
- *Pyrogenium 7 C*, 5 granules per day, and *Naja 4 C*, 5 granules only once, in addition to the remedies for a closed fracture. Do not touch the injury until a doctor arrives.

Frostbite
(See Also Chilblains)

Above all, avoid exposing frost-bitten areas to sources of direct heat and do not rub frozen limbs with snow or wet cloths. The best thing to do is imitate the Eskimos, who warm up frozen flesh through contact with warm human skin. Hot drinks will also help.

If there is any burning, apply a *Calendula* ointment dressing.
- *Secale cornutum 4 C*. 2 granules four times per day.

Genital Injuries

It's always a good idea to consult a doctor in cases of genital injury, to make sure there is no internal damage.
- *Arnica 15 C*. 10 granules immediately. For haematoma.
- *Hypericum 15 C*. When intense pain is felt in the soft parts: labia, testicles or glans.

Grief
(See Also Depression)

Grief is not a physical trauma, strictly speaking. However, people can be classified as emergency cases because of the emotional trauma involved. After all, psychological wounds are more painful and take longer to heal than a lot of physical wounds.

Use one of the following remedies:

- *Ignatia 7 C*. 10 granules only once.
- *Kali phosphoricum 7 C*. 10 granules only once.

Haemorrhage
(See the section Haemorrhage in the chapter
on the Circulatory System)

If the haemorrhage is caused by a wound, use *China 4 C,* 2 granules every hour, with *Arnica 15 C,* 10 granules administered as quickly as possible.

Apply *Calendula* ointment. Prepare a dressing with one teaspoon of *Calendula tincture* in a glass of boiled and cooled water.

Head Injuries

These cases go beyond the scope of family medicine. Consult a doctor as soon as possible, especially if there is any vomiting or convulsions.

Administer 10 granules every two hours of the appropriate remedy:

- *Arnica 15 C*. For all cases where individuals remain conscious and have contusions.
- *Cicuta virosa 15 C*. Cases go into convulsions and lose consciousness.
- *Hypericum 15 C*. When concussion is a possibility.
- *Helleborus 15 C*. If patients become drowsy, suffer from mental confusion, or fall into a coma.
- *Natrum sulphuricum 7 C*. For the after-effects of a head injury, to be administered during convalescence to avoid possible delayed complications.

Headaches

Chronic headaches are signals being sent to you by the body (see Migraines). When you resort to drugs, you're a little like a driver who shoots a hole in the dashboard because she/he doesn't like to see the warning signals flashing!

Consulting a doctor is usually necessary to determine the cause of headaches and find an appropriate remedy. Of course, we're not talking about the occasional headache that everyone has from time to time, after working too hard, or drinking or eating too much.

A trick to get rid of an occasional headache is to apply an onion or horseradish compress to the neck, calves or soles of the feet.

Internal treatment: 3 granules of the appropriate medication every half an hour, or more often if need be. Reduce the frequency as soon as there is any improvement.

- *Actaea racemosa 7 C*. Pain is centred around the neck and nape.
- *Belladonna 7 C*. The head is congested and pain is pulsing.
- *Gelsemium 7 C*. Pain is situated in the forehead; eyelids are heavy, eyes close on their own.
- *Iris versicolor 7 C*. Pain is accompanied by vision problems.
- *Kali phosphoricum 7 C*. For headaches following intense mental effort.
- *Nux vomica 9 C*. For headaches associated with digestive problems and nausea.

Heat (Exposure to)

For direct exposure to the sun for prolonged periods (see Sunstroke).

After excessive exposure to a source of heat, people feel general discomfort; they are drowsy and thirsty, and sometimes develop fever.

Avoid sudden changes of temperature - cool the person down gradually. Loosen clothing and administer cool compresses. If the person is thirsty, add a pinch of sugar and salt to a glass of cold water.

- *Glonoinum 4 C*. 2 granules, followed fifteen minutes later by:
- *Belladonna 4 C*. 2 granules, followed fifteen minutes later by:
- Lachesis 5 C. 2 granules.

Then alternate *Glonoinum* and *Belladonna* every two hours.

Hysterics

This occurs after intense psychological stress or shock (real or imagined). Administer 3 granules of the appropriate remedy, every quarter of an hour until the crisis subsides.

- *Actaea racemosa 15 C*. 5 granules. When fits are linked to the menstrual cycle.
- *Ignatia 7 C*. After some emotional trauma, causing grief.
- *Moschus 7 C*. For those who tend to over-dramatize and faint a lot.

Indigestion

For simple cases where people eat too much, administer *Nux vomica 7 C* and *Antimonium crudum 7 C,* alternating 3 granules of each every ten minutes. Consult the section on Indigestion in the chapter on Digestive Disorders.

Inflammation

If inflammation (oedema) is sudden and intense, use 5 granules of *Aconitum 7 C* or *Belladonna 5 C* immediately, and repeat every four hours. For cases of chronic inflammation, administer 2 granules *of Kali muriaticum 5 C* every day.

Inflammation of joints: the joint is red, hot and swollen. If there is no improvement after 3 days, consult a doctor.

4 granules every two hours:

- *Apis 7 C*. Inflammation appears suddenly and has a pink colour; cold aggravates the condition.
- *Belladonna 7 C*. Inflammation is red, hot and very sensitive to touch.
- *Bryonia 7 C*. Inflammation is hot; moving the affected joint causes more pain.

Injuries

Cases often require the presence of a doctor. All kinds of injuries can be soothed by applying cold compresses. In all cases, use:

- *Arnica 15 C*. 10 granules immediately.

Insanity
(See Nervous Breakdown)

For cases of religious mania or exaltation, administer *Melilotus 7 C*. 2 granules per day.

Insect Bites

As a preventive measure, use *Ledum palustre,* 3 granules twice a day.

You can destroy wasp or bee venom by holding a lighted cigarette close to the bite, being careful not to burn the skin.

After being bitten, alternate *Ledum palustre 7 C,* 10 granules every hour, with one of the following remedies:

- *Apis 15 C.* If the bite results in swelling (oedema).
- *Hypericum 7 C.* For intense pain.

Then administer 3 granules once a day of *Hepar sulphuris 15 C* if the bite suppurates.

Insomnia
(See Also Sleep Insomnia in the
Chapter on Psychological Disorders)

For cases of occasional insomnia, administer one of the following remedies, depending on the circumstances.

3 granules before going to bed, repeated as required:

- *Aconitum 15 C.* When insomnia is caused by fear, for example after seeing a very gruesome horror film.
- *Arnica 15 C.* For those who are physically fatigued.
- *Coffea 7 C.* For people kept awake by intense emotion (especially elation).
- *Nux vomica 7 C.* For insomnia due to over-eating, mental fatigue or work worries.

Intoxication

Refers here to intoxication caused by inhalation of coal gas, carbon monoxide, etc.

Start by giving artificial respiration, or give patients pure oxygen if it is available. Slide 2 granules of *Carbo vegetabilis* under the tongue every two hours.

Migraines

For persistent cases, consult a doctor.

Use compresses made with fresh onion or garlic, cabbage or even horseradish, which you apply to the nape of the neck, to soothe the pain. Another method is to shower the nape and spine with hot water (shower the abdomen if the migraine is associated with digestive problems). You can also take footbaths in herbal water, with wild thyme, mother of thyme, juniper, or other aromatic herbs.

3 granules every fifteen minutes, spacing out the doses more as symptoms improve:

- *Actaea racemosa 7 C*. Severe pain in the eyes, accompanied by sight problems; symptoms are more intense during menstruation.
- *Bryonia 7 C*. Pain becomes more intense towards evening; the slightest movement of the head or eyes aggravates the pain.
- *Gelsemium 7 C*. The face is red and congested; migraines are preceded by sight problems; pulse is slow, and people are not thirsty; they tremble, appear exhausted and pass large amounts of urine.
- *Iris versicolor 7 C*. For migraines affecting the eyes; people experience foggy vision and suffer from nausea and vomiting.
- *Melilotus 7 C*. The face is congested and red; bleeding from the nose, or the start of periods soothes the pain.
- *Nux vomica 7 C*. For migraines linked to digestive problems, often occurring after people over-eat; usually only one side of the head is affected; pain gets worse towards evening; the tongue is coated; exposure to noise or light may result in vomiting.
- *Sanguinaria 5 C*. A general remedy often prescribed for migraines and simple headaches.
- *Silicea 7 C*. For those suffering from chronic headaches, whose nervous system is exhausted.

Muscular Fatigue

Massage affected areas with *Homeodora (Calendula)* cream.

- *Arnica 5 C.* For general muscular fatigue.
- *Phytolacca 5 C.* 2 granules once every two days. For muscular fatigue accompanied by cramps.
- *Arnica 5 C, Crataegus 4 C* and *Rhus tox 5 C,* alternating 2 granules of each, three times per day. For muscular fatigue suffered by athletes.

Nausea

(See Also Indigestion and Nausea
in the Chapter on Digestive Problems)

Unless otherwise indicated, take 3 granules of the appropriate medication per hour, then space out the doses as the symptoms begin to improve.

- *Chelidonium 5 C.* Pains are felt in the region of the liver (see section); stool is discoloured.
- *Cocculus 6 C.* For nausea accompanied by dizziness.
- *Colchicum 6 C.* The smell of food is enough to cause nausea.
- *Ipecac. 5 C.* For persistent nausea that is not soothed by vomiting.
- *Iris versicolor 7 C.* Burning vomiting and diarrhoea accompany the sensation of nausea.
- *Phosphorus 7 C.* 3 granules three times per day. For nausea accompanied by migraine headaches.
- *Symphoricarpus 7 C.* The slightest movement aggravates the feeling of nausea.

Nervous Breakdown

When someone close to us has a nervous breakdown, starts "cracking up" (which seems to be more and more common in these troubled times), we are sometimes at a loss as to how to react, torn between our own fear of the unknown, and our desire to see the person regain his or her health.

Find a quiet place to talk, and try to be understanding, until a doctor can be consulted. Give supplements of vitamins B_1, B_2, B_3, C, D, and G.

- *Arnica 15 C.* When depression results from some emotional or mental shock.

- *Ambra grisea 15 C.* People seem numb and indifferent, not reacting to what is going on around them.
- *Ignatia 15 C.* After suffering from grief; these people become withdrawn and seek solitude; the more you try to console them, the more depressed they seem to become.
- *Kali bromatum 15 C.* People are apathetic, suffer from memory loss, have sluggish reflexes and seem insensitive to physical pain.

Nervousness
(See Also Anxiety)

When you feel yourself getting nervous, take a five-minute break. Gather your thoughts (you can do this almost anywhere), concentrate on your breathing (especially on the moment of transition between inhaling and exhaling) until you feel your pulse return to normal.

Meditation is an effective way to control your nerves. There are numerous techniques and teachers, and you don't necessarily have to adopt a whole belief system to practise meditation.

3 granules every three hours, spacing out the doses when there are signs of improvement.

- *Aconitum 7 C.* For nervousness accompanied by fever.
- *Arsenicum album 15 C.* For nervousness accompanied by agitation.
- *Asa foetida 6 C.* People are nervous and irritable; they experience frequent mood changes, are hypersensitive to pain, suffer from shortness of breath and palpitations.
- *Borax 9 C.* For timid, hypersensitive children, who get agitated and anxious for no reason.
- *Coffea 7 C.* For those who get over-excited.
- *Rhus toxicodendron 7 C.* When nervousness is accompanied by aches and pains, or various skin disorders (herpes, shingles, chicken-pox, etc.)
- *Spigelia 7 C.* For nervousness characterized by palpitations.
- *Valeriana 7 C.* For cases of hypersensitivity and over-excitability; people are physically agitated, and experience frequent mood swings.

Neuralgia

Neuralgia refers to pain centred along a nerve pathway. For localized pain, refer to the appropriate section.

- *Aconitum 5 C.* Pains occur after exposure to cold dry wind or draughts, and are characterized by a prickling, tingling sensation.
- *Arnica 15 C.* 3 granules every ten minutes. When pain appears suddenly, with no apparent cause.
- *Arsenicum album 4 C.* 2 granules every eight hours. For burning pain accompanied by excitation; pain tends to get worse at night.
- *Belladonna 5 C.* 2 granules every half an hour. Searing pains get worse in the evening and the middle of the night, but are soothed by rest and heat; also for pain that affects the region under the eyes.
- *Chamomilla 5 C.* 2 granules every two hours. Very intense pain is accompanied by extreme nervousness and agitation (which is very unpleasant for others, as well as for the patient).
- *China 5 C.* 2 granules per hour. Pain is aggravated by the slightest touch or draught.
- *Dulcamara 7 C.* Pains occur after exposure to damp cold.

Facial Neuralgia

Administer *5 C* of the appropriate medication, two or three times per day:

- *Aconitum.* Prickling, tingling pains appear after exposure to dry cold wind.
- *Actaea racemosa.* Pains are very intense and come in spasms.
- *Arsenicum album.* Burning pains are aggravated by heat; people are sometimes agitated, sometimes prostrate.
- *Belladonna.* Facial muscles twitch spasmodically.
- *Bryonia.* Pain is aggravated by movement, and soothed by rest and hot compresses.
- *Coffea.* Pains spread to the ears and forehead, and are soothed by cold.
- *Colocynthis.* Gnawing pains accompanied by shivering, often brought on by a fit of rage.
- *Iris versicolor.* Pain is situated below the eyes.
- *Kalmia.* Shooting pains (like those from an electric shock) with a tingling sensation in the teeth and the tongue.
- *Rhododendron.* Pains are aggravated by cold.
- *Rhus tox.* After exposure to damp cold; the jawbone cracks.

Nightmares (Night Terrors)

Be careful about the stories you read to your children before they go to bed, or the TV programmes they watch. Avoid subjects like monsters, beasts, ghosts and violence in general.

- *Kali bromatum 7 C* and *Stramonium 7 C*, 2 granules around six o'clock in the evening on alternate days.

Nosebleed

If bleeding is very profuse, or if it lasts longer than half an hour, see a doctor.

Place 2 granules of *China 4 C* under the tongue if the nosebleed was caused by a blow. Get patients to breathe deeply and slowly, while pinching the nostrils. Cool the skin, especially the forehead, with a damp cloth. If people are congested after a heavy meal, or in an overheated room, bring them to a well-ventilated, cool place.

Be careful about stopping an occasional nosebleed which only lasts a few minutes, especially if people suffer from hypertension. In these cases, the nosebleed acts as a safety valve for the body, releasing excess pressure. For these cases, give 2 granules of *Melilotus triiodatus 5 C,* followed an hour later by 2 granules of *Crotalus 5 C.*

After a blow or accident:

Apply cold water compresses to the nape of the neck, changing them often. Get patients to take a few deep breaths, then pinch the nostrils together, and get them to lean forward.

- *China 4 C.* 2 granules immediately in all cases, alternated with 2 granules of *Arnica 5 C* every fifteen minutes. Repeat the treatment as long as the nosebleed lasts.

Add one of the following remedies, depending on the case:

- *Aconitum 4 C.* 2 granules. For those who are congested and anxious; the pulse is strong.
- *Hamamelis 4 C.* 2 granules. If the flow of blood is very black.
- *Ipecac. 4 C.* 2 granules. Repeat every thirty minutes if the nosebleed (epistaxis) persists; pulse is rapid and weak, and individuals feel nauseous.
- *Pulsatilla 4 C.* 2 granules twice a day. For pre-menstrual nosebleeds.

Oedema

For temporary swelling caused by a blow, a fall, or a shock, administer 2 granules of *Apis 5 C* every two hours.

For oedema accompanied by urticaria, add 2 granules of *Urtica arens 4 C*, twice a day. People should eat onions and drink onion wine (300 grams of raw, ripe onion, 300 grams of white liquid honey, and 600 grams of good white wine - steep for eight days and filter).

Overwork
(See Also Weakness, Fatigue)

In this age of unparalleled technological progress, it is surprising that people are overworked as much as they are. The reason probably lies in our insatiable desire for material gain. People compete fiercely for money and position, without appreciating the difference between ensuring a secure and comfortable lifestyle for themselves and their families, and getting caught up in a cruel race for possessions, which is so injurious to both physical and mental health.

For people doing mental work, *Pollen* and *Pollavena* (a combination of pollen and oat flowers) are excellent natural fortifiers, allowing them to work longer and more efficiently without getting tired.

A tablespoon of *Lehning's* vegetable tonic, taken half an hour after meals, is another effective fortifier.

- *Ignatia 30 C*. 2 granules every two or three hours. For overworked, nervous people.
- *Natrum muriaticum 7 C*. 5 granules every 2 weeks. When fatigue is accompanied by vision problems and headaches. Recommended for students (including schoolchildren).
- *Sulphur 9 C*. 10 granules every ten days, alternated with *Adrenaline 9 C*. For business people who are very tense, and only sleep a few hours a night.

Pains
(See Also Neuralgia)

In all cases, use 10 granules *of Arnica* 30 C immediately. Considering the vast number of possible causes of pain, you should look up specific sections of this book, which describe symptoms and remedies in detail. Make a note of the frequency and the times when pains are most intense - this can help doctors make a more accurate diagnosis and lead to a more speedy recovery.

3 granules every two hours, unless otherwise indicated:

- *Aurum 5 C.* For back pains.
- *Belladonna 5 C.* For burning pain.
- *Bellis perennis 5 C.* 2 granules every two hours. For cases where *Arnica* does not soothe pain in the thumb.
- *Ferrum muriaticum 5 C.* For pains in the shoulders, especially if they are persistent.
- *Kali carbonicum 5 C.* For prickly pain.
- *Ledum 5 C.* 2 granules every two hours. For serious bruising of the ankles.
- Rhus tox 7 C. 5 granules twice a day. For muscular pains after sudden exertion.
- *Ruta 7 C.* 5 granules immediately. For pain in the wrists and hands. If pain persists, take *Calcarea carbonica 5 C,* 2 granules every two hours.

Palpitations (Emergency)
(See Also Palpitations in the Chapter on Circulatory Disorders)

When palpitations begin, take *Spigelia 7 C,* 3 granules every ten minutes, and space out doses as the symptoms improve. Alternate *Spigelia* with 3 granules of one of the following medications:

- *Aconitum 7 C.* When palpitations are accompanied by anxiety.
- *Aconitum 15 C.* For palpitations caused by a scare.
- *Coffea 7 C.* When coffee is the cause of palpitations.
- *Ignatia 7 C.* After an emotional shock or tragic event.
- *Strophanthus 4 C.* For intermittent palpitations, or palpitations triggered by alcohol, coffee, tea or tobacco abuse.

Paralysis

For sudden paralysis in one or more limbs: while waiting to see a doctor, give *Arnica 5 C,* 2 granules every fifteen minutes, alternating with 2 granules of *Belladonna 5 C.* After three hours, continue alternating the remedies, but only every half an hour.

Facial Paralysis

Consult an acupuncture specialist. While waiting, administer 2 granules of the appropriate remedy every two hours:

- *Aconitum 5 C*. For paralysis caused by exposure to cold.
- *Causticum 5 C*. When the skin is whitish and the condition is soothed by humidity.
- *Cocculus 5 C*. When facial paralysis is accompanied by cramps and facial contractions.
- *Dulcamara 5 C*. For paralysis that occurs in a damp climate or location.

Parasites

For cases of intestinal parasites, consult the section on Parasites in the Chapter on Digestive Disorders.

For external parasites (lice, crabs, fleas, etc.) spray Xylol, mixing equal parts of *Xylol* with pure alcohol.

- *Ignatia 7 C*. 10 granules only once. To soothe itching, with *Dolichos pruriens 4 C*, 3 granules four times per day.

Poisoning

Contact your nearest anti-poison centre or accident and emergency unit as quickly as possible.

1. When people have swallowed some highly toxic poison, and a doctor has already been alerted: get the person to spit and vomit. Administer *Ipecac. 7 C*, 1 granule diluted in a little warm water. Then make the person drink milk and powdered charcoal. Use a laxative like sodium sulphate or castor oil. Vinegar, lemon juice and carbohydrate juices (potatoes) may also work as an antidote when nothing else is available.

2. Individuals are intoxicated from an overdose of medication or some drug:
   - *Nux vomica 7 C*, 10 granules only once.
   - *Thuja 30 C*. For those who have taken an overdose of homeopathic medication.

3. For cases of food poisoning; these people are vomiting or suffering from

diarrhoea, or both.

- *Arsenicum album 7 C.* 2 granules twice a day. For cases of poisoning due to rotten food or contaminated drinking water. Combine with *Veratrum album 7 C* if poisoning occurs after eating mussels.
- *Pyrogenium 7 C.* 3 granules twice a day. For all cases.

Post-operative Shock
(See Also Surgery)

Even when surgery is successful and everything goes according to plan, it is still a traumatic event for the body, which homeopathy can help to soothe.

- *Arnica 8 C.* 5 granules to be administered immediately.

Taking thermal cures or going to a spa for mud baths and relaxation can also go a long way towards soothing post-operative shock.

Scabies

Scabies is caused by a minuscule parasite, and usually starts in the folds and furrows of the skin. Treatment is primarily external.

Bathe with black (tar) soap and apply *benzyl benzoate* (or *Ascabiol)* lotion, which you keep on the body for 24 hours. Complement external treatment with *Psorinum 9 C,* 5 granules every two weeks.

Scars

When scars are hard, apply *Homeodora* cream. To help scars heal more quickly:

First carefully clean the wound, then administer:

- *Arnica 7 C.* 2 granules in the morning, followed by *Symphytum 7 C,* 2 granules around noon, then *Calendula 7 C,* 2 granules at around six o'clock in the evening.

Painful scars:

- Arnica 7 C or Calendula 7 C or Graphites 7 C.

Sore Throat
(See Also Tonsillitis, and Laryngitis in the Chapter
on Respiratory Disorders)

If a simple sore throat is ignored, it can develop into tonsillitis, with all the associated complications that involves. So it's a good idea to treat a sore throat right away - in the long run it will save you time and energy.

External Treatment

Make sure the throat is effectively protected from the cold - a woollen scarf is not a luxury in cold weather. Patients should rub camphor on their neck before bed, and sleep with a scarf. This can cure a sore throat in a couple of days. But if fever appears, it's a good idea to consult a doctor.

You can also bathe a sore throat with *Molkosan, a* powerful disinfectant made from acidic whey which destroys disease-carrying germs that tend to collect on the surface of the tonsils. At the first sign of a sore throat, get the person to gargle with salt water.

Apply compresses, alternating cabbage leaves with clay. Drinking *Solidago* infusions helps the body to eliminate toxins. You can also gargle three times a day with 20 drops of *Phytolacca tincture* dissolved in a glass of tepid water.

Internal Treatment

- *Lachesis 12 C.* 2 granules, alternated with *Aconitum 5 C,* 2 granules, every four hours: the face is red (but goes pale when patients sit down); people are anxious and agitated; coughing causes a prickly sensation in the throat.
- *Belladonna 5 C.* 2 granules every four hours if the condition does not improve. The face is red, eyes are shiny, pupils dilated; patients perspire from the head, and have a sharp, dry cough that irritates the throat.

Sores
(See Also Tetanus)

Use *Calendula tincture* instead of iodine to bathe the sore; it will accelerate healing and reduce risk of infection.

Prepare dressings with sterile gauze and change once or twice a day (make sure you wash your hands and disinfect them with alcohol or ether before changing a dressing).

Wet dressings should be boiled in water for half an hour before applying. To prevent the dressing from adhering to the wound, coat it with the following mixture (use a knife blade which has been sterilized in a flame to spread the ointment): 1 granule of *Calendula tincture* and 1 granule of *Hypericum tincture,* mixed with one ounce (28 g) of vaseline.

Internal Treatment:

- *Calendula 5 C.* 2 granules four times per day, accompanied by 3 granules every hour of one of the following remedies (spacing out doses as symptoms improve):
- *Echinacea 6 C.* For wounds or sores that turn livid purple and bluish.
- *Hepar sulphuris 15 C.* For suppurating wounds (consult the section on Abscess).
- *Hypericum 5 C.* For intensely painful wounds.
- *Ledum palustre 5 C.* For wounds caused by needle or nail pricks.
- *Staphysagria 5 C.* For cuts.

Spitting Blood

When people suddenly start spitting blood (haemoptysis) a doctor should be consulted. But since fast action is sometimes required, you should know what to do while waiting to see a doctor.

Cases are classed as haemoptysis only if people cough up or spit blood. If not, you may be dealing with a simple nosebleed.

- *Aconitum 6 C.* 2 granules. Especially if the blood is bright red and frothy. Follow up with 2 granules of *Millefolium* 6 C. Then alternate between *Aconitum* and *Millefolium,* 2 granules per hour.
- *Arnica 30 C.* 2 granules in the morning and in the evening before going to bed.

Sports (Accidents)

Physical activity is essential for good health. However, keen sportspeople are susceptible to a host of minor or more serious injuries. Consult the following sections in case a problem arises: Muscular Strain, Contusions, Aches, Cramps, Sprains, Muscular Fatigue, Tendinitis, Tennis Elbow.

Sprains

Consult a doctor. Acupuncture can numb pain as well as an injection of local anaesthetic. While waiting to see a doctor, administer *Arnica 15 C,* 10 granules, immediately after the sprain occurs.

External Treatment

Bathe the affected joint in hot water - mix a teaspoon of *Calendula tincture* or *Arnica tincture* in a litre of water. Repeat once or twice per day. Massage patients regularly (throughout convalescence); prepare a dressing with *Calendula ointment,* and get patients to rest the injured joint.

Note: Osteopathy can be very helpful in such cases, and can also be used to treat a chronic joint problem (like a bad knee, for example).

Internal Treatment

- *Rhus tox* 6 C. 2 granules every three hours. When pain is aggravated by rest; the sprain is accompanied by stiffness of muscles and tendons.
- *Ruta* 6 C. 2 granules every three hours. If intense pain is felt at one or two points around the joints.

Stage Fright

Take the appropriate medication as a preventive measure: 10 granules the evening before and 10 granules the morning of the performance (speech, presentation, etc.) Take 3 more granules if the feeling of stage fright persists or reappears.

- *Argentum nitricum 7 C.* People are anxious, impatient, and suffer from diarrhoea.
- *Gelsemium 7 C.* People feel paralyzed and need to urinate constantly.
- *Ignatia 7 C.* Stage fright is characterized by confusion, and mental and physical agitation.

Stitch in the Side

Various factors can cause recurring stitch or twinges in the side, including pneumonia, pleurisy, tuberculosis, a fractured rib, hepatic colic, shingles and others. A doctor should be consulted in order to identify and cure the cause.

For occasional stitch, an easy way to relieve the pain is to lean forward and touch the ground, then stand up straight, then lean forward again, repeating the process as long as necessary.

- *Ceanothus 5 C.* 3 granules immediately. Repeat after ten minutes, if necessary.

Strains (Muscular)

Muscle strain occurs after excessive exertion or a false movement, and is characterized by intense pain and redness caused by blood spreading around the affected area.

Apply compresses soaked in *Calendula tincture* (one teaspoon dissolved in a cup of water that has been boiled and cooled).

- *Arnica 15 C.* 10 granules as soon as possible, then 3 granules every two hours. As soon as there is an improvement, start spacing out the doses.

Sunburn (Emergency)
(See Also Tanning, Sunstroke)

For cases of severe, extensive sunburn or sunburn in infants, it would be better to consult a doctor.

Protect burns with gauze or sterile bandages. Take 3 granules per hour of the appropriate remedy until there is some improvement, and then space out the doses.

- *Apis 15 C,* when there is inflammation.
- *Belladonna 7 C,* if the only symptom of sunburn is red skin.
- *Cantharis 7 C,* when blisters develop.

Surgery
(See Also Post-operative Shock)

Homeopathy can be used to help prepare the body for surgery, and to calm apprehension on the eve of an operation.

- *Aconitum napellus 7 C.* 10 granules two days before the operation, to calm people down, and 2 granules per day of *Gelsemium sempervirens 5 C* with *Ignatia 5 C.*
- *Arnica 7 C* and *China 5 C.* Administer after surgery, alternating 3 granules of each every two hours.

- *Raphanus 5 C.* 3 granules, three times per day after surgery to the abdominal area, until normal digestion and elimination of gas is established.

Synovia (Effusion of)

If effusion occurs spontaneously, it must be examined by a doctor. When caused by an accident like a fall or blow, administer the following treatment:

External treatment:
- Apply compresses soaked in a teaspoon of *Calendula tincture* dissolved in a glass of boiled and cooled water.

Internal Treatment:
- *Arnica 7 C.* 2 granules every 48 hours, and *Apis mellifica 5 C,* 2 granules twice a day.

Tendinitis

Drink a lot of pure water and apply ice packs to the affected area.
- *Rhus tox 15 C.* 3 granules five times a day for a week, as soon as pain begins.

Tennis Elbow (Epicondylitis)

This affliction affects keen tennis players, and is a form of tendinitis.
Drink pure (distilled) water in large quantities, and apply ice packs.
- *Rhus tox 15 C.* 3 granules three times per day for a week, as soon as pain starts.

Tension
(See Also Hypertension in the Chapter
on Circulatory Disorders)

There is a way to reduce tension other than taking a holiday, which has proved very effective in many cases: eat a wholemeal rice diet - some spectacular improvements have been seen with this regime. To make the diet more effective, take *Viscasan* drops (prepared with mistletoe) to improve the performance of your digestive system and *Arterioforce (Hawthorn* and *Arnica).* Also take garlic wine (if you can find it) to stimulate the vascular system.

Tetanus

Tetanus (or the bacterium responsible) is present in soil and faecal material, and usually enters the body through a wound.

The incubation period usually lasts about a week, but may be shorter. Initial symptoms include contraction of the jaw muscles, causing people to clench their teeth, and increasing pain; pulse becomes rapid and temperature is slightly above normal (between 99° and 100°F, 37.5-37.8°C).

If affected people do not have access to anti-tetanus serum for one reason or another, wash the wound and dress it with *Hypericum tincture*. Also administer:

- *Hypericum 4 C.* 2 granules four times a day for seven days.

Toothache

There are few things more unpleasant than a severe toothache. If the pain does not subside, if it comes back frequently or the tooth has a cavity and starts to turn black, a dentist must be consulted.

A good way to soothe pain from a toothache is to insert half a clove of garlic between the gum and inside of the cheek.

- *Chamomilla 7 C, Hypericum 7 C,* and *Magnesia carbonica 7 C.* 3 granules every two hours, alternating. As soon as there is an improvement, space out the doses.

Note: Also see the section on Teeth in the Chapter on General Disorders.

Travel

Take your emergency first aid kit along (see Appendix) while travelling. This will help you deal with unexpected situations in unfamiliar places, until you can find specialized help.

Travel Sickness

This disorder can be extremely unpleasant, and homeopathy is an excellent way to control it. When in doubt about which medication to use, take 3 granules of each, alternating every quarter of an hour. Space out the doses as soon as there is any improvement.

- *Cocculus Indicus 7 C.* 3 granules. When discomfort is aggravated by cold air (opening the window in a car, for example), or by looking at objects passing by.
- *Petroleum 7 C.* When closing the eyes or breathing fresh air eases the discomfort.
- *Tabacum 5 C.* 3 granules. When the condition improves in fresh air.

Vertigo
(See Also Travel Sickness)

- *Conium maculatum 7 C.* 3 granules every half an hour, spacing out doses as improvement occurs. For all cases.

Vomiting
(See Also Indigestion, Travel Sickness and Nausea)

Space out doses as improvement occurs:

- *Chelidonium 7 C.* 3 granules every hour. For cases where there is pain in the liver region and stool is discoloured.
- *Iris versicolor 5 C.* 3 granules every hour. When vomit is burning, accompanied by burning diarrhoea.
- *Phosphorus 7 C.* 3 granules three times per day. Vomiting is accompanied by migraines and liver pains.

Weakness
(See Also Fatigue, Overwork)

After a period of intense activity or emotion, you may feel drained and empty. Your resistance is low and you become more and more irritable.

If you find that you're always annoyed and impatient at work, your body may be warning you of an imminent breakdown. You may be a candidate for "burn-out" (the plague of modern urban living, from which people do not always recover). Rest as soon as you can. If you wait too long before doing something, you may not have a chance.

- *Avena sativa 1 X* (1st decimal dilution). 20 drops in a glass of water before the two main meals of the day.

Wounds

(See Also Accidents, Cuts, Contusions, Fractures)

Apply cold in the form most appropriate to the circumstances.

- *Arnica 30 C.* 10 granules as quickly as possible.

APPENDIX

EMERGENCY FIRST AID KIT

This section is designed to help you organize your own homeopathic "home pharmacy" so that you will be prepared to deal with most situations. Of course, for rare or infrequent disorders, you will have to obtain appropriate remedies from a homeopathic pharmacist. Keep adding them to your own collection when the treatments are completed.

Don't be surprised if dosages indicated on the remedies differ from those suggested in this section. In homeopathy, it is an accepted fact that the right remedy will be effective whatever dosage is administered, from *4* C to *15 C*.

Stock your first-aid kit with one container of granules of each of the following:

- Aconitum 5C and 7C
- Allium cepa 5C
- Antimonium crudum 5C
- Antimonium tartaricum 5C
- Apis 7C
- Argentum nitricum 5C
- Arnica 5C, 7C and 15C
- Arsenicum album 5C
- Belladonna 5C
- Bryonia 5C and 7C
- Cactus 5C
- Calcarea carbonica 5C
- Calendula 5C
- Calendula mother tincture
- Calendula ointment
- Carbo vegetabilis 5C
- Chamomilla 7C
- Chelidonium 5C
- China 5C and 7C
- Coccus cacti 7C
- Coffea 7C
- Cuprum 5C
- Drosera 5C
- Ferrum phosphoricum 4C

- Gelsemium 5C
- Glonoinum 5C
- Hepar sulphuris 5C
- Ignatia 5C and 7C
- Ipecac. 5C
- Kali bichromicum 5C
- Lachesis 5C
- Lycopodium 5C
- Mercurius solubilis 5C
- Nux vomica 5C
- Oscillococcinum 200
- Opium 5C
- Pulsatilla 5C
- Pyrogenium 5C
- Rhus toxicodendron 5C
- Sulphur 5C
- Veratrum album 5C

Add materials for making dressings and compresses: cotton wool, sterile gauze, gauze pads, sterile tape.... and, of course, your *Family Encyclopaedia of Homeopathic Medicine!*

Bibliography

- **Homeopathy**
Optima
1988
Brunton Nelson

- **Discovering Homeopathy: Medicine for the 21st Century**
North Atlantic Books
1991
Ullman Dana

- **Homeopathy and the Medical Profession**
Croom Helm
1988
Nicholls Phillip A.

- **Science of Homeopathy**
Grove PR
1980
Vithoulkas George

- **Genius of Homeopathy**
B Jain
1981
Close Stuart

- **Homeopathy in Practice**
Beaconsfield Publishers Ltd
1982
Borland Douglas

- **Everyday Homeopathy**
Beaconsfield Publishers Ltd
1997
Gemmell David M.

- **Homeopathy as Art and Science**
Beaconsfield Publishers Ltd
1990
Hubbard Elizabeth Wright

- **The Complete Book of Homeopathy**
Fine Communications
1997
Weiner Michael

- **A Beginner's Introduction to Homeopathy**
Keats Publishing
1987
Cook Trevor M.

- **The Family Health Guide to Homeopathy**
Celestial Arts
1993
Barry Dr. Rose

- **Healing Homeopathy Remedies**
Dell Publishing Co
1996
Bruning Nancy Pauline

My Personal Notes

Here are the symptoms I've got :

_____

_____

_____

_____

My homeopathic remedies :

☐ _____

_____

☐ _____

_____

☐ _____

_____

☐ _____

_____

Here are the symptoms I've got :

_____

_____

_____

_____

My homeopathic remedies :

☐ _____

_____

☐ _____

_____

☐ _____

_____

☐ _____

_____

Here are the symptoms I've got :

_____

_____

_____

_____

My homeopathic remedies :

☐ _____

_____

☐ _____

_____

☐ _____

_____

☐ _____

_____